The Diet Cure

THE Diet Cure

**The 8-Step Program to Rebalance
Your Body Chemistry and End Food Cravings,
Weight Problems, and Mood Swings—Now**

JULIA ROSS, M.A.

Viking

VIKING
Published by the Penguin Group
Penguin Putnam Inc., 375 Hudson Street,
New York, New York 10014, U.S.A.
Penguin Books Ltd, 27 Wrights Lane,
London W8 5TZ, England
Penguin Books Australia Ltd, Ringwood,
Victoria, Australia
Penguin Books Canada Ltd, 10 Alcorn Avenue,
Toronto, Ontario, Canada M4V 3B2
Penguin Books (N.Z.) Ltd, 182–190 Wairau Road,
Auckland 10, New Zealand

Penguin Books Ltd, Registered Offices:
Harmondsworth, Middlesex, England

First published in 1999 by Viking Penguin,
a member of Penguin Putnam Inc.

3   5   7   9   10   8   6   4   2

LIBRARY OF CONGRESS CATALOGING-IN-PUBLICATION DATA
Ross, Julia.
The diet cure : the 8-step program to rebalance your body chemistry and end food cravings,
weight problems, and mood swings—now / Julia Ross.
p.   cm.
Includes index.
ISBN 0-670-88593-2
1. Diet—Health aspects.   2. Diet—Physiological aspects.   3. Diet therapy—Physiological aspects.
4. Food—Health aspects.   5. Nutritionally induced diseases.   6. Nutrition—Health aspects.   I. Title.
RA776.5.R685   1999
615.8'54—dc21   99-19180

This book is printed on acid-free paper.

Printed in the United States of America
Set in Minion
Designed by Jaye Zimet

I dedicate this book
to
F.L.R., my spirit of truth

and to the nutritionists and counselors
who have helped create The Diet Cure

and to the women and men, the girls and boys
whose struggles inspired us to find a better way.

AUTHOR'S NOTE

If you have a known or suspected medical condition, or are taking medication of any kind, or have specific health concerns, you should consult a qualified health care provider before following any of the suggestions in this book. Supplement and pharmaceutical dosages are meant to be guidelines only, and dosage and results will vary according to the specific needs of each individual. The dietary guidelines, too, need to be tailored to each individual. Because this book cannot respond to individuals' needs and circumstances, as we do in our clinic, you should ask a qualified health care professional to help you assess and apply *The Diet Cure*. Although we did our best to provide sound and useful information, we cannot and do not promise results to a reader, nor can we or do we accept liability to anyone who may use the book.

CONTENTS

Part I
Identifying the Eight Imbalances   1

Part II
Correcting Your Imbalances   115

Part III
Your Master Plan for the Diet Cure   239

ACKNOWLEDGMENTS

For someone like me, who is not as generous with praise as I should be, I am so happy to have this chance to express my gratitude and appreciation to Frances Lillian Ross, my mother, partner, and pal, whose brilliant sense of language made me love to speak and to write.

I am also most grateful to Helen Jones, courageous author and long-time friend, who believed in me when I needed it most; to Barbara Madore, whose early support made our clinic possible; to Dean and Liz Lieth, kindred spirits whose generosity took us over the top; and to the valiant and beautiful Eileen Hinkson.

I am also grateful to the following people for providing key steps in my understanding of eating disorders and nutritional therapy: Alex Schauss, Ph.D., Lynn Elliott-Harding, R.N., Joan Matthews-Larson, Ph.D., Krispin Sullivan, C.N., and William Timmons, N.D.

To my inspired and adorable agent, Faith Hamlin, at Sanford J. Greenburger Associates in New York and her associate Nancy Stender; to the winged feet of Nancy Peske, editor par excellence; to the exceptional vision of my editor at Viking, Janet Goldstein, and her colleagues Barbara Grossman and Susan Petersen, who ordained the happy fate of this book, I give many thanks.

I am more than fortunate to have had around me colleagues, friends, and family who made it possible for me to finish this book despite the death of my mother on December 9, 1998. The contributions of my dear friend Genie Dreyfus, which included daily support, computer and conventional research, and an intuitive ability to turn my illegible prose into computer clarity, are too numerous to catalogue. She and her remarkable husband, Jared, put together most of the wonderful information in chapters 20 and 21 from their own experience as master cooks (and master writers!). Another dear friend, Colleen Heater, did the great research on essential support for chapter 21 and held my hand throughout the writing process. Timothy Kuss, the head of my clinic's nutritional program since 1992, has been the mastermind behind so many of our successful nutritional strategies. He compiled the material for three of the book's most complex chapters and reviewed all of the supplement protocols for me. He is one of four superb clinicians who comprise the board of advisers for this book. I would like to thank the other three as well: Daniel Amen, M.D., with his extraordinary understanding of brain function; Kenneth Blum, M.D., my mentor in amino acid therapy; and Richard Shames, M.D., without whose care many of our clients would not have found their Diet Cures.

Many thanks to the wonderful Clara Felix, editor of the *Felix Nutrition Letter;* and to health editor Nancy Faass for reviewing parts of the manuscript for accuracy; and to Sharna Rose, chef extraordinaire, who provided many scrumptious recipes out of her personal enthusiasm for *The Diet Cure.*

Because of the enormous clinical and administrative gifts of my unique and lovely assistant, Maria Dorio, Recovery Systems has gone on without me too often these past months. Thank you, Maria and our patient clients. Special thanks to writer Amy Kauffmann, whose electric account of her eating disorder and addiction was cut along with two huge chapters that are going to make a great sequel to *The Diet Cure.*

Finally, I want to salute my two beloved brothers, Fred and Robert, their loving wives, Margo and Kay, and the stalwart, darling Kass.

The board of advisers for this book includes:

◆ *Daniel Amen, M.D.,* a clinical neuroscientist, psychiatrist, and the medical director of the Amen Clinic for Behavioral Medicine in Fairfield, California. He is a nationally recognized expert in the field of brain imaging and its clinical applications. He is the author of more than 250 articles, 15 books, and a number of audio and video programs. His most recent book is *Change Your Brain, Change Your Life* (New York: Times Books, 1998).

◆ *Kenneth Blum, Ph.D.,* a professor of pharmacology and biological studies at the University of Texas and University of North Texas. Dr. Blum has published 300 studies and 9 books on genetics, neurochemistry, and brain nutrition. His most recent book is *To Binge or Not to Binge: Overeating and the Addictive Brain* (Psychiatric Genetic Press, 1999).

◆ *Richard Shames, M.D.,* a graduate of Harvard University and the University of Pennsylvania, is an alternative and integrative medicine pioneer. Dr. Shames is the author of three books, including a forthcoming book from William Morrow on the hidden epidemic of thyroid dysfunction. He is on the faculty of the University of California Medical School in San Francisco and is an expert in wholistic approaches to the diagnosis and treatment of metabolic and weight dysfunctions.

◆ *Timothy Kuss, Ph.D.,* is a clinical nutritionist, consultant, and author. Dr. Kuss has written two books and numerous articles in health publications. He is an adjunct faculty member in nutrition at John F. Kennedy University in Orinda, California.

8 Steps to the Diet Cure

This is not going to be like any diet book you have ever read. I won't mention calories except to forbid you to eat too *few!* I won't tell you to tune in to your "real" appetite because I know that if you could have you would have long ago. I won't tell you to discipline yourself because I know that your weight and eating habits are not the result of laziness, gluttony, or because you don't *want* to exercise or eat well.

Many of you are trapped inside a body that is malfunctioning. Your body needs help. Years of dieting, psychotherapy, and the best pep talks about accepting your body as is can't help much when what you really need is a biochemical overhaul.

Usually, the clients that come to Recovery Systems, the clinic that I direct, have already tried therapy. If they haven't, or they need more counseling, we provide that service. We educate them about their health and encourage them to accept the body that their genes have programmed for them. But when that body is a wreck, psychological and educational approaches just aren't enough. Fortunately, we have now learned how to identify and repair the underlying physical imbalances that have been neglected for so long.

We used to think that dieting was the cure. Many of us still hope that the next diet will really "do it." But more of us have begun to suspect, or to be outright convinced, that dieting has actually become a bigger problem than weight gain.

We know now that dieting leaves us in worse shape than before we started. Our health, energy, mood, and weight have all deteriorated because of dieting. *And yet we can't quit.* We know no other escape from the weight gain that was triggered by our last diet! What we really need now is to be cured of dieting. We have to find an entirely new way to deal with our weight.

You're about to learn it.

I discovered this "miracle" diet cure while I was out desperately looking for a cure for alcohol and drug addiction! At that time I was the director of a large outpatient treatment complex in the San Francisco Bay Area, the Henry Ohloff Outpatient Programs. We provided intensive counseling for addicted adults and adolescents and their families in three counties. In 1986 I began hearing that certain nutritional supplements could stop addicts' cravings for alcohol and even for cocaine. I asked my staff nutritionist to research these nutrients and to start offering them to our addicted clients. These supplements worked right away, dramatically reducing our clients' drug and alcohol cravings. Much to our surprise, they also cured the insatiable cravings for sweets that our clients typically suffered.

In early 1988, I opened my own outpatient treatment program. Staffed with nutritionists and counselors, Recovery Systems, in Mill Valley, California, is five minutes north of San Francisco. Initially, my clients at Recovery Systems were food addicts and others concerned about eating disorders and serious weight problems. Compulsive overeating and bulimia were their most common complaints. Some anorectics came to us, too, as well as many people without any eating disorders, but with weight gain that was intractable. If these sound like tough problems, you're wrong. We rarely failed to help even our most severely impaired clients, because we had the secret nutrient weapons. We used the same nutrients with them that I had used with my former drug- and alcohol-addicted clients. They stopped food cravings even more effectively than drug cravings, and had the delightful side effect of eliminating mood swings, too.

As the word spread, we began to get many clients who did not have full-blown eating disorders or major weight problems, but were looking for an escape from yo-yo dieting, low energy, moodiness, and a tendency to eat too much bread and frozen yogurt. You can imagine how easy it was for us to help them, having already discovered nutrients that were powerful enough to "cure" the cravings and mood problems of bulimics and drug addicts. These miracle nutrients are called amino acids.

Amino acids are the key to the Diet Cure. They are stronger than willpower and more effective and safer for most people than drugs like Prozac and Fen-Phen. Available in every health food store in America, these isolated protein fragments are the miracle foods that your brain uses to make its most powerful pleasure chemicals: serotonin—your natural Prozac; dopamine/norepinephrine—your natural cocaine; endorphin—naturally stronger than heroin; and GABA—naturally more relaxing than Valium. A brain that is fully stocked with these natural mood enhancers simply has no need for a sugar high.

What's more, you don't have to wait weeks or months to see changes in your body. My clients consistently report that within twenty-four hours after taking amino acids, their moods lift and their food cravings disappear. Like them, you will no longer need to diet because you will have stopped overeating—*naturally.* These benefits soon become permanent. After three to twelve months you won't need the amino acids and other corrective supplements anymore. Instead, you will be permanently freed from cravings and able to follow the Diet Cure's sensible eating suggestions for life.

THE EIGHT STEPS

At Recovery Systems, we have discovered eight steps to overcoming the physical, *bodily* handicaps that can lead directly to food cravings, emotional eating, low energy, and weight gain. Some of these steps correct problems that the body has developed on its own, while others correct problems that have been inadvertently brought about through eating habits. The good news is that these eight steps can correct all imbalances, whatever their source.

Step One: Correcting BRAIN CHEMISTRY IMBALANCES, which cause anxiety, depression, and "emotional" eating.

Step Two: Ending LOW-CALORIE DIETING, which results in problems with eating, mood, energy, and weight by depleting the whole body and brain.

Step Three: Balancing UNSTABLE BLOOD SUGAR, which causes moodiness and cravings for sweets and starches and can lead to adrenal exhaustion.

Step Four: Repairing LOW THYROID FUNCTION. Usually overlooked, low thyroid function is a common cause of weight and energy problems.

Step Five: Overcoming ADDICTIONS TO FOODS YOU'RE ALLERGIC TO. These "allergy-addictors" can trigger powerful cravings for foods, along with many other problems, such as congestion, headache, and constipation.

Step Six: Calming HORMONAL HAVOC, which can induce food cravings and weight gain, particularly during PMS and menopause.

Step Seven: Eradicating YEAST OVERGROWTH, which can be triggered by antibiotics or cortisone, causing bloating and powerful cravings for sweets and starches.

Step Eight: Fixing FATTY ACID DEFICIENCY, which can cause cravings for rich, fatty foods.

Most of these imbalances, if they continue, can result in serious health problems. Whether you must take one, two, or all of these steps, you will be able to overcome your handicaps; you do *not* have to accept them. This book is a repair manual. It will help you to find and fix the physical malfunctions that have caused your particular eating, mood, weight, or health problems. Then you will be able to drive away in your refurbished body and crave, binge, starve, and obsess no more. The best news is that by using the techniques recommended in this book, you will be able to stop cravings and start to feel better in a matter of days, or even hours! Having crossed this bridge, you can continue on your way to optimum health without having to struggle with your own body's messages to feed it sugar and junk food.

HOW TO USE THIS BOOK

The first step is to fill out the Quick Symptom Questionnaire, which follows this introduction. It will reveal which of the imbalances you probably have. Each of the eight biochemical imbalances has a chapter in part 1 devoted to helping you recognize its symptoms. In part 2, you will find eight chapters that give you specific information on taking the steps to correct each of the imbalances discussed in part 1, including exactly which easy-to-find supplements and foods to use.

Once you have diagnosed your particular imbalances and know what steps you need to take to correct each one, turn to part 3. There you'll find many ways to make your Diet Cure easy, including a master supplement scheduler, menus and recipes, a food-mood log, and help in finding a wholistic health professional, if you need one. The last chapter will take you through your first twelve weeks and set you on the road to a permanent cure.

It will take you a few weeks to study this book and to design your supplement and food plan. But as soon as you start to follow your plan, you will see and feel the effects. Within twenty-four hours your mood and food

Kate's Story

One of our clients, Kate, had all eight imbalances to correct. Her story illustrates how these imbalances can intertwine and how she was able to address them all and return to good health.

A creamy-skinned blonde who wrote children's books, Kate had suffered from chronic childhood earaches caused by an allergy to dairy products. As a result, she was given many courses of antibiotics, which created an intestinal yeast overgrowth, causing her to overeat sweets and gain weight. Her mother put her on a diet when she was 8 years old.

Kate's energy had never been robust, but it dropped even lower, and she began to gain more weight after she started her period. This was partly the result of a low thyroid problem she had inherited from her mother and maternal grandmother. There was diabetes in the family as well, and Kate's inherited tendency to unbalanced blood sugar was intensified by her early overeating of sweets. Consuming sweets also contributed to her severe PMS: Before her periods, Kate's food cravings were at their worst. By age 15 she had become a perpetual yo-yo dieter, gaining more weight and eating more after every diet. As the child of an alcoholic father, she had inherited mood problems, which she soothed by eating. Her Swedish father had also passed on his genetic need for special fats—so Kate also craved rich, fatty foods as well as sweets and starches.

What happened to Kate, who had every imbalance that we address in the *Diet Cure*? Just one week after starting on the nutritional supplements and active foods, she lost interest in her Reese's peanut butter cups and her pasta alfredo. Her PMS and yeast overgrowth were gone in three months. By that time her thyroid had been tested and treated, raising her energy and allowing her to exercise moderately four times a week. Because she was actually enjoying healthy food, and plenty of it, she did not feel deprived without her sweets, and it was easy for her to continue with her improved diet permanently. She lost forty-five pounds in the first year, stayed there for six months, and then lost her last thirty pounds in nine months. She said that she even enjoyed her six-month plateau, because she had never been able to keep weight off before, in the thirty years she had been dieting.

If, like Kate, you have multiple imbalances to overcome, you will be taking many supplements for several months. However, because they work so quickly, and are only needed temporarily, you will be able to tolerate them. After all, you have probably done much harder things—like eat nothing but hard boiled eggs for months! And this time your efforts will go toward building, not stripping, your health. Remember this: a healthy, balanced body cannot have chronic mood and weight problems.

problems should be notably improved, if not completely eliminated. Within three to twelve months you will be able to eliminate all but a few supplements for good.

You'll soon be used to eating for health and pleasure, neither starving nor bingeing, and enjoying permanent freedom from weight gain. As your body responds to special supplements and activating foods, you will become energized, craving-free, and a regular, happy exerciser. You will watch your body acquire its real, ideal shape and weight at a nice, steady pace.

The Quick Symptom Questionnaire

My goal in this book is to stop your food cravings, address your eating and weight problems, and eliminate your mood swings and negative obsessions about your body. But first we have to determine what is causing these problems.

Our clinic asks clients to fill out an extensive symptom questionnaire so that we can isolate the causes of their problems. The questionnaire here is similar to the one I administer at Recovery Systems. Its eight key sections will help you to identify your particular physical imbalances. Circle the number next to any symptom that applies to you and follow the directions at the end of each section to calculate your score. If you are uncertain about whether you might have a particular imbalance, please turn to the more complete symptom lists found in the corresponding chapters.

1. Is depleted brain chemistry the problem?

4   Sensitivity to emotional (or physical) pain; cry easily

4   Eat as a reward or for pleasure, comfort, or numbness

4   Worry, anxiety, phobia, or panic

4   Difficulty getting to sleep or staying asleep

3   Difficulty with focus, attention deficits

2   Low energy, drive, and arousal

4   Obsessive thinking or behavior

4   Inability to relax after tension, stress

3   Depression, negativity

4 Low self-esteem, lack of confidence
4 More mood and eating problems in winter or at the end of the day
3 Irritability, anger
4 Use alcohol or drugs to improve mood

Total Score _____ If your score is over 10, please turn to chapter 1.

2. Are you suffering because of low-calorie dieting?

4 Increased cravings for and focus on food; overeating
4 Regain weight after dieting, more than was lost
3 Increased moodiness, irritability, anxiety, or depression
3 Less energy and endurance
3 Usually eat less than 2,100 calories a day
3 Skip meals, especially breakfast
3 Eat mostly low-fat carbohydrates (bagels, pasta, frozen yogurt, and others)
2 Constantly think about weight
2 Use aspartame (NutraSweet) daily
2 Take Prozac or similar serotonin-boosting drugs
2 Have become vegetarian
3 Decreased self-esteem
4 Have become bulimic or anorectic

Total Score _____ If your score is over 12, please turn to chapter 2.

3. Are you struggling with blood sugar instability and stress?

4 Crave a lift from sweets or alcohol, but later experience a drop in energy and mood after ingesting them
3 Dizzy, weak, or headachy, especially if meals are delayed
4 Family history of diabetes, hypoglycemia, or alcoholism
3 Nervous, jittery, irritable on and off throughout the day; calmer after meals
3 Crying spells
3 Mental confusion, decreased memory

3 Heart palpitations, rapid pulse
4 Frequent thirst
3 Night sweats (not menopausal)
5 Sores on legs that take a long time to heal
4 Crave salty foods
4 Often feel stressed, overwhelmed
4 Dark circles under eyes
4 More awake at night

Total Score _____ If your score is over 12, please turn to chapter 3.

4. Do you have unrecognized low thyroid function?

4 Low energy
4 Easily chilled (especially hands and feet)
4 Other family members have thyroid problems
4 Can gain weight without overeating; hard to lose excess weight
3 Have to force yourself to do even moderate exercise
4 Find it hard to get going in the morning
3 High cholesterol
3 Low blood pressure
4 Weight gain began near the start of menses, a pregnancy, or menopause
3 Chronic headaches
3 Use food, caffeine, tobacco, and/or other stimulants to get going

Total Score _____ If your score is over 15, please turn to chapter 4.

5. Are you addicted to foods you are actually allergic to?

3 Crave milk, ice cream, yogurt, cheese, or doughy foods (pasta, bread, cookies, among others) and eat them frequently
3 Experience bloating after meals
4 Gas, frequent belching
3 Digestive discomfort of any kind

3   Chronic constipation and/or diarrhea

4   Respiratory problems, such as asthma, postnasal drip, congestion

3   Low energy or drowsiness, especially after meals

4   Allergic to milk products or other common foods

3   Undereat or often prefer beverages to solid food

3   Avoid food or throw up food because bloating after eating makes you feel fat or tired

4   Can't gain weight

3   Hyperactivity or manic-depression

3   Severe headaches, migraines

4   Food allergies in family

Total Score _____ If your score is over 12, please turn to chapter 5.

6. Are your hormones unbalanced?

4   Premenstrual mood swings

4   Premenstrual or menopausal food cravings

4   Irregular periods

3   Experienced a miscarriage, an abortion, or infertility

4   Use(d) birth control pills or other hormone medication

3   Uncomfortable periods—cramps, lengthy or heavy bleeding, or sore breasts

4   Peri- or postmenopausal discomfort (e.g., hot flashes, sweats, insomnia, or mental dullness)

3   Skin eruptions with period

Total Score _____ If your score is over 6, please turn to chapter 6.

Note: Some men experience "male menopause" as a result of hormonal imbalance. Men, please see the box on page 79 if you are experiencing weight gain and emotional stress.

7. **Do you have yeast overgrowth triggered by antibiotics, cortisone, or birth control pills?**

    4   Often bloated, abdominal distention
    3   Foggy-headed
    2   Depressed
    4   Yeast infections
    4   Used antibiotics extensively (at any time in life)
    4   Used cortisone or birth control pills for more than one year
    4   Have chronic fungus on nails or skin or athlete's foot
    3   Recurring sinus or ear infections as an adult or child
    3   Achy muscles and joints
    3   Chronically fatigued
    4   Rashes
    3   Stool unusual in color, shape, or consistency

Total Score _____ If your score is over 13, please turn to chapter 7.

8. **Do you have fatty acid deficiency?**

    4   Crave chips, cheese, and other rich foods more than, or in addition to, sweets and starches
    4   Have ancestry that includes Irish, Scottish, Welsh, Scandinavian, or coastal Native American
    3   Alcoholism and depression in the family history
    3   High cholesterol, low HDL levels
    4   Feel heavy, uncomfortable, and "clogged up" after eating fatty foods
    4   History of hepatitis or other liver or gallbladder problems
    4   Light-colored stool
    4   Hard or foul-smelling stool
    4   Pain on right side under your rib cage

Total Score _____ If your score is over 12, please turn to chapter 8.

After you have finished tallying your symptoms in the questionnaire and reading the corresponding chapters, you will create your own master plan for the Diet Cure. This plan will include supplements, foods, and special support. When your Diet Cure master plan is completed, you will be ready to launch into week one, Detox Week.

If you have any questions about your scores, check the more detailed symptoms lists within the first eight chapters. Even if you have only a few key symptoms in a section, they may well indicate an imbalance that you should explore.

Part I

Identifying the Eight Imbalances

ONE

Depleted Brain Chemistry

The Real Story Behind "Emotional" Eating

Almost everyone who has ever come into my office has felt like a failure at weight loss. They say they just don't seem to have the willpower to stay on a diet anymore or, even if they did, they can't stick to the maintenance part of the plan. Mostly, this is because they crave sweets or breads and can't do without them for long. They start with "just a little" and end up eating a lot more than they feel they should. Often their spouses or other family members criticize them, saying, "Why don't you try harder?" "If you'd just limit yourself to one . . . ," which only serves to make them feel even worse about themselves. "I guess they're right," these women and men would think, "I just don't have enough self-discipline." Yet oddly, these same people are usually doing well in every other aspect of their lives. They are effective at work, they keep the bills paid and the checkbook balanced, they organize their children's lives beautifully. They mastermind professional projects while keeping their households and personal and creative lives functioning. They are models of willpower.

It's this issue of willpower that usually begins my counseling sessions. "So why can't I lose weight?" my clients ask. I point out that they usually *have* lost weight—dozens, sometimes hundreds of times. Truly, there is nothing harder than dieting. Starvation by any name—famine, drought, or Optifast—is a frightful ordeal. Most of those critical spouses and family members could never stand the course of even *one* diet.

So if it's not lack of willpower, what *is* wrong with you? Are you an emotional basket case who can't get by without comfort food? That implies that if you had more strength, you could power through your problems without overeating. Should you feel ashamed of yourself for needing emotional sustenance from foods? No! I hope to help you understand that you are using food as self-medication, and why. *It's not because you are weak willed, it's because you're low in certain brain chemicals.* You don't have enough of the brain chemicals that should naturally be making you emotionally strong and complete.

These brain chemicals are thousands of times stronger than street drugs like heroin. And your body *has* to have them. If not, it sends out a command that is stronger than anyone's willpower: "Find a druglike food or a drug, or some alcohol, to substitute for our missing brain chemicals. We cannot function without them!" Your depression, tension, irritability, anxiety, and craving are all symptoms of a brain that is deficient in its essential calming, stimulating, and mood-enhancing chemicals.

WHY ARE YOUR NATURAL MOOD-ENHANCING CHEMICALS SOMETIMES DEFICIENT?

Something has interfered with your body's ability to produce its own natural brain drugs. What is it? It's obviously not too unusual, or there wouldn't be so many people using food to feel better, or taking Prozac for depression relief. Actually, there are several common problems that can result in your becoming depleted in your feel-good brain chemicals, and none of them is your fault!

✦ *You may have inherited deficiencies.* We are learning more all the time about the genes that determine our moods and other personality traits. Some genes program our brains to produce certain amounts of mood-enhancing chemicals. But some of us inherited genes that undersupply some of these vital mood chemicals. That is why some of us are not emotionally well balanced and why the same emotional traits seem to run in families. If your mother always seemed to be on edge, and had a secret stash of chocolate for herself, it should come as no surprise that you, too, need foods like candy or cookies to calm yourself. Parents who have low supplies of naturally stimulating and sedating brain chemicals often produce depressed or anxious children who use food, alcohol, or drugs as substitutes for the brain chemicals they desperately need.

✦ *Prolonged stress "uses up" your natural sedatives, stimulants, and pain re-*

lievers. This is particularly true if you have inherited marginal amounts to begin with. The emergency stores of precious brain chemicals can get used up if you continually need to use them to calm yourself over and over again. Eventually your brain can't keep up with the demand. That's why you start to "help" your brain by eating foods that have druglike effects on it.

✦ *Regular use of druglike foods such as refined sugars and flours, and regular use of alcohol or drugs (including some medicines), can inhibit the production of any of your brain's natural pleasure chemicals.* All of these substances can plug into your brain and actually fill up the empty places called receptors, where your natural brain drugs—the neurotransmitters—should be plugging in. Your brain senses that the receptors are already full, so it further reduces the amounts of neurotransmitters that it produces. As the amounts of these natural brain chemicals drop (remember, they can be thousands of times stronger than the hardest street drugs), more and more alcohol, drugs, or druglike foods are needed to fill newly emptied brain slots. This vicious circle ends when these substances you ingest are unable to "fill the bill" any longer. Now your brain's natural mood resources, never fully functional, are now more depleted than they ever were, and you still crave your mood-enhancing drugs—whether it's sugar or alcohol and cocaine.

✦ *You may be eating too little protein.* In fact, you almost certainly are if you've been dieting or avoiding fatty foods, many of which are high in protein, too. Your brain relies on protein—the only food source of amino acids—to make all of its mood-enhancing chemicals. If you are not getting enough protein, you won't be able to manufacture those crucial chemicals. A little later in this chapter and in chapter 18, you'll learn about complete and incomplete proteins, and what is "enough" protein for you. Simply put, eating the equivalent of three eggs, a chicken breast, or a fish or tofu steak at every meal might get you enough protein to keep your brain in repair.

EATING FOR ALL THE WRONG REASONS

At Recovery Systems, we treat people who use food to remedy a variety of emotional problems. Here are the stories of some typical clients.

✦ Brenda ate because she needed an energy boost. She needed sweets first thing in the morning to get her going and throughout the rest of the day to keep her going—especially during her three P.M. energy dip at work.

✦ Sharon ate at night to get to sleep. She couldn't fall asleep by ten or eleven o'clock, even on nights when she was not upset. Being upset made it worse. But a few bowls of cold cereal with milk and sugar would unravel her tension pretty reliably and help her fall asleep.

✦ Monica ate for comfort. She needed a treat to get through the day. A pastry in the morning, chocolate throughout the day, and a rich dessert after dinner made her life worth living, especially on bad days.

✦ Paul ate because he was depressed. He ate more in the wintertime and during his lonely nights. Breads, pastas, and late-night bowls of ice cream were his antidepressants.

✦ Brandon ate when he was angry. He stuffed himself with candy bars to keep from losing his temper, or after he'd finally exploded inappropriately, again.

✦ Dinah ate to numb her painful memories. She had been sexually assaulted often as a child, and food had become her ally, something she could always count on to soothe her and literally kill the pain.

✦ Andrea "got high" by starving. When she ate, it not only made her feel fat and bloated, but she lost her elevated mood.

Our counselors found that with clients like these, no amount of therapy seemed to stop this "emotional" eating. I wondered if there could possibly be a physiological cause for this intractable overeating? Eventually, I would find my answer, but it would come from an unexpected source.

THE PHYSICAL CAUSE
OF EMOTIONAL EATING

In the late 1970s, I was the supervisor of a large San Francisco alcoholism treatment program. Our clients were very serious about getting sober, and we gave them the most intensive treatment available anywhere. Yet they could not stop drinking. Eighty to ninety percent relapse rates were standard then, and still are, in the alcohol- and drug-addiction fields.

As I studied these heartbreaking relapses, I began to see a pattern. Our clients had stopped drinking, but they had quickly developed a heavy addiction to sweets. Sugar is almost identical to alcohol biochemically. Both are highly refined, simple carbohydrates that are instantly absorbed, not needing digestion (complex carbs, like whole grains, need time to be digested). Both sugar and alcohol instantly skyrocket blood sugar levels and temporarily raise levels of at least two potent mood chemicals in the brain.

This high would be followed by a low, of course. So, just as when they were using alcohol, our clients who had switched to eating large amounts of sugar were moody, unstable, and full of cravings. Since alcohol usually works even faster than sugar does, at some point, caught in a particularly low mood, they would break down and have a drink to get some relief. One drink would become a full-blown relapse.

In 1980, when I became the director of the program, I began hiring nutritionists to help solve this disturbing relapse problem. They suggested to our clients that they quit eating sweetened foods, foods made from re-fined (white) flour, and caffeine, and that they eat more whole grains and vegetables. Unfortunately, these nutritional efforts didn't pay off. For rea-sons that we understood only later, our clients just couldn't stop eating the sweets and starches that eventually led them back to alcohol. For six years we struggled for a solution. Then, in 1986, we found one.

The solution came from Dr. Joan Mathews Larson, the director of a nutritionally oriented alcoholism-treatment center in Minneapolis, Min-nesota. This brilliant pioneer, the author of *Seven Weeks to Sobriety*, intro-duced me to a technique that was quickly eliminating her alcoholic clients' cravings and raising her center's long-term success rate from 20 percent to 80 percent! The technique involved the use of specific amino acids that could rapidly feed the addicted brain exactly the type of protein that it needed to naturally fill up its empty mood-chemical sites. The results were spectacular. No longer did alcoholic clients need sweets or alcohol to feel good! Amino acid therapy revolutionized the work at our clinic, too, dra-matically raising our success rates with alcohol- and drug-addicted clients. Moreover, we were able to successfully treat clients with other addictions as well. In fact, our most spectacular successes were with food-addicted clients. *Ninety percent of the compulsive overeaters we have treated with amino acid therapy have been freed from their addiction within forty-eight hours.*

USING AMINO ACIDS TO END EMOTIONAL EATING

When psychological help does not clear up emotional eating, we need to look at the four brain chemicals—neurotransmitters—that create our moods. They are:

1. dopamine/norepinephrine, our natural energizer
2. GABA (gamma amino butyric acid), our natural sedative

3. endorphin, our natural painkiller
4. serotonin, our natural mood stabilizer, sleep promoter, and mind-focusing chemical

If we have enough of all four, our emotions are stable. When they are depleted, or out of balance, what we call "pseudo-emotions" can result. These false moods can be every bit as distressing as those triggered by abuse, loss, or trauma. They can drive us to relentless overeating.

For some of us, certain foods, particularly ones that are sweet and starchy, can have a druglike effect, altering our brains' mood chemistry and fooling us into a false calm, or a temporary energy surge. We can eventually become dependent on these druglike foods for continued mood lifts. The more we use them, the more depleted our natural mood-enhancing chemistry becomes. Substituting amino acid supplements for these drug foods can have immediate and dramatic effects.

Toni, a 26-year-old Native American, was referred to our clinic because she was exhausted, profoundly depressed, anxious, and suffering lifelong trauma from the physical and emotional violence of her family.

Toni drank alcohol and ate sweets to cope. She went regularly to her scheduled counseling sessions but was unable to rouse herself to communicate with her counselor. She had volunteered to come to Recovery Systems, hoping that a new approach would help. Toni had already been through three long-term treatment programs for alcohol addiction. Clearly, she was motivated to solve her problem.

When we saw Toni's condition, the nutritionist and I conferred and decided to give her amino acids on the spot. I asked her to tell me one thing: What was the worst thing she was experiencing at that moment? She said, "I'm soooo tired." Her slumped body and still, dull eyes confirmed this.

Our goal? To treat her lack of energy and depression by raising her levels of the neurotransmitter norepinephrine, the body's natural energizer. We gave her our smallest dose—500 milligrams of L-tyrosine. While we waited and hoped for an effect, I spoke about how and why amino acids can be helpful.

After about ten minutes, Toni said, "I'm not tired anymore."

"Great!" I said. And then I asked my next question: "What is the worst thing you are experiencing, now that your energy is better?"

She answered by bending over and grasping herself around the stomach. "I'm really uptight."

We then gave Toni the smallest dose of GABA—100 milligrams—a natural Valium-like chemical along with 300 milligrams of L-taurine. We suspected that together these supplements would help relieve her tension and allow her to relax—and they did. She stretched her legs out in front of her and then stood up, got a glass of water, and went to the bathroom. While she was gone, her counselor came in and happened to tell me that Toni was in a lot of emotional pain because of the chronic alcoholic violence in her family. When her family members drank alcohol, they all became different people, vicious and cruel. And they had never been able to stay away from alcohol.

When Toni returned, I asked her, "Can we give you something to help you endure the emotional pain that you are in?" She said yes, so I gave her a supplement containing 300 milligrams DL-phenylalanine and 150 milligrams L-glutamine. (DL-phenylalanine is the amino acid used to alleviate emotional pain.)

In ten minutes I asked Toni how she was feeling, and she smiled and said, "Just right."

I was incredulous. How could these small amounts really be helping her? Our European American clients usually need two to four times as much of each type of amino acid to get such dramatic effects.

I asked if she would like any more of any of the aminos I had already given her for energy, relaxation, or pain relief. Her answer: "Just right," and a shake of her head.

By this time Toni's eyes were sparkling. Weeks later her counselor reported that by continuing with the amino acids she had first used in our office, Toni was actually talking for the first time in their counseling sessions, was being praised at work, and was being noticed for the first time by men.

Mood Foods: How Amino Acids Feed Your Brain

The four key mood chemicals (neurotransmitters) are made of amino acids. There are at least twenty-two amino acids contained in protein foods. High-protein foods, such as fish, eggs, chicken, and beef, contain all twenty-two, including the nine amino acids that are considered essential for humans. Other foods, such as grains and beans, have some but not all of the essential nine aminos, so they need to be carefully combined to provide a complete protein (for example, rice and beans, or corn and nuts).

If you are eating three meals a day, each meal including plenty of protein (most people with eating and weight problems are doing neither), your positive moods and freedom from cravings can be maintained. But

Amino Acids Help Post-Optifasters

In a study published in October 1997, University of Texas researcher Dr. Kenneth Blum and colleagues monitored two groups of dieters for two years after they had completed a medically monitored fast. The fasters had used the product Optifast, a powdered nutritional drink containing various vitamins and minerals, which dieters use to replace one, two, or even three meals a day. In Dr. Blum's study, 247 Optifast graduates were divided into two equal groups. One group took a formula consisting of three amino acids, the other group took no amino acids. As we know from Oprah Winfrey's highly publicized experience with Optifast, and from the 1992 Senate investigation of Optifast and Nutrisystems, a quick regain of weight after a liquid fast is to be expected in more than 90 percent of cases. However, this did *not* happen to Dr. Blum's amino acid–taking group.

At the end of two years, the amino acid takers showed:

✦ a twofold decrease in percent overweight for both males and females;

✦ a 70 percent decrease in craving for females and a 63 percent decrease for males;

✦ a 66 percent decrease in binge eating for females and a 41 percent decrease for males;

✦ and the experimental group regained only 14.7 percent of the weight they lost during fasting while the control group regained 41.7 percent of their lost weight.

most people need to kick-start the brain's repair job, using certain key amino acids. This will allow you to actually enjoy eating protein and vegetables instead of cookies and ice cream. After a few months, you will be getting all the aminos you need from your food alone and won't need to take amino acids as supplements any longer.

Restoring depleted brain chemistry sounds like a big job—but it isn't. Three of the four neurotransmitters that color all your moods are made from just a single amino acid each! Because biochemists have isolated the key amino acids, you can easily add the specific ones that may be deficient. These "free form" amino acids are instantly bioavailable (in other words they are predigested), unlike protein powders from soy or milk, which can be hard to absorb. Hundreds of research studies at Harvard, MIT, and elsewhere (some of which date back to the early part of this century) have confirmed the effectiveness of using just a few targeted amino acid "precursors" to increase the key neurotransmitters, thereby eliminating depression, anxiety, and cravings for food, alcohol, and drugs.

Stopping Carbohydrate Cravings

It may sound impossible, but you can stop your food cravings almost instantly with just one amino acid supplement. Any absence of fuel for your brain's functions is perceived correctly by your body as a code-red emergency. Powerful biochemical messages then order you to immediately eat refined carbohydrates to quickly fuel your brain. There are only two fuels that the brain can readily use:

1. glucose, which is blood sugar made from sweets, starches, or alcohol
2. L-glutamine, an amino acid available in protein foods (or as a supplement, carried in all health food stores).

L-glutamine reaches the starving brain within minutes and can often immediately put a stop to even the most powerful sweet and starch cravings. The brain feeds on L-glutamine instead of glucose and is satisfied. Don't be intimidated by the strong effects of supplementation. L-glutamine is a natural food substance; in fact, it's the most abundant amino acid in our bodies. It serves many critical purposes: stabilizing our mental functioning, keeping us calm yet alert, and promoting good digestion.

Restoring Energy and Focus

When your brain is adequately fueled with its back-up emergency supplies of L-glutamine, you are ready to rebuild your four key neurotransmitters, starting with dopamine/norepinephrine, your natural caffeine. Without this natural brain stimulant, you can be slow and tired and have a hard time concentrating. You don't sparkle and can't stay on track mentally. It's hard to get things done and you can feel dull and sometimes just want to stay in bed. Your physical as well as your mental energy drops without adequate norepinephrine. The amino acid that provides this jet-fuel is the nutritional powerhouse L-tyrosine. L-tyrosine produces thyroid hormones and testosterone as well as norepinephrine. Like L-glutamine, L-tyrosine goes to work in minutes to perk you up.

Enhancing Your Ability to Relax

The next key mood-enhancing chemical is GABA (gamma amino butyric acid), our natural Valium. GABA acts like a sponge, soaking up excess adrenaline and other by-products of stress and leaving us relaxed. It seems to drain the tension and stiffness right out of knotted muscles. GABA can even smooth out seizure activity in the brain. My colleague, Elliott Wagner, a specialist in drug detox, taught me that GABA can even give relief to heroin addicts going through the severe anxiety of early withdrawal. Think what it can do for garden variety stress and uptightness!

How Effective Are L-tyrosine and GABA?

A few years ago a young couple came into my office for help with a big problem. She had discovered that her husband was using speed (methamphetamine) on a daily basis. Her father had just died of alcoholism, and she had come home from the funeral to discover her husband with his drugs laid out on the kitchen table. She was distraught and furious (and she had a tendency to be tense and edgy, anyway). She told him he had three days to assemble a recovery plan or move out. He threw his drugs away and made an appointment to see me. He told me that he had started to use speed on the road as a performer when his energy had started to sag years before. Now, years later, he was always tired unless he was on speed. He'd been secretly using it daily for years. When he got to me, he had used no speed in two days, and he was exhausted, trying hard to stay awake.

As they sat together, the husband was slumped dejectedly back into his chair, and his wife was ramrod straight on the edge of hers. I left to consult briefly with our nutritionist and came back with 1,000 milligrams of L-tyrosine for the husband and 500 milligrams of GABA for his wife. Within twenty minutes, the wife was sitting back, relaxed and smiling, while her husband was straight-backed and alert. Correcting their brain chemistries helped enormously in getting their marriage back on track: He left the next day for an inpatient treatment program that I referred him to, she went home with her GABA. It is now five years later, and he has not used drugs since. He is back on stage and his energy is fine without drugs, largely because of the L-tyrosine that he used for six months to rebuild his own brain energy system. His wife relaxes with her GABA whenever she needs to.

WHEN FOOD IS COMFORT

For many people, overeating helps compensate for a depletion of the natural pain relievers, the endorphins. Life's pain can be unendurable without adequate amounts of these buffer chemicals. Some of us (for example, those of us from alcoholic families) may be born with too little natural pain tolerance. We are overly sensitive to emotional (and sometimes physical) pain. We cry easily. Like our alcoholic parents, we need something to help us endure our daily lives, which seem so painful. Others of us use up too much endorphin through trauma and stress. We just run out, especially if we were born short on endorphins to begin with. When our comfort chemicals run low, many of us turn to comfort foods.

If you need food as a reward and a treat, or to numb your feelings, your natural pleasure enhancers, the pain-killing endorphins, are probably in short supply. Foods that elevate your endorphin activity can easily become addictive. If you "love" certain foods, those foods are firing a temporary surge of endorphins—the "love" chemicals that are thousands of times stronger than heroin. Endorphins can do more than kill pain, they provide the sensation of pleasure, too. ("That chocolate truffle tasted so good.") Orgasm releases a surge of endorphins. Euphoria, joy, the "runner's high"—these are all feelings produced by endorphins. Some people have so much natural endorphin that they smile all the time and get great pleasure from everyday life. Of course, we all endure suffering and loss. But, with enough endorphins, we can bounce back.

For anorectics and bulimics, the trauma of starving and vomiting can trigger an addictive endorphin high, because trauma of any kind can set off an automatic burst of soothing endorphins. You may know of people who felt no pain for hours after a terrible physical injury. Runners don't get their big endorphin high until they have run past "the wall of pain." At that point, they have run too far!

Raising Serotonin, Our Natural Prozac

Low serotonin can be the easiest deficiency of all to develop. Very few foods are high in the amino acid tryptophan, which is the only nutrient that the body can use to make serotonin. According to a 1997 *Lancet* study, tryptophan is one of the first nutrients to be depleted by weight-loss dieting. If, in addition to dieting, you inherited low serotonin levels and experience a lot of stress, your levels can fall low enough to set off a major eating disorder or serious emotional disturbances.

Restoring your serotonin levels can be a life-or-death matter. Suicides and violent crimes are closely associated with deficiencies of serotonin. The fatal obsessions and self-hate of bulimics and anorectics are clearly linked to low serotonin levels.

Do you have any obsessions that might be caused by low serotonin levels? The women I have worked with who report obsessive behavior tend to be "neat-niks" and suffer from negative obsessing about their physical appearance, while the men are often "neat-freaks," although they also complain about troubling sexual fantasies they can't stop. As we all know, anorectics (who are low in serotonin) are driven to obsessive control of their food intake. Obsessive fears and phobias are common among people with low serotonin levels.

It may be a difficult adjustment for you to begin to see symptoms like control, fear, and low self-esteem as biochemical problems, not just psychological ones. But the success of drugs like Prozac has already alerted us to the biochemical nature of many symptoms that don't respond to psychological help alone.

Drugs like Prozac are called serotonin reuptake inhibitors (SSRIs) because they keep whatever serotonin we have active. But they do not actually provide *additional* serotonin. For this reason, most people using SSRIs often continue to have some low-serotonin symptoms. Before there were SSRIs, the pharmaceutical compound L-tryptophan was commonly used to increase serotonin levels. For more than twenty years, psychiatrists and health food stores enthusiastically recommended it for relieving depression and food cravings and normalizing sleep without side effects. Many people found that their symptoms were eliminated permanently after only a few months of L-tryptophan use.

In 1989 a series of bad batches of L-tryptophan, which killed forty people and made many more very sick, prompted the Food and Drug Administration (FDA) to stop all U.S. sales. One Japanese company, Showa Denko, had produced all of these batches, which, it was found, were contaminated because they had eliminated three filter systems that they'd been using for years—just why they chose to take away these safety filters is a question that remains unanswered. Showa Denko has never made tryptophan again. Despite evidence that no other manufacturer has ever made a problem batch, the FDA recommended for years that L-tryptophan not be used as a supplement. (Interestingly, they have made no effort to stop the sale of infant formulas, most of which contain L-tryptophan.)

With L-tryptophan unavailable, SSRI drugs like Prozac, Zoloft, and Redux have become our primary tools for combating the crippling symptoms of low serotonin. Unfortunately, these drugs provide only temporary and incomplete benefits, and often have uncomfortable or dangerous side effects. Fortunately, in 1996, many compounding pharmacies began providing L-tryptophan again, by physician prescription, and a new version of tryptophan called 5HTP (5-hydroxytryptophan) became available over the counter in 1998 without FDA opposition.

Whatever mood-enhancing brain chemicals you have in short supply, they can be replenished quickly, easily, and safely. Chapter 9 will give you detailed information on how to create an amino supplement plan individualized for your unique brain chemistry needs.

TWO

Malnutrition Due to Low-Calorie Dieting

The Number One Cause of Overeating, Weight Gain, Bulimia, and Anorexia

Have you ever dieted? Do you skip meals for any reason? Do you try to eat fewer than 2,500 calories a day? If so, you may actually be suffering the effects of malnutrition.

America is on a killer diet. You are probably one of the millions of Americans who are cutting more than calories to fit into the thin-body ideal. Despite the fact that dieting has a mere 2 percent long-term success rate, its lure continues to be irresistible. We are dieting more frequently, more radically, and at younger ages every year. In 1964 a Harris poll found that 15 percent of adults were dieting. By 1992, 70 percent of women and 50 percent of men were dieters, as were 80 percent of seventh-grade girls.[1]

THE CALORIE CONTROVERSY

Unfortunately, low-calorie dieting does not add up to permanent weight loss, but to starvation. Your body can't tell the difference between Jenny Craig's prepackaged meals and concentration-camp fare. The consequences of depriving yourself of food are always the same, whether the deprivation is voluntary or not.

If you have been a "serious" dieter, your average daily food intake in calories may have dropped below the amount provided at the dreaded

Nazi camp at Treblinka: 900 per day. When I give this figure to female high school and college students they gasp. They think of 900 calories as generous and regard 2,500 calories per day as "gross." You may agree with them. Yet the United States Department of Agriculture (USDA) standards indicate that 2,500 calories is the *minimum* amount of calories an adolescent or adult woman needs to get the *minimum* amounts of life-sustaining nutrients such as iron. Men need at least 2,800 calories a day; their greater muscle mass and higher testosterone levels give them a naturally higher metabolism than women. (But it's not just the calories you need; eating 2,500 to 2,800 calories of junk food and popping vitamins won't protect you from malnutrition, either. You need plenty of vegetables, fruits, proteins, and fats, as well as healthy carbohydrates, for your body to function properly.)

Frankly, uniform caloric recommendations don't seem to exist. Even the *Nutrition Desk Reference* (NDR), a hefty 672-page tome last updated in 1995, offers no comment on calories at all. The 1985 *NDR* uses a phrase that's found everywhere: "If the daily caloric intake is 2,000 . . ." You'll notice that the serving sizes on almost all packaged foods are based on a mysterious "2000" calories. Does it refer to the millennium? I have not been able to find a book by dietitians, physicians, or nutritionists that made any attempt to justify this 2,000-calorie-a-day mystery figure.

Fortunately, the World Health Organization (WHO) has solved our problem through its experience with worldwide starvation. It has established that *starvation begins under 2,100 calories per day.* It uses this calculation as a basis for determining the organization's guidelines for emergency food aid.

There are two things that nutrition experts all agree on:

1. *Junk-food calories are no good.* Sugar, white flour, and junk fats, while high in calories, are health hazards that offer nutritional depletion instead of nourishment. Unfortunately, they account for most of our calories, yet they do nothing to supply the essential food and nutrients our bodies need. Obviously, junk foods are the worst promoters of unneeded weight gain.

2. *U.S. women don't eat enough food.* Half eat fewer than 1,500 calories per day. All sources agree: this is not enough food to keep our calorie furnace going. The more food we eat, the faster we burn calories (unless we have a thyroid impairment). Are you skipping meals, cutting calories whenever you can, and eating too much fast food? It's that easy to move into malnutrition. Like so many of us, you are probably too rushed to prepare fresh, whole foods—something you will learn, in chapters 18, 19, and 20, is crucial and not as difficult as you may think.

Fast and packaged foods you choose for convenience contain few nutrients. Most of the essential vitamins and minerals you need have been destroyed in processing (such as the refining of sugar or flour) and are not adequately supplied by the few synthetic nutrients that may be added back in.

We all need nutrient-rich calories. They do not add unneeded weight even if we eat lots of them. Please, try to stop counting calories or fat grams. If you follow your individualized Diet Cure program and eat foods that make you feel strong and energetic, you'll be doing fine; you will lose unneeded pounds and settle into your body's own ideal weight. Chapter 18 will give you the details of how to get the *best* calories. How many calories just doesn't seem to matter much. I've never had a problem with clients eating too many calories, only too few, as long as the calories were high quality. The truth is that low-calorie dieting is surprisingly dangerous. This chapter will explain how low-calorie, low-fat, and even vegetarian diets may have harmed you.

A FEW OF THE HEALTH CONSEQUENCES OF LOW-CALORIE DIETING

+ Heart disease, including loss of heart muscle (congestive heart failure) and sudden death syndrome (yes, people have died from very low-calorie dieting)
+ Gallstones, requiring removal of the gallbladder, caused by liquid fasting and diets under 800 calories a day (20 percent of liquid dieters develop gallstones and must have their gallbladders removed)
+ Increased risk of developing diabetes
+ Weakness, loss of endurance
+ Risks related to using tobacco to kill appetite (lung cancer, heart disease, emphysema, among others, and consequent health damage)
+ Decreased sexual interest
+ Mental dullness (lower scores on intelligence tests)
+ Stroke, caused by diet pills
+ Decreased life expectancy[2]

Dieters and Drugs

Dieters know that hunger pangs can be powerful, and rather than listen to their bodies' cries for more food they often pacify themselves with drugs that will silence those pleas. Some of these drugs seem relatively benign at first; however, dieters can become more and more dependent on them. For years, dieters have recognized the power of cigarettes in squelching hunger. The vast majority of fashion models smoke and cigarettes are often packaged for women with subtle messages about being "long" and "slim." Many people have come to rely on caffeine, either in coffee, colas, or over-the-counter diet pills. Amphetamines can be an alluring appetite suppressant as well.

Then, too, sometimes people indulge in drugs to alter their moods and perceptions, to loosen up and feel better about themselves, or for an energy pickup (a need you'll experience quite often if you aren't eating right). Often they think that since their use is "casual," they don't have to worry about the physical toll these drugs are taking on them, much less the possibility of addiction. I truly hope that if you are using any of these drugs, you are not yet addicted to them. Ask yourself the following:

✦ Am I drinking more caffeine—either as coffee or in diet sodas—or more alcohol to satisfy my need for more food?
✦ Have I ever used harder drugs to stifle hunger pangs?
✦ Am I using more diet drugs, such as Dexatrim or Ephedra, or stronger stimulants to stay thin?

If you answer yes to any of these, you're skating on thin ice. I can't tell you when the ice will crack underneath you, but I can tell you that you'll need to get help escaping from the danger zone of addiction once you've entered it. It will be important to find therapeutic support in the form of counseling and 12-step programs. You should also read chapters 1 and 9 on brain chemistry, since brain chemistry imbalances are responsible for cravings for street (and pharmaceutical) drugs. And read *Seven Weeks to Sobriety*, by Joan Mathews Larson, which gives detailed information on effectively using nutrition to escape addiction.

THE LEGACY OF THE 1960S: THE DIETING AND JUNK-FOOD GENERATION GROWS UP MALNOURISHED

The malnourishment of the typical American started with the baby boomers, who grew up after World War II and missed the food shortages and famines of the wars and the Great Depression. With plenty of food available, and with access to vitamin-fortified grains and milk and iodine-enriched salt, they grew up with no fear of malnutrition and its related diseases. They didn't worry about pellagra (caused by vitamin B_3/niacin deficiency) and beriberi (caused by B_1/thiamin deficiency), which were real threats to previous generations, killing and crippling millions worldwide. Perhaps as a result, the boomers easily fell for the Twiggy look, popularized by the famous emaciated model who appeared in the magazines of the early 1960s. The thin, "boyish" look for women was suddenly in, while natural womanly curves and body fat were out. Starving—low-calorie dieting—was now sophisticated and glamorous. Dieting has since grown into a deadly serious (and immensely profitable) enterprise. *Today, more than half of adult women in the United States eat fewer than 1,600 calories a day.* Men have latched on to the dieting craze, too, especially young men and gay men.

Dieting is particularly dangerous because of other starvation factors that are at work. USDA household food consumption surveys in 1965 showed that three basic nutrients were seriously deficient in American food: vitamins A, C, and B_6. By 1990 adequate amounts of thirteen basic nutrients had been lost to the typical American diet: vitamins A, C, B_6, thiamin, riboflavin, and folic acid; and the minerals calcium, iron, magnesium, zinc, copper, manganese, and chromium![3]

Diseases of malnutrition that haven't been seen in generations are starting to crop up again. Scurvy, a severe vitamin C deficiency marked by a rash and bleeding into the skin and mucous membranes, is normally seen only in countries in which starvation is common. But in 1993, a 14-year-old girl in Detroit was diagnosed with full-blown scurvy. It wasn't that she wasn't eating, it was that she had junk-food malnutrition. Though high in calories, her entire diet consisted of burgers, shakes, fries, candy, and soda pop.

Children and Teens Begin Dieting in Large Numbers

I am particularly concerned about people who dieted as children. A 1981 report on levels of twelve basic nutrients found that dieting girls 15 to 18 years old were seriously deficient in eleven of them! Why? Largely because since the 1960s, young girls have become regular dieters. Like so many of them, did you begin to diet because you were terrified by the weight gain that is normal in puberty? Prepubescent girls' bodies are only 10 to 15 percent fatter than boys, but they are genetically programmed to eventually develop twice as much fatty tissue in their breasts, hips, thighs, and stomachs. As your body grew natural and healthy curves in your teens, did you start dieting as a way of life? Did dieting become totally confused with normal eating for you, as it has for most American girls, and for perhaps most American adults as well?

The fact is that when children and teens diet, their fat cells double in size and increase in number. Their already naturally escalated fat production can double, sending them off on a lifetime of unnecessary dieting.

As the first baby boomers' children, born in the 1960s, reached puberty in the 1980s, a bizarre and tragic consequence of dieting was becoming apparent. A new wave of eating disorders, directly linked to low-calorie dieting, was building toward what has become an epidemic in the '90s. A significant 1991 study identifying the risk factors for developing an eating disorder found that a history of dieting and being born after 1960 topped the list.[4]

Skipping meals, food restricting, low-calorie dieting, fasting, excessive exercise, and using diet pills are common among high school and college-age girls. It is not a big step from these "casual" dieting practices to bulimia and anorexia. More and more young women, and increasingly more men, are crossing this invisible line every day.

ANOREXIA AND BULIMIA: THE DIRECT CONSEQUENCES OF NUTRIENT RESTRICTION

Has deliberately skipping meals evolved into occasional all-day fasting and eventually become compulsive fasting—or anorexia? You may have found how easily you can get rid of the food consumed during a "pig-out" by vomiting or taking diet pills or laxatives. The use of these purging methods can become more frequent as bulimia and addiction to diet pills and laxatives take over.

The high school and college girls that come to my lectures report that 60 to 80 percent of all the girls at their schools binge, purge, and starve on a regular basis. It is discussed openly; there is no real stigma left. In fact, many girls *want* to be anorectic. They are disappointed if they can't throw up and become bulimic. In a 1995 University of Michigan study, 86 percent of the 557 incoming freshmen women were dieters. Three percent were bulimic. Within six months, an additional 19 percent of the dieters had become bulimic. In total, 22 percent of freshmen girls were bulimic within six months of entering college. Although this study ended at six months, we can assume a continued increase in bulimia and the emergence of anorexia among these dieting students over time.

Puberty and adolescence are especially dangerous times for under-eating because the body is still growing. During this critical period, rapidly developing bodies already require at least 2,500 high-quality calories per day, yet many girls, if not most, at this age try to limit themselves to fewer than 1,000 calories a day, and often those are junk-food calories. This starvation dieting can quickly develop into compulsive eating, bulimia, and anorexia. In fact, two 14-year-old anorectic girls came to the Recovery Systems clinic recently. Their eating disorders had started after their very first diets.

As with anorexia, bulimia is rooted in the dieting mentality. Miranda's story is a sadly typical one. A 24-year-old beauty with a well-proportioned and muscular body, Miranda found herself close to the upper weight limit for her height. (Muscle is heavier than fat.) She had never dieted in her life, but when she went to flight attendant training school, she noticed that most of the other trainees were regular dieters. At the school, which served fast food, she did not get her usual nutritious food or her usual exercise. She found herself gaining a little weight. Concerned that she might go over the weight limit, she began skipping meals. Soon her starving had turned to bingeing and vomiting. By the time she left the training, only two months later, she had developed unbearable sweet cravings and was bingeing and purging at least once a day. Even back home on her exercise program and healthy diet, she could not shake the cravings. Her bulimia progressed. Miranda came to our clinic at age 27, obsessed and miserable, bingeing and purging three to five times per day. I'm happy to say that, through using the supplements outlined in chapter 10 and following the Diet Cure plan, many bulimic women like Miranda have been able to return to their original weight and health.

Why is it so easy to become a bulimic? One reason is that both bingeing and vomiting can trigger waves of the potent brain chemicals—the endorphins. The release of these natural heroin-like brain chemicals helps establish the powerful compulsions that bulimics are helpless to fight. When we develop false ideas about what we "should" weigh and begin dieting, we open ourselves up to the possibility of developing an eating disorder, just as Miranda did.

A growing number of women—and men—are forced by the dieting mentality into the danger zone of anorexia. They have literally lost their appetites as well as weight. No longer protected by healthy rebound food cravings, they never get to the point where they "just *have* to have a cheeseburger." When very low-calorie dieting becomes a way of life, so does the descent through the levels of starvation.

A few months into her first-ever diet, 14-year-old Courtney developed most of the symptoms of full-blown anorexia. She was chronically sick with colds and flu, lost her period, and was too weak to exercise. She quit going out with her friends and just stayed at home. She developed radical mood swings that included irritability, hysteria, and insomnia. Soon it became easy for her to starve: an apple could last her all day.

Courtney's symptoms are classic signs of malnutrition. In the concentration camps, the starving prisoners made tiny amounts of food last all day, too. How do the starving survive? How do anorectics endure working out for hours each day in the gym, like the Nazi's slave laborers?

Most of the anorectics that I have worked with *actually get high on starvation*. Anorexia triggers the same kind of powerful high that opiates like heroin give to drug users. How do we know? When anorectics are given drugs that prevent opiates from affecting them, they go into a sudden withdrawal, just as heroin users do. Their highs are cut off. It turns out that anorectic starvation, like bulimic vomiting and bingeing, is a traumatic experience that can stimulate a deep survival mechanism; the release of endorphins, the powerful, natural druglike chemicals that allow us to experience pleasure. They also kill pain and ease stress. If your body has become addicted to these natural opiates and you resume normal healthy eating, you will miss the endorphin highs. Like laboratory monkeys who pull the lever that gives them heroin in preference to food or drink until they die, an anorectic will ferociously defend her refusal to eat for powerful biochemical reasons. Bulimics binge and refuse to keep food down with a similar ferocity for the same reasons. This obsessive behavior is actually caused by nutritional deficiencies—which, thankfully, we now know how to address.

How Vitamin and Mineral Deficiencies Can Lead to Anorexia

Let's take just two vitamin and mineral deficiencies commonly caused by low-calorie dieting and trace their course as they trigger the symptoms of eating disorders.

Vitamin B₁ (thiamin). Easily depleted by undereating, this is one of the nutrients that your body cannot make itself, so you must get B_1 from foods, primarily the whole foods that chronic dieters and people with eating disorders rarely eat enough of: beans, whole grains, seeds, meats, and vegetables.

Common Early Symptoms of Thiamin Deficiency

+ Loss of appetite
+ Reduced weight
+ Abdominal discomfort
+ Constipation
+ Chest pain
+ Anxiety
+ Sleep disturbance
+ Fatigue
+ Lack of well-being
+ Depression
+ Irritation

At some point in your dieting, your B_1 levels may have dropped into the danger zone. You were still the same person, but one day you had just enough B_1, the next day you didn't, and the symptoms of anorexia began to erupt like sores do on the skins of people with vitamin C deficiency. Anorexia actually just means "loss of appetite." When a condition such as vitamin B_1 deficiency kills your appetite, you eat less, particularly if you are dieting to begin with. Suddenly dieting becomes easy. You aren't fighting a normal appetite anymore. You lost it when you lost too much vitamin B_1 from dieting. We literally are what we *don't* eat. You can't control what is lost in a diet. It isn't just your body fat that gets lost, it's your muscle and bone, and brain tissue, too. Anorectics have empty spaces that show up on brain scans where they have literally lost brain weight.

Zinc. The mineral zinc is hard to find in foods, even when we are not dieting. Red meat, egg yolk, and sunflower seeds are high in zinc. But these are fatty foods, and red meat has a bad name, so they are not likely to be included in dieters' meals. According to eating disorders specialist and nutrition researcher Alex Schauss, Ph.D., study results from Stanford University, the University of Kentucky, and the University of California at Davis agreed that most anorectics, and many overeaters and bulimics, were zinc deficient.[5] The influential mineral zinc is the second most abundant trace element in the body. *A classic symptom of zinc deficiency is loss of normal appetite.* Without enough zinc, the body can register only extreme sweetness, saltiness, or spiciness as having any taste. Simple, healthy food becomes unappetizing. In anorectics, little or no appetite remains at all. Other common zinc-deficiency symptoms are apathy, lethargy, retarded growth, and interrupted sexual development. One five-year study, reported by Dr. Schauss, showed an astounding 85 percent recovery rate for anorexia in patients given zinc supplementation. It concluded: "The zinc supplementation resulted in weight gain, better body function and improved outlook."[6] At Recovery Systems we, too, have had success using zinc (along with other nutrients) to help stop the cravings of overeaters and bulimics as well as the appetite loss of anorectics. Clients report that junk foods actually begin to be repellent and sweets "too sweet" once they have taken enough zinc.

It's especially important for teens to get enough zinc. During puberty, reproductive development is at its height. Zinc is crucial for reproductive function as well as appetite, immune function, and mental clarity. If dieting reduces the supply of zinc and other minerals at this nutrient-demanding growth stage, not only can appetite disappear but eventually a girl's menstruation may taper off, along with her mental function, as an eating disorder sets in. In boys and men, zinc is a key ingredient in sperm and protects against prostate problems as well as weak immunity.

Fortunately, these deficiencies are easily addressed with supplements and foods. In chapter 10 you will find specific nutritional suggestions to help you if you are anorectic or bulimic.

IS THERE AN IDEAL WEIGHT?

I know that finding the ideal weight is a dilemma for most women—and increasing numbers of men—in this country and abroad. How can you accept a body that you feel is socially unacceptable? It's heartbreaking that so many people are caught in this terrible bind. On the one hand, the food industry urges us to eat unhealthy foods that are addictive and make it impossible to stay at an optimal weight. On the other hand, the diet and fashion industries torture us with images of bodies that most people really should not have, that can be created only by starving or "carving" (resorting to plastic surgery and liposuction).

There are as many ideal weights as there are people. You may have heard of the three body types known as ectomorph (thin), mesomorph (medium, muscular build), and endomorph (stocky). In India, these same three types have been recognized for six thousand years and are called *pitta, vata,* and *kaffa.* Many studies warn us that it is actually more dangerous to have a low weight for your body type than a heavier weight. In his book *Big Fat Lies,* exercise physiology professor Glen A. Gaesser makes it clear that fitness (that is, good health status) has little or nothing to do with low weight. Heavy people who are fit live three times longer than thin, unfit people.

As you put together your own Diet Cure, keep in mind that the average healthy woman worldwide, between 20 and 50 years old, is five feet four inches, weighs 145 pounds, and has almost 29 percent body fat. The average man has 11 percent body fat at age 20 and 26 percent at age 60. Weight charts are not an accurate gauge of healthy body weight, either: the numbers on these charts have been yo-yoing for years as various groups fight over what is "normal" weight. For example, if you are a five-five woman, according to the Metropolitan Life Insurance Company chart of 1959, depending on your frame (measured at your elbow) you could be between 111 and 143 pounds and be considered healthy. In 1983 those numbers were bumped up—now you could weigh between 117 and 155. Then again, the U.S. Department of Agriculture (USDA) currently says that the healthy weight range for a five-five woman is 114 to 150, depending not on your frame but on your age. Meanwhile, the task force of the National Institutes of Health says that, based on body mass, a five-five woman is overweight if she's above 144 pounds, though until last year their figures said you could have weighed as much as 156.

So what *should* you weigh? It is your body's job to maintain its genetically programmed features, including its weight. Try to alter that weight at your peril. Researchers at the prestigious Rockefeller Institute examined some formerly obese women from Overeaters Anonymous who had reduced to "normal" weights. They looked "normal," but had symptoms usually seen in women with anorexia nervosa: Their fat cells were shrunken, they no longer menstruated normally, their pulses were fifty to sixty beats per minutes instead of the normal seventy to eighty, their blood pressures were abnormally low, and they were always cold. In addition, cruelly enough, they burned 25 percent fewer calories than their heights and weights indicated that they should be burning. They literally were semistarved, and had to stay that way to maintain socially acceptable weights.

DIETING: THE NUMBER ONE CAUSE OF WEIGHT *GAIN*

Up to 83 percent of those who start formal weight loss programs drop out because: (1) they can't stop eating; (2) they can't lose weight; or (3) they continue to gain weight while sticking to their diet plan! More than 60 percent of all dieters are neither overweight nor overeaters to begin with.[7] But after enough dieting attempts, dieters progressively gain more weight and are apt to become overeaters. Those who are already compulsive eaters know that they tend to lose all control after a monitored fast or more gradually lose control after less extreme diets. More than 95 percent of dieters gain back any weight they lose within two years after a diet. But many have gained more than they ever lost to begin with. It is typical for dieters to become progressively heavier than they ever would have been had they never dieted. Has rebound weight gain set off a panic that propelled you into more dieting, more rebound weight gain or, eventually, into an eating disorder?

The Flame Goes Out: Why Dieters Gain Weight

One reason dieters gain weight is because when they diet, they do not get enough protein and calories to build and maintain muscle tissue. Instead of using carbohydrates to make glucose, the body's "fuel," your dieting body starts burning muscle instead, just as someone in an isolated cabin might run out of firewood and have to burn furniture for warmth. Sure, the fuel "works," but you really don't want to get this point. Since muscles burn calories and keep your metabolism high, this loss of muscle slows down your system and causes the calories you eat to turn into fat rather than be burned as energy by your body. This is why it's important to keep your muscles toned through moderate exercise.

Loss of muscle mass isn't the only reason for rebound weight gain after a diet. After the trauma of dieting, your body, which wants to return to its ideal weight, adds extra pounds to protect against what it correctly perceives as the danger of future famines (in other words, more diets!). It does this by lowering the flame of metabolism: levels of T3, the thyroid hormone that raises your metabolic thermostat, begin to drop within hours of calorie deprivation and continue to fall until the body receives more calories. Why? Because the body knows it is starving. This is a law of nature. Rats that are allowed to feed only two hours per day, rather than eat freely all day as they normally do, end up 30 percent heavier.

Let me offer a specific example of how dieting causes weight gain. Francine, a 40-year-old cashier, came to Recovery Systems five years after starting a medically monitored fast that included a mere 400 calories plus one hour of exercise per day. Within a year on that diet, she dropped from her top weight of 300 pounds to 150 pounds. At the end of the year, she was taken off the fast. By the time we met her she had gone from 150 to 500 pounds. It had taken her thirty years to gain 300 pounds gradually, but only four years to gain 350 additional pounds by dieting. In fact, she went on the fast two more times during this period, with no weight loss at all!

Francine, like many people who diet, began with a slow-burning metabolism. As a child she had been heavy and had lower energy than her sisters. She had a low-functioning thyroid gland. Through medical testing, medication, and nutritional support, we turned up her metabolic flame so that her calories began to burn at a normal rate and she slowly began to lose weight once and for all.

Rebound Overeating: The Dieter Becomes a Food Addict

We know that one half to two thirds of people who begin dieting are not overeaters. This includes those with significant weight problems. But what about the rest? One third to one half of those on formal diet programs do eat compulsively, and may have developed food cravings as strong as any alcoholic's or drug addict's cravings.

Some people have been food cravers since childhood and are most easily catapulted into binge eating by dieting. Others probably never craved, hid, or stole food in their lives until they began to diet. But after a diet, they may have discovered that the body had a second way of preserving its ideal weight: it didn't just burn calories more slowly, it also fought back against starvation by escalating food cravings until they were strong enough to overwhelm the will to diet. These powerful cravings may not stop when weight is regained. This is why I call dieting Russian roulette. We don't know which diet will trigger food cravings that will not stop. Chapter 1 explained that the brain chemistry of overeating is very similar to that of alcohol and drug addiction. As you crave and consume more refined carbohydrates (sweets and starches), these "drug foods" can create a false high in the brain. You may have become helplessly dependent on junk foods that you began to overeat only because of a diet.

One of my clients, Sharon, a 49-year-old physical therapist, had uncontrollable food cravings that had suddenly erupted four years previously, after the first of six medically monitored fasts she had endured. A runner, she'd quit smoking and went from 170 pounds up to 225. On the first fast, she lost 100 pounds but gained it back in six months. Within that first year she lost her gallbladder and got cancer. The next year Sharon began another fast, and over the years found that with each fast she developed more cravings and weight gain until she reached 250 pounds. Sharon had never been a compulsive eater in her life until she began to fast, and she had never before experienced quick weight gain. The good news is that her cravings and weight gain stopped in the first week on our program.

If you are an overeater, you may consume thousands of calories of sugar, starch, and fat, and yet be almost as malnourished as a bulimic or anorectic. Healthy, whole foods rarely inspire binges. Fish, chicken, beef, beans, vegetables, whole grains, fruit: all these sources of real nourishment are missing from most compulsive overeaters' diets. The empty calories in junk food are like black holes, using up valuable nutrients. For example, the mineral chromium, deficient in almost all our diets, is further depleted by eating sweets. Chromium is critical for preventing blood sugar swings. Without it, your sweet cravings can grow ever stronger. Other valuable vitamins and minerals are wasted and lost in the stress of trying to digest junk food. As you start to overeat junk food after a diet and to undereat *real* food, especially vegetables and protein, you become even more malnourished. With junk-food eaters, starvation is real—it just may not show.

Adrenal Exhaustion

By now you know that dieting turns down our metabolic thermostat. But yo-yo dieting can also exhaust our health guardians, the adrenal glands, which protect us from all stress and help the thyroid regulate our weight. Anything that threatens us forces them into action, and too much inner or outer stress can wear them out. Here are two top adrenal exhausters:

✦ *hunger:* skipping meals, undereating, fasting
✦ *refined sweet and starchy foods:* the things we eat between diets, or after we've "been good" all day, like frozen yogurt, ice cream, bread, cookies, or pasta.

(For more on adrenals, see chapter 3.)

HIDDEN RISKS OF LOW-CALORIE DIETING

Low-calorie dieting doesn't just lead to weight gain. It can also cause major nutritional deficiencies: overconsumption of carbohydrates, diabetes, and addiction to artificial sweeteners and drugs like tobacco and appetite suppressants. Let's see if you might be suffering from any of these common problems caused by not eating enough good food.

Fat Deficiency

It's hard to think of fat as a nutrient because for years we have all been hearing so much about fat as a health hazard. While we fear and vilify fat, we have forgotten how essential it is to our health. Here are some real fat facts for you:

✦ A Harvard study of forty thousand nurses found that the 20 percent with the lowest fat intake had the highest rate of cancer.
✦ Eskimos had normal cholesterol levels for thousands of years on a diet containing 75 percent sea animal fat.
✦ Mediterraneans, too, are notably free of heart disease, although they consume diets containing 40 percent fat (mostly from olive oil).
✦ Scandinavians, the Celtic Irish, and north coast Native Americans, among others, have high genetic requirements for the fats that they traditionally got from their original fish-based diets. Depression and alcoholism are two conditions that they suffer now that their diets are much lower in fish and the natural fats that fish contain.
✦ We all need the essential fat-soluble vitamins A and E that low-fat diets jeopardize. Some of the most dramatic functions of vitamins A and E are to maintain our immune system and our eyesight and to protect against stroke and liver disease.
✦ Every cell in the body is protected by a lining of fat.
✦ The brain is 60 percent fat.

The fact is, fats (or fatty acids, as they are biochemically known) play an essential role in our entire body's function. Our recent low-fat mania has yielded many adverse results.

The Low-Fat Experiment That Failed. You may remember that in the 1970s the Pritikin Institute, the nation's first low-fat diet center, electrified

the country. Nathan Pritikin's program was designed for people with severe and chronic health problems, primarily heart disease. His therapeutic
diet became mainstream before any long-term evaluation of the Pritikin
approach had been done. The extraordinary media attention that the Pritikin Diet quickly received eventually led to what has become a national fat
phobia.

Former Pritikin Institute nutritionist and respected health writer Ann
Louise Gittleman tells us in her book, *Beyond Pritikin*, that there was indeed an initial weight loss and health gain for those who came to the Pritikin Institute. But later many of these same people, on the same low-fat
regimen, gained back at least as much weight as they had lost. Although
their heart problems cleared up, they began to regain unneeded weight
and developed new health problems, such as arthritis, chronic yeast infections, and increased PMS, apparently as a result of their low-fat, high-carb
diets. Our current nationwide low-fat experiment has produced the same
effect: fat consumption has dropped (the average American now consumes
34 percent of their calories as fat)[8] yet weight has gone *up* over the past ten
years. Instead of eating fats, we're overeating carbohydrates. For millions
who do not have heart disease, and who never overate fat to begin with,
low-fat high-carb dieting has become a menace.

Fat Deficiency Causes Fat Cravings. Although many of our clients have
avoided fat, overeating sweets and starches instead, many are addicted to
fatty foods like cheese, butter, and potato or corn chips. When we add certain oils to their diets, they lose interest in rich foods and their weights
drop. Low-fat dieting depletes our bodies of *essential* fatty nutrients. In reaction, our bodies signal us via cravings to eat more fats. But the kinds of
fats in the junk food that we binge on in response to those cravings do
not satisfy our fundamental nutritional needs, and we actually put on
weight as we become fat deficient. When we eat the specific fats we need,
which we can get from certain fish or plants, our fat cravings cease. (If this
sounds like you, turn to chapter 8 to see if you have fatty acid deficiency).

Fatty foods, such as avocado, salmon, and olives, are profoundly nourishing. A handful of nuts a day actually cuts the risk of heart disease.

Protein Deficiency

Low fat often means low protein. What are the healthy foods that you may be avoiding because of their fat content?

- ✦ eggs
- ✦ fish
- ✦ chicken in the skin
- ✦ red meat
- ✦ tofu
- ✦ nuts
- ✦ seeds
- ✦ cheese
- ✦ avocado
- ✦ oils

Take a close look. Many of the best sources of protein have become suspect. When you throw this baby out with the bathwater, you are moving toward protein malnutrition. Remember, protein is the only food that can be used to create new muscle. Also, since brain and mood chemicals can be made only from protein, moods and thinking can deteriorate without enough of this mind fuel. Like most dieters and eating disorder sufferers, you may be avoiding protein-rich foods because they also contain fat. "I don't want to use up my calories for the day on a steak, because it's too fatty!" you tell yourself. "I'd rather use them on ice cream." Protein is a food that few people crave (a hallmark of a healthy food!), so it's easy to dispense with.

Protein Malnutrition Causes Brain-Power Outage. As the activity of the brain shrinks with dieting, the brain's mental and emotional stability can falter—even fail. (You can recognize brain chemistry deficiency by its very specific symptoms, such as depression, anxiety, irritability, obsessiveness, and low self-esteem.) My clients who are dieters or have eating disorders always suffer from mood problems, caused primarily by protein malnutrition. The four brain chemicals that dictate your moods are all derived from the amino acids in protein foods. Even nondieters who tend not to eat enough protein can suffer from low-protein brain drain.

Tryptophan Depletion: The Path to Depression, Low Self-esteem, Obsession, and Eating Disorders

Serotonin, perhaps the most well known of the brain's four key mood regulators, is made from the amino acid L-tryptophan. Because few foods contain high amounts of tryptophan, it is one of the first nutrients that you can lose when you start dieting. A new study shows that serotonin levels can drop too low within seven hours of tryptophan depletion. Let's follow this single essential protein (there are nine altogether) as it becomes more and more deeply depleted by dieting, to see how decreased levels of even one brain nutrient might turn you toward depression, compulsive eating, bulimia, or anorexia.

In his best seller, *Listening to Prozac*, Peter Kramer, M.D., explains that when our serotonin levels drop, so do our feelings of self-esteem, regardless of our actual circumstances or accomplishments. These feelings can easily be the result of not eating the protein foods that keep serotonin levels high. As their serotonin-dependent self-esteem drops, girls tend to diet even more vigorously. "If I get thin enough, I'll feel good about myself again!" Tragically, they don't know that they will never be thin enough to satisfy their starving minds. Extreme dieting is actually the worst way to try to raise self-esteem because the brain can only deteriorate further and become more self-critical as it starves. More and more dieters worldwide are experiencing this miserable side effect of weight reduction on the brain.

When tryptophan deficiency causes serotonin levels to drop, you may become obsessed by thoughts you can't turn off or behaviors you can't stop. Once this rigid behavior pattern emerges in the course of dieting, the predisposition to eating disorders is complete. Just as some low-serotonin obsessive-compulsives wash their hands fifty times a day, some young dieters may begin to practice a constant, involuntary vigilance regarding food and the perfect body. They become obsessed with calorie counting, with how ugly they are, and on how to eat less and less. As they eat less, their serotonin levels fall farther, increasing dieters' obsession with undereating. As their zinc and B vitamin levels drop low as well, their appetite is lost. This can be the perfect biochemical setup for anorexia.

What so many therapists and others have observed as the central issue of "control" in anorexia often comes down to this: just as vitamin C deficiency (scurvy) results in an outbreak of red spots, so does tryptophan (and serotonin) deficiency result in an outbreak of the obsessive-compulsive behavior that we call "control." There may be psychological elements in the picture, too, but a low-serotonin brain is ill equipped to resolve them.

Tryptophan, Serotonin, Compulsive Overeating, and Bulimia

For reasons we don't entirely understand, some dieters whose serotonin levels drop lose self-esteem and become obsessed with weight loss, but do *not* lose their appetites. On the contrary, their appetites expand. In the late afternoon and evening, especially in winter and during PMS (low serotonin times for all of us), they can become ravenous and binge on sweets and starches.

One of our clients ate regular breakfasts and lunches but dreaded her evenings, when she would binge on ice cream and cookies, whether she had eaten a normal dinner or not. Terrified of weight gain, she would throw up as soon as she ate.

In one study, bulimics were deprived of the single protein tryptophan. In reaction, their serotonin levels dropped and they binged more violently, ingesting and purging an average of 900 calories more each day.[9] In another study, adding extra tryptophan to the diet reduced bulimic binges and mood problems by raising serotonin levels. Most recently, an Oxford researcher, Katherine Smith, reported that even years into recovery, bulimics can have a return of their cravings and mood problem after only a few hours of tryptophan depletion. She concluded, "Our findings support suggestions that chronic depletion of plasma tryptophan may be one of the mechanisms whereby persistent dieting can lead to the development of eating disorders in vulnerable individuals."[10]

Note that most compulsive eaters do not vomit. They keep it all down. But dieting can lower their serotonin levels, too, causing the same wild cravings and self-hate that bulimics suffer.

As we trace the fate of only one depleted nutrient, tryptophan, and the brain chemical made from it, serotonin, you can again see how easily a dieter can develop an eating disorder. If you consider how many other critical brain and body chemicals are depleted through dieting, you have a more profound appreciation of the dangers you are risking on low-calorie diets.

We have just looked at the important nutrients that we *lose* on low-fat diets. Now let's talk about what foods are left to eat. The foods that contain no fat fall into one category: they are all carbohydrates.

THE LOW-FAT HIGH-CARB RECIPE FOR FOOD ADDICTION AND DIABETES

Carbohydrate foods made from white flour, like pasta, bagels, and bread, are likely to be your first choice on a low-fat diet. You will probably also consume lots of sweets. While it's true that grains in their natural, whole form contain some protein, vitamins, minerals, and fats and unrefined sweets, like fruit and sugarcane, contain valuable nutrients, you probably eat the refined, stripped forms of these sweet and starchy carbohydrates. Most low-fat dieters reach for cookies, muffins, pastries, pasta, cereal, and similar foods made from a combination of white flour and white sugar. A nationally known addiction researcher, Forrest Tennant, M.D., draws the biochemical parallel between the effects of eating these "high" carbohydrate foods and the elevating effects of alcohol and cocaine. Pointing out that these "foods" can trigger powerful brain chemical releases, he calls alcohol the ultimate carbohydrate drug. Refined from high-carbohydrate foods like grains and grapes, alcohol contains three more calories per gram.[11] When we ask sweet and starch addicts how these foods affect their moods, like alcoholics they often say their "drugs" makes them feel "energized," "comforted," or "relaxed." Over time it takes more carbohydrates to deliver the druglike effect, leading to stronger sweet cravings, more and bigger binges, and faster weight gain. If you are bulimic, you probably began vomiting at this stage to empty out so you could quickly start bingeing again. You may also have started to alternate between periods of abusing alcohol and abusing food. All of the adverse health consequences of high-fat diets can result from low-fat, high-carbohydrate diets as well. But there is one added risk: diabetes. Many of us fear developing diabetes but don't realize that most diabetes, or chronically high blood sugar, can be caused just by eating too many carbohydrates. Rates of diabetes have risen parallel to average weight gain over the past ten years. Although as a nation in the last ten or so years we have dropped our consumption of fat, our consumption of carbohydrates has risen. Additionally, each of us now eats more than one hundred pounds of sugar or corn syrup every year, on average, in contrast to the twenty-five pounds we ate in 1900.

Because refined carbohydrates made from sugar and white flour rapidly increase insulin levels, they can permanently exhaust the pancreas (the insulin-producing organ), causing diabetes. Another factor that contributes to diabetes is mineral malnutrition. Eating sugar in large quantities can cause mineral loss, most notably chromium, which is particularly important for blood sugar regulation. Chromium protects from the cravings and overeating that are triggered when blood sugar levels are unstable.

Diabetes is the ultimate eating disorder that can result from low-fat dieting. Diabetic food addicts are unable to stop eating carbohydrates, especially the simple ones (sugars), even though they know that these sweets are literally killing them.

The Artificial Sweetener Trap

Billie drank a pot of black tea from a lovely handmade tea pot in a special corner overlooking her garden. She sweetened each cup with several packets of NutraSweet (aspartame). She was a compulsive eater, so she felt that using a diet sweetener was a good, healthy choice for her. When I asked her to give up her black tea because of its caffeine content, she wept. So I relented and said, "Okay, keep the tea for a week. Just stop using Nutra-Sweet." She happily agreed. Two days later I got a phone call from her. "I hate black tea!" she said. She thought it was the tea she craved, but she had actually been an aspartame addict for years, without even knowing it. She experienced the longest drug withdrawal cravings I have ever seen when she stopped using her NutraSweet. For months, she could not satisfy her thirst with any liquid because her body so sorely missed the aspartame.

Most dieters, and even many of you who are not serious dieters, use diet drinks and diet foods to avoid high-calorie sweeteners. Before coming to me, my clients have typically been drinking quarts of diet soda, even cases of it, every day, bingeing on junk food and washing it down with diet Cokes. Artificial sweeteners contribute to compulsive eating for some users. You may have noticed that your cravings for sweets and fatty foods, and your weight, have increased along with your aspartame use. Several studies have confirmed this ironic fact in both animals and humans.[12] In 1996, Richard Simmons, the diet and fitness guru, announced that he had given up diet sodas after years of addiction and suddenly lost ten pounds!

The amino acid phenylalanine, which is a component of aspartame, can be very stimulating, especially when combined with caffeine. Aspartame's ingredients compete with tryptophan. They block its conversion into our fog-clearing and mood-enhancing chemical serotonin. This is one way that aspartame impedes recovery for those of you who are anorectics and bulimics, even when you try to begin eating normally again. Artificial sweeteners can also make you feel bloated and fat, further discouraging real food consumption. You may avoid healthy food or purge it.

So far, more than ten thousand aspartame users have reported over one hundred adverse symptoms, compiled by the Food and Drug Administration (FDA). They include everything from menstrual changes, weight gain, and headaches to severe depression, insomnia, and anxiety attacks.

Aspartame is not the only chemical sugar on the market you should avoid. Saccharin is not only linked with cancer but, like aspartame, can cause an increase in the consumption of sweets.[13]

VEGETARIANS' SPECIAL CHALLENGES AND RISKS

Vegetarian diets can lead to malnourished states and, eventually, to eating disorders, even when the vegetarian had no intention of reducing weight by eliminating meat. Flesh foods—like red meat, poultry, and fish—are high-protein foods that contain all of the essential amino acids. Avoiding these foods can weaken many crucial body functions, including muscle and brain strength. Both are dependent on adequate protein. It is possible to get enough protein from vegetarian sources, but it takes careful study and planning. Many vegetarians eat little but carbohydrates and become quite addicted to sweets.

What may be most difficult to get from a vegetarian diet is iron. Twenty percent of women generally are iron deficient. Iron deficiency is a particularly common problem among female athletes. Iron status is also closely linked with mental and emotional functioning. When dieting depletes iron levels, the result is the mental and emotional fog so characteristic of eating disorders. Very similar symptoms result from zinc deficiency, which is also easy for vegetarians to develop. Red meat is one of the few reliable and easily digestible sources of both zinc and iron (it's harder to metabolize the zinc and iron found in foods like raisins, kale, and spinach).

Fifty percent of anorectics are vegetarian. One of my favorite colleagues, sports medicine specialist Al Loosli, M.D., treats many female high school and college athletes who are vegetarian. According to Dr. Loosli, these vegetarians often suffer from loss of periods, bone mass deterioration, bone fractures, general weakness, and lowered endurance. Many of them have full-blown eating disorders.[14]

Many of my vegetarian clients have supplemented with iron and zinc successfully, and increased protein from plant sources. Others have reluctantly added fish to their diets several times per week and felt much stronger. Still others have had to accept that their bodies were not built to thrive on a vegetarian diet and have added back red meat and poultry. Several recent books, most notably *Eat Right for Your Type*, by Dr. Peter J. D'Adamo, have linked blood type with optimal diet and found that blood type O, in particular, may require animal protein. In chapter 10 you will find specific suggestions for how to be a vegetarian without becoming depleted in iron, zinc, and protein. Don't get me wrong: I applaud the idealism of vegetarians. These cautionary remarks are not meant to discourage those of you who are vegetarian but to alert and strengthen you.

Whatever problems you've developed as a result of restricted eating, please read chapter 10, "Nutritional Rehab for the Ex-Dieter," to immediately address your most important nutritional needs. Next, part 3 of *The Diet Cure* will help you to develop, perhaps for the first time, a wholistic plan for using food, supplements, exercise, and other support that will allow you to recuperate from the effects of low-calorie dieting and reach your own ideal *healthy* weight.

THREE

Unstable Blood Sugar

Carbohydrate Addiction, Hypoglycemia, Diabetes, and Adrenal Exhaustion

---

A Special Note Regarding Insulin-Dependent Diabetes

If you are diabetic and taking insulin, you will need to monitor your insulin levels often and work very closely with your M.D. to keep your levels optimal. Insulin levels can and should come down as your diet improves once you start taking the supplements. Otherwise, your sugar-free diet will drop your glucose levels too low.

You probably know by now whether your own insulin-producing capacity has become irreversibly damaged. If so, you will not be able to stop your medicine, but you will "manage" it much more easily. I highly recommend *The Diabetes Solution*, by Richard K. Bernstein, as a guide to managing severe diabetes with a diet like the one we recommend (higher protein than the usual diabetic diet) and excellent, practical suggestions for exercise and medication.

You already know that junk carbos like candy and cookies are nutritionally worthless, at best. And you may also have discovered that they are powerfully addictive. If you could stop eating them permanently, on your own, you probably wouldn't be reading this chapter. You have tried "just saying no." You have probably stopped eating them for short periods during a diet, but I want you to be able to walk away from them, for life, *easily*. And I don't mean you should shift over to health-food cereals, granola bars, and honey-sweetened cookies. Although these products do contain some real food, their first ingredient is usually a sweetener such as brown sugar, fruit juice concentrate, or honey.

Some people successfully quit sugar in a roundabout way by gradually substituting healthier and healthier foods. But weaning yourself from sugar usually takes years, if it works at all. Many people are so sensitive to concentrated carbohydrates that they really can't do this. They can't stop eating dried fruit any more than others can stop eating Oreos. Brown sugar and honey, like their refined white cousin, can be highly addictive substances.

There's a much faster, easier, and healthier way for you to lose your interest in sweets. In fact, most of you can be freed from your sugar cravings in just twenty-four hours.

THE BLOOD SUGAR BLUES

Your body and brain are built of protein, water, fat, minerals, and vitamins. Like auto parts that must be made from solid materials (metal and rubber), body parts—muscles, hormones, nerves, bones—can be made only from water and solid foods like protein, minerals, and fat. Without them, your body doesn't have the building blocks to replenish itself and replace worn-out cells. Carbohydrates have a very different function. They are the fuel that your body uses. Yes, they're important, but just as you cannot build an engine or a tire out of gasoline, you cannot make muscle or hormones or bones out of carbos. Imagine a car that did not get its oil replaced or its tires repaired. How far could it go on gasoline alone?

Your body does need high-quality carbohydrate "gas," but the amount depends on how much "driving" your body is doing. Athletes and fast metabolizers need more carbohydrates. Less-active people need fewer. And not just any carbohydrate will do the job. You need *high-quality* ones, like vegetables, beans, and brown rice; not low-quality carbohydrates, highly sweetened with sugar, or starchy ones like white bread or bagels and pasta, which are converted into sugar in seconds in your mouth. If you are a carbo junkie, you are frequently running low on glucose, the blood sugar fuel made from carbos that keeps your brain and body going.

But if glucose is made from carbohydrates and you are regularly eating lots of sweet and starchy carbos, how can you be running so low on blood sugar? Paradoxically, it's *because* you are eating so many high-carbohydrate foods! Your body can't tolerate the amount of carbohydrates in highly processed foods like candy, cookies, or even bagels, especially if you eat your carbohydrates without lots of balancing protein, fiber, and fat. If you had lox and cream cheese on your bagel, you'd be all right. If you ate a salmon steak every time you had a candy bar, you'd probably be okay, too! But you don't, of course. And some people are so sensitive to sweets that no matter what they eat with them (even if they eat a full meal), they'll get a headache and feel irritable after the initial pleasure injection wears off.

So what happens to all sweets and starches you eat? They turn into blood sugar (glucose) at exactly the same rate—in seconds!—while still in your mouth, shocking and alarming your whole system. "Get rid of it, fast!" shrieks your body. Out rushes insulin, made by your pancreas, for just such occasions, from whatever protein you are eating. Insulin knocks every bit of that glucose high out of your bloodstream and quickly stores it as fat, where it gathers in your body, crowding your muscles, and clogging your arteries. As you gain excess fatty weight around your middle from consuming too many carbohydrates, insulin gets less effective. The more carbos you eat, the more fat you store in your abdomen, and the more insulin you need. Meanwhile, your pancreas is running out of protein to meet the escalating demand for insulin, because you aren't eating much protein. You're filling up on carbs and sweets instead. Often, the end result of all this is diabetes—when, in a sense, your gas tank just fills up with sugar.

The Adrenals Rush to Help

But before you get to that point, while you still have plenty of insulin, your problem is that, too often, you don't have enough sugar in your blood. Your insulin has taken too much. At this point your two adrenal glands, your emergency stress team, are mobilized to handle the situation. Blood sugar that drops too low for even a few minutes can drop you into a coma, because your brain is particularly vulnerable to any absence of blood sugar. So, like firemen with a safety net, the adrenal hormones are sent out to "catch" your blood sugar before it falls too low. They boost it with emergency stores of a special sugar called glycogen.

If this stressful scenario repeats itself too often, your adrenals will get overwhelmed. That's because they are simultaneously taking care of all of the other stresses that are occurring both inside and outside of you. So, sooner or later, your adrenals will be unable to "make the save" as effectively. You'll start feeling worse, faster, after your sweet or starchy highs. As you feel the increasing need to raise your blood sugar back up, you'll run to the nearest candy machine more often. This low blood sugar, or hypoglycemic distress, is by far the most common problem that we see at our clinic.

Common Symptoms of Low Blood Sugar
(Hypoglycemia), in Order of Frequency

✦ Craving sweets
✦ Nervousness
✦ Exhaustion
✦ Faintness, dizziness, tremors, cold sweats
✦ Depression
✦ Drowsiness
✦ Headaches
✦ Digestive disturbances
✦ Forgetfulness
✦ Insomnia
✦ Constant worrying, unprovoked anxiety
✦ Confusion
✦ Internal trembling
✦ Heart palpitations, rapid pulse
✦ Muscle pains
✦ Numbness
✦ Indecisiveness
✦ Asocial or aggressively antisocial behavior
✦ Crying spells
✦ Lack of sex drive (women)
✦ Allergies
✦ Lack of coordination
✦ Leg cramps
✦ Lack of concentration
✦ Blurred vision
✦ Muscle twitching and jerking
✦ Itching and crawling skin sensations
✦ Sighing and yawning
✦ Unconsciousness[1]

IS YOUR BLOOD SUGAR RISING?

If you are in the first, hypoglycemic stage of the blood sugar roller-coaster ride, then much of the time your pancreas is still hardy, punching out the insulin to stop sugar shock. But you may be beginning to show signs of impending diabetes: your pancreas can't keep up the pace and release enough insulin indefinitely. Your pancreas was built for the occasional shock, not for daily or hourly carbo overload.

Eventually your pancreas will falter in its job of keeping up your insulin supply. As a result, your blood sugar can eventually rise too high, for too long, too often. You become diabetic. People with the more common Type II diabetes have all been hypoglycemic first, then they became addicted to refined carbohydrates to the point that their pancreas's blood sugar–coping capacity was exhausted.

All of our diabetic or prediabetic clients would love to manage their blood sugar problem with diet and exercise, and they try, but they cannot. They are unable to eat healthy food because they are too heavily addicted to carbohydrates. Realistically, their cravings for carbs have to be dealt with before they can begin to exercise and eat in a more healthy way.

Diabetes[2]

How do you know if you are diabetic? Keep in mind that you're more likely to get it if you have a family history of Type I or Type II diabetes. And the most common symptoms are increased thirst and urination, vision problems (such as failing eyesight), and fatigue. If you have any of these symptoms, please see your doctor for diabetes testing.

Common Symptoms of Diabetes

+ Lowered resistance to infection
+ Boils and leg sores
+ Lesions and cuts take a long time to heal
+ Overweight
+ Crave sweets, but eating sweets does not relieve symptoms
+ High sugar in urine and blood
+ Extreme systemic acidity
+ Severe itching
+ Rapid weight loss
+ Constant hunger
+ Elevated cholesterol[3]

HOW DID YOU GET CARBO ADDICTED?

Most low and high blood sugar is caused by addiction to sweets and starches. How did you get addicted? It could have started with any or all of the imbalances that I discuss in this book: brain chemical imbalances, dieting, food allergy, hormonal imbalances, yeast overgrowth, or, as we'll see later in this chapter, too much stress.

But your first problem may be that you were born or now reside in the United States. Diseases of sugar addiction like hypoglycemia and diabetes are almost unknown in countries that are too "primitive" to produce the fancy packaged carbos that contain no nutrients. In the United States, we each consume more than one third of a pound of sugar per day! That is a big habit, and it's getting bigger. And this doesn't include the junk food starches like bagels, pasta, and cold cereal that the body can't distinguish from sugar.

The Pima, a Native people who live both in the United States and in Mexico, are among the most vulnerable people in the world to "carbo-drugs" (as I like to call them). In the United States, where they have unlimited access to junk carbohydrates, they have the highest rate of obesity and diabetes in the world. But the Mexican Pimas, who still eat mostly whole corn, beans, vegetables, fruit, eggs, chicken, and meat, do not have diabetes.

Every ethnic group that comes to the United States (except the English, who may eat as poorly as we do) experiences a drastic reduction in health with the first and certainly by the second generation from exposure to our "diet."[4] That's because essentially we have stopped eating food here: we mostly eat chemicals and carbo-drugs. Products made from them are cheap, overly available, and addictive—of course we eat them! And then we can't stop. Some of us, like the Pima, are addicted more easily. (Fortunately, the very quality that makes Native Americans so vulnerable to the carbo-drugs, sugar, white flour, and alcohol also makes them respond instantly to the nutritional supplements that I describe in chapter 11.)

A California Native tribal member came to me at age 47 with diabetes so bad that he had become impotent and lost his wife. He had such low energy that he could hardly get up in the morning or stay awake after dinner to visit with his children. Worse, he was losing his eyesight. He knew he had to do something about his health—quickly. I offered him two doses (four capsules) of a multiple vitamin-mineral formulation designed to stop blood sugar swings. The next day he reported that after taking the first two capsules the night before he had stayed alert until ten P.M. (he usually

Any Doubts About How Addictive (and Destructive) Sugary Foods Can Be?

Many clients have told me that they got hooked the very first time they got a high from ice cream, sodas, or cookies. Personally, I think of refined sugar as a drug. When white sugar was first introduced to Europe in the sixteenth century, it was kept under lock and key, because of its potency. It was worth its weight in silver and they even called it "crack"! Just because sugar is legal, cheap, and easily available doesn't mean that it isn't destructive. Remember, cocaine was once the key ingredient in Coca-Cola, and available to adults and children all across America.

dozed from seven o'clock on), that he woke up alert (unheard of!), and that after taking the second two capsules, he had felt fine all the next day (also rare). Within two months, he was no longer impotent. Now, I have rarely seen people of other ethnic backgrounds respond this quickly and dramatically to supplements designed to balance blood sugar levels. But people of all ethnicities do respond to this same approach—it just takes days rather than hours.

If you have chronic low blood sugar, or are diabetic, staying on a good diet and getting some moderate exercise works miracles. Blood sugars even out quickly, and health, energy, and weight normalize fast. Simply staying away from sugary foods can usually stop symptoms like headaches, dizziness, and irritability immediately.

So why don't people with unbalanced blood sugar "just do it"? Most people suspect that it's because diabetics and hypoglycemics are too self-indulgent and have no willpower, or that they just don't care. But they're wrong. Their only problem is that they are up against a biochemical power much stronger than they are. They are caught in the jaws of a relentless biological mechanism that demands that they continue to eat carbos.

Fortunately, it's easy to disarm this biochemical monster. All we typically need are one mineral, an amino acid, and a few vitamins. These natural substances can turn the killer into a pet in just a few minutes. (In chapter 11, you'll get the exact details of this monster-killing protocol.)

Although most of our clients have been hypoglycemic, we have also worked with many Type II diabetics, as well as a few Type I diabetics. We have been able to help them all successfully avoid toxic carbos. But they do typically need extra help beyond what the usual supplements and food can give, if (1) they are diabetic and the damage to their insulin-producing pancreas has been too great, or (2) their adrenal glands have become too exhausted by stress and sugar.

ARE YOU OVERSTRESSED? DO YOUR ADRENALS NEED HELP?

Because almost everyone who comes to Recovery Systems has a low blood sugar problem, we are very familiar with the symptoms of hypoglycemia. But it took years for us to realize that many of the symptoms of hypoglycemia are identical to the symptoms of adrenal exhaustion.

As explained earlier, the adrenals are your stress-defense team. One of their primary duties is to "handle" any blood sugar slumps. In case of a sudden "emergency," like the blood glucose drop after insulin has made a sugar sweep in reaction to a Snickers bar, the adrenals release adrenaline, which is why eating sweets can make you very nervous, jittery, and irritable. That jolt of adrenaline is intended to get you out of a potentially dangerous fix by forcing a release of a backup fuel supply called glycogen. It's hard work for the adrenals each time they have to perform this emergency procedure. And if you eat sweets a lot, especially without balancing them with protein, you are going to exhaust them eventually. This is true if you diet a lot, too, because your blood glucose is always low when you diet. Dieting is a big strain on the adrenals. There is no greater strain than impending death, which is what the adrenals perceive starvation dieting to be (the adrenals become wildly active during anorexia). But *any* extreme or prolonged stress will overtax them.

The Stages of Stress Exhaustion

No matter how much stress we endure, we have just two little glands to fight it for us: the adrenal glands. In periods of profound stress—a divorce, drug addiction, low-calorie dieting, an eating disorder, a major illness or injury—we can go into adrenal overdrive. Our adrenals can get stuck in the "on" position, pushing our whole system into chronic "fight or flight" mode. The chemicals the adrenals release to accomplish this are adrenaline and cortisol: adrenaline is needed for short blasts (when you're approached by a mugger or an angry boss); cortisol is used for the longer-lasting stresses (like an illness or a divorce). As this state of adrenal alarm

> A 1995 story on stress, reported in the *New York Times*, included the interesting results of a survey showing that 68 percent of those questioned felt stressed most or all the time.[4]
>
> A survey of more than 1,000 adults found that 79 percent of women and 69 percent of men reported stress eating of sweets, particularly chocolate.[5]

progresses other systems try to compensate: The thyroid turns down its hormonal activity in an attempt to reverse the adrenal overdrive. This can make us tired and heavy as our metabolic rate eventually slows. DHEA and other adrenal hormones alter their functions, too, in an attempt to balance out cortisol's systemic rampage. This is the first stage of stress exhaustion. Often we don't get the relaxation and rest that would allow us to repair and rebound. So we get sick more often, or have trouble sleeping. In the second stage we start running too low on cortisol and feel tired and stressed too often. In the third stage we are quite low most of the day, in cortisol, DHEA, thyroid, and other hormones, like testosterone, estrogen, and progesterone. In this stage we are always tired and cannot cope with stress at all well.

Where are you in the stages of adrenal stress exhaustion? First, see if you have the following typical symptoms.

Common Symptoms of Adrenal Exhaustion

✦ Sensitivity to exhaust fumes, smoke, smog, petrochemicals
✦ Inability to tolerate much exercise, or you feel worse after exercising
✦ Depression or rapid mood swings
✦ Dark circles under the eyes
✦ Dizziness upon standing
✦ Lack of mental alertness
✦ Tendency to catch colds easily when weather changes
✦ Headaches, particularly migraines, along with insomnia
✦ Breathing difficulties
✦ Edema (water retention)
✦ Salt cravings
✦ Trouble falling asleep or staying asleep
✦ Feeling of not being rested upon awakening

✦ Feeling of tiredness all the time

✦ Feeling of being mentally and emotionally overstressed

✦ Low blood sugar symptoms

✦ Need for caffeine (coffee, tea, and others) to get you going in the morning

✦ Low tolerance of loud noises and/or strong odors

✦ Tendency to startle easily

✦ Food or respiratory allergies

✦ Recurrent, chronic infections, such as yeast infections

✦ Lightheadedness

✦ Low tolerance for alcohol, caffeine, and other drugs

✦ Fainting

✦ Tendency to get upset or frustrated easily, quick to cry

✦ Tendency to get a second wind (high energy) late at night

✦ Low blood pressure

✦ Haven't felt your best in a long time

✦ Eyes sensitive to bright light

✦ Feeling of being weak and shaky

✦ Constant fatigue and muscular weakness

✦ Sweating or wetness of hands and feet caused by nervousness or mood swings

✦ Ability, sometimes, to relieve paranoia and depression by eating

✦ Frequent heart palpitations

✦ Chronic heartburn

✦ Vague indigestion or abdominal pain

✦ Low blood pressure

✦ Alternating constipation and diarrhea

✦ Infrequent urination

✦ Sweet cravings

✦ Lack of thirst

✦ Clenching and/or grinding of teeth, especially at night

✦ Chronic pain in the lower neck and upper back

✦ Inability to concentrate and/or confusion, usually along with clumsiness

✦ An unusually small jawbone or chin; lower teeth crowded, unequal in length or misaligned

✦ A chronic breathing disorder, particularly asthma

✦ An excessively low cholesterol level (below 150mg/dl)

✦ Bouts of severe infection

As you're considering these symptoms,[6] consider the other stressors, beyond too many carbos, that may have led you to adrenal exhaustion. What has your emotional, financial, and work stress level been? Did your parents or other family members cope well with anxiety and troubles? A weak adrenal response to stress can be passed on genetically. This is often the case in addictive families where tranquilizing drugs, like alcohol and tobacco, are used when stress becomes too overwhelming.

Alcohol, Coffee, Tobacco, Salt, and Your Adrenals

Alcohol is a super sugar that can be enormously stressful to the adrenals. Coffee (especially with sugar) can spike your blood sugar, too, then crash it, so it too is hard on your adrenals. Cigarettes, which are liberally laced with sugar (up to 90 percent!), can have the same effect.[7] Yet most smokers describe tobacco as "calming." Somehow, tobacco seems to counter the effects of the adrenaline that carbos, caffeine, and stress all stimulate. The more "calming" tobacco you need, the more concerned you should be about the condition of your adrenal glands.

Do you crave salty foods such as chips, pretzels, or olives? Especially when you crave salty as well as sweet foods, you can be sure that your adrenals are overworked, because they are in charge of keeping levels of salt (as well as the glucose levels) in your system balanced.

The adrenals can become really overwhelmed and worn out if you alternate dieting and overeating sweets and starches. That leaves them less able to help you with illness, trauma, allergies, injury, and daily stress. High doses of pharmaceutical cortisone (such as prednisone) can also shut your own adrenals down.

In chapter 11, I'll give you the details on exactly what to take to restore your adrenal function. If your supplements and improved diet do not relieve your symptoms of adrenal exhaustion, you must test your adrenal function with an accurate, inexpensive, convenient, and painless saliva test. It is all too easy to become stressed beyond what simple remedies can handle. Depending on the stage of adrenal exhaustion that your symptoms and test results show you to be in, you can take adrenal-restorative supplements, natural hormones, or medications to quickly rebuild your stress-coping capacity.

Then you can look at your lifestyle and de-stress it. You'll need to be careful not to overexercise—that demands too much of your adrenals. Learn to give in to relaxation at least twice a day. Breathe quietly. Get plenty of rest. Learn yoga or other stretching-to-relax exercises or just make the time to participate in your favorite relaxing activities (see chapter 21 for more advice on how to relax) and get whatever counseling you might need to help you de-stress. Be nice to yourself—everything depends on it.

Leanne's Story

Leanne was a client who suffered unknowingly from adrenal burnout. After fifty years of overeating sweets and many years of smoking tobacco (she quit alcohol when she turned 40), Leanne, an office manager, was one hundred pounds overweight and an oversensitive powder keg. She blew up at everything. She tried to relax, but she could never seem to slow down. Her adrenal-stress profile (obtained through a saliva test) showed her dangerously low in the essential stress-coping chemicals cortisol and DHEA. The lab technicians retested her specimen three times because they could not believe her score.

Why was Leanne so stressed? Her addiction to sweets started when she was a little girl, and she had a genetic thyroid problem, so she gained weight easily. By age 7, she was enduring regular diets and was being dragged to the scale and reviled, beaten by her parents because she did not (could not!) lose weight. Leanne had even tried living at a weight loss center for months at a time. Until she finally "gave up" in her 40s, she had tried every diet and fast imaginable. Starvation dieting had stressed her out, she said, as had her heavy sugar and tobacco (and former alcohol) use. Constant family criticism and inner self-hate stressed her terribly as well.

A few days after she began using nutritional supplements, Leanne stopped overeating sweets. She had no trouble eating well and was finally chocolate-free. She lost forty-five pounds in her first year. In counseling, Leanne was able to detach from her early abuse and stop hating herself. She became less irritable. But, after a year and a half, she felt that she was still too easily stressed, and her weight had not dropped for six months, though this was the first time in her life that she had not regained weight after a weight loss. We decided to test her adrenal function. Before we got the results, we had given her extra nutrients to support her adrenals. But after we got the results, we agreed with her doctor that she needed more aggressive care. In addition to prescribing DHEA, he put her on three small daily doses (2.5 to 5 milligrams) of hydrocortisone per day. (Because she had high-normal blood pressure, she could not use the licorice extract that we usually use to treat adrenal breakdown.) In short order, she was feeling stronger and less reactive. She could really relax at last, and she began to lose weight again. After six months, she was able to go off of the medication entirely. Her own adrenals had rested up and were working again on their own.

Leanne is a good example of someone whose adrenals are too worn out to be restored by an improved diet and supplements alone. I suspect that many of you are in this category because of the terribly high stress levels that we are all living with these days. I consider the adrenal saliva tests (which you can even order yourself) and treatments among the most exciting new developments in health care in this decade.

Why? Not just because restoring our adrenals makes us feel more relaxed and more capable of dealing with challenges of all kinds, which is grand. Or that normalizing the adrenals helps optimize weight by turning up the thyroid and metabolic rates, which is wonderful. No, the best part of this discovery is that it prevents the degeneration of our physical health that will inevitably ensue if we don't salvage our adrenal function. The adrenals govern the immune system but they can't do a good job distracted by stress duties. The adrenals are also supposed to regulate our sex hormones and manufacture them when the ovaries flag in perimenopause and menopause. But they cannot support us through menopause if stress has exhausted them. Restoring the adrenals can literally save our lives as well as the quality of our lives. Chapter 11 will describe exactly what is involved in adrenal restoration.

Now it's time go into action with the specific supplements, foods, and tests that you'll use to treat the blood sugar and adrenal blues. If you are panicking about changing your entire eating style, don't forget that you can always go back to sweets. As the rabbis say, "Your health is the most important thing. You can always kill yourself later." Just turn to chapter 11, and try my advice for killing your sweet tooth instead.

FOUR

Unrecognized Low Thyroid Function

Tired, Cold, and Overweight

"Overweight people are lazy gluttons." If there's any myth I wish I could debunk, it's that one, because it causes so much unnecessary guilt and shame. I have never met people who try harder at anything than the people who come to our clinic for help in losing excess weight. No one volunteers for unneeded weight gain. I *do* see many people who are too tired to exercise, or even to cut up vegetables. They always say, "I'm just lazy. I'm not trying hard enough." But over the years I've seen that their "laziness" miraculously disappears as a result of a successful restoration of their thyroid function. As for gluttony, like everyone else, I used to think that weight gain was always the direct result of overeating. But then I learned how to help people stop overeating by eliminating low-calorie dieting, increasing the quality of their food, and using amino acids and other nutrients. Some of my clients immediately lost the weight they needed to lose, but others either lost very, very slowly or not at all. They did immediately quit gaining additional weight, but they were frustrated to be eating so well, so effortlessly, with little or no weight loss. Inevitably, their thyroid was the problem.

If you have a thyroid disorder that has forced you to gain weight, you have probably been subjected to ridicule, humiliation, hatred, and contempt for years, even for life. And yet you have tried everything to stop the weight gain. You have been willing to pay almost anything to lose weight.

You are disciplined. You may be keeping your calories at starvation levels on a daily basis, while forcing yourself to exercise despite your low energy, trying to prevent more weight gain, even if you have lost hope of ever losing weight. Still, your doctors tell you that you aren't trying hard enough. You are tired and easily chilled. Your body seems unable to burn calories briskly, to keep your weight at appropriate levels for your body type. Sounds like a thyroid problem—yet in your annual physicals you are told, "Your thyroid has always tested normal."

Some of my heaviest clients are not food cravers or overeaters at all. They eat normally. In fact, many of them chronically *under*eat, because moderate eating, even combined with exercise, has resulted in continued weight gain! Some of them actually gain weight on starvation diets or medically monitored fasts. When I looked into the research on this, I found that fully half of people entering formal weight-loss programs do not overeat. The dropout rate for these programs runs as high as 85 percent,[1] partly because so many dieters just cannot lose weight by cutting calories.

As you learned in chapter 2, dieting (or starvation) may have triggered your weight increase, shutting down your thyroid, causing calories to be stored rather than burned. For most of you, dieting just makes an already sluggish thyroid even more sluggish. But identifying and correcting a low-functioning thyroid can make all the difference.

How do you know your fatigue and weight gain are due to a thyroid problem? There are other key signals that this gland is the culprit: constantly having cold hands and feet (do you wear socks to bed?) is one. Having gained weight after a big hormonal shift such as getting your first period; having an abortion, miscarriage, or baby; or entering menopause is another. Having family members with thyroid problems also is a big red flag.

To help you further understand why your thyroid isn't functioning properly, let's look at how it is supposed to work.

THE FUNCTION OF THE THYROID

Where is your thyroid? It sits like a butterfly in the throat on your vocal cords just under your Adam's apple.

What does your thyroid do? This remarkable master gland affects every cell in your body, regulating cell metabolism like a thermostat. Your body needs a constant level of heat to perform its functions vigorously. There's a huge difference in how your cells function, depending on whether they are cold or warm. When your thyroid function is low (what is called a "sluggish" thyroid), it doesn't produce enough active hormones, or your own immune system is fighting your thyroid and preventing the hormones from getting to the cells, so your whole system becomes more inert. And that is the way you tend to feel if your thyroid is not able to do its heating and energizing job well. Literally, every part of your body, from your skin to your heart, head to toe, is diminished when the thyroid is not functioning well. Because the thyroid regulates the burning of calories, your weight tends to go up as your thyroid function goes down.

SYMPTOMS AND CAUSES OF LOW THYROID FUNCTION

First, and most important, if you suspect you may have a thyroid problem, look at your symptoms and your history carefully, *yourself.* I have found that nothing is more important than your sense about how your own body is working—or *not* working. At the Recovery Systems clinic, we always look first at symptoms of thyroid problems instead of relying on one or more fallible tests, as most medical doctors do. Our doctors do a physical examination of the thyroid, and they test reflexes, review a home temperature log, and order blood tests (among other tests). Yet if symptoms strongly suggest there may be a thyroid problem, the doctors may ignore test results entirely and try a monitored trial of medication, if nutritional strategies don't seem to help. Keep in mind as you look at this list of symptoms that you don't have to have all of them, but if you have several that are severe, you should definitely read this chapter.

Most Common Symptoms and Risk Factors of Low Thyroid Function

✦ Uncomfortably heavy since childhood
✦ Family history of thyroid problems
✦ As a child, played quietly rather than physically
✦ Weight gain began when you got your period, had a miscarriage or an abortion, gave birth, began menopause, or after a starvation diet
✦ Low energy, fatigue, lethargy, need lots of sleep (more than eight hours), trouble getting going in the morning

+ Tendency to feel cold, particularly in hands and feet
+ Tendency to excessive weight gain or inability to lose weight
+ Hoarseness, gravelly voice
+ Depression (including postpartum)
+ Low blood pressure/heart rate
+ Menstrual problems, including excessive bleeding, severe cramping, irregular periods, severe PMS, scanty flow; early or late onset of first period (before 12 or after 14 years old); premature cessation of menstruation (amenorrhea)
+ Reduced sexual drive
+ Poor concentration and memory
+ Swollen eyelids and face, general water retention
+ Thinning or loss of outside of eyebrows
+ Tend to have a low temperature
+ Headaches (including migraines)
+ High cholesterol
+ Lump in throat, trouble swallowing (e.g., pills)
+ Slow body movement or speech

Less Common Symptoms of Low Thyroid Function

+ Goiter; enlarged, swollen, or lumpy thyroid (look at the base of your throat, under your Adam's apple)
+ Coarse, dry hair
+ Bulging eyes
+ Infertility, impotence
+ Weak, brittle nails
+ Anemia, low red-cell count
+ Adult acne, eczema

In addition, low thyroid function can cause these symptoms,
which may be more common in older women:

+ Dry, coarse, or thick skin
+ Pale skin
+ Hypoglycemia
+ Constipation
+ Hair loss
+ Labored, difficult breathing

+ Swollen feet
+ Nervousness, anxiety, panic
+ Enlarged heart
+ Premature graying
+ Gallbladder pain
+ Pain in joints
+ Autoimmune conditions often associated with thyroiditis: diabetes, rheumatoid arthritis, multiple sclerosis, lupus, Addison's disease, allergy, candida, and pernicious anemia
+ Angina
+ Heart palpitation, irregular heartbeat
+ Muscle weakness
+ Atherosclerosis
+ Strong-smelling urine
+ Tongue feels thick
+ Vision, eye problems
+ Excess ear wax

Sluggish Thyroid, Sluggish Mood

If your thyroid has been sluggish, you have probably not been able to get the complete benefits from the foods you have consumed or even the nutritional supplements that you have taken. This low thyroid malnutrition may have been going on for years, leading to depression. Depression is not necessarily caused by low thyroid. But whenever I see depression, particularly when the client wants to sleep all day, has trouble getting up in the morning, has a low libido, and is generally tired and apathetic, I investigate the thyroid.

At the clinic, we became particularly aware of low thyroid depression because it would not respond to our amino acids, which are usually so helpful so quickly. If I suspect that low thyroid is the cause of their depression, I often suggest they start taking the amino acid L-tyrosine immediately. I have learned that if they don't feel more energetic in ten to fifteen minutes, or only have a brief or subtle response, they are likely to need medical treatment for a thyroid problem. Once the thyroid is running well, the depression lifts.*

---

*If you have depression characteristic of low serotonin, and your thyroid function is low, you may not respond to tryptophan or 5-HTP until your thyroid is repaired.

How Could Your Thyroid Develop a Problem?

For most people, there is more than one trigger for low thyroid function.

Genetics. This may be the most common cause of thyroid problems. You may have relatives who have been diagnosed and treated for low thyroid. More often, and more tragically, they may never have been properly diagnosed or treated. Review this chapter's symptom questionnaire with your relatives in mind, and interview your family members. You may be surprised by what you learn.

Brid, one of our clients, took her 70-year-old mother, Mae, to her M.D. after she herself had been successfully treated by him for severe problems caused by thyroiditis (a surprisingly common allergic reaction to her own thyroid). Brid had, as a result of her thyroid allergy, energy, sleep, and mood problems. She knew Mae had been disabled by similar symptoms since age 35 (after she had given birth to two children). Indeed, Mae reported that she was deeply exhausted, anxious, and had suffered extreme weight gain. She had a nodule on her thyroid that could be seen across the room.

When I asked her whether she'd ever been tested for thyroid function, she said she had been given the standard thyroid blood test (TSH) many times and that the results were always in the normal range. No other test had been given to her, nor had a doctor ever examined her thyroid. But when Brid's M.D. tested Mae more thoroughly, her scores on another kind of thyroid test were astronomically high, indicating that she definitely had a thyroid problem. Now that Mae has been successfully treated she is happy, energized, and at her normal weight. What's more, it turned out that Mae's mother (Brid's grandmother) had had almost identical symptoms, down to a thyroid nodule that visibly protruded from the same spot in her throat!

Low-Calorie Dieting and Nutrient-Deficient Diets. These also reduce thyroid function, as well as other body functions. Slowing down the thyroid early on in the process of starvation actually helps the body hold on to its nutritional resources until the ordeal (the famine, or diet) is over. Within hours of restricting calories, the thyroid will slow down and remain slow until the restriction is lifted. The resulting slowdown of calorie burning results in the familiar postdiet rebound weight gain.

Hormonal Events. When your menstrual period first began, did you begin to diet, fast, and skip meals in an effort to stop sudden excessive breast development or general weight gain? Until I ask clients what was going on when their dieting started, many have never taken their first hormonal body changes seriously. "I just started dieting at around fourteen," they say, as if this had no significance. But the beginning of adolescent body changes is often the crucial moment when thyroid problems begin. Dieting at this point can further depress your thyroid, which has probably already begun to falter, causing excessive weight gain and early breast development. If this happened, and you continued with yo-yo dieting, your thyroid could not rebound.

Hormonal events throw many vulnerable people into low thyroid states. Even if you passed through puberty normally, a miscarriage, abortion, or pregnancy may have depressed your thyroid function. "I never lost all of the weight after my last baby" is a common complaint of our clients whose thyroids gave out after giving birth. Postpartum depression is the next possible signal from a troubled thyroid. The final hormonal trigger, often confused with what we, probably mistakenly, assume is natural aging, is the menopausal thyroid sag.

Vegetarian Diets. Eating a vegetarian diet can cause you to become pale and listless because the body lacks iron, which is needed for vigorous thyroid function, along with other nutrients like selenium and zinc. These nutrients are found plentifully in red meat but are more difficult to get from foods on a vegetarian eating plan, especially if you are a vegan (no fish, chicken, or milk products).

Anorexia. People with anorexia typically have low thyroid function. If they have no major genetic thyroid problem, anorectics usually bounce back just by being given more food and supplements—particularly certain minerals and the amino acid L-tyrosine—that the thyroid needs to make its hormones.

Physical Injury or Severe Illness. Thyroid function is also slowed down by these conditions. A 1995 study of adverse effects of physical injury on thyroid reviewed the convincing evidence and described a new study showing that head injuries often adversely affected the thyroid. One of our trusted medical advisers on the thyroid, Richard Shames, M.D., says that whiplash, which drastically affects the throat (where the thyroid sits), often seems to affect thyroid function. The shock of a major illness can also depress your thyroid's effectiveness.

The Adrenal Link

Many of my clients seem to have exhausted adrenal glands as well as malfunctioning thyroids. If you have been under continual stress, your adrenals may be contributing to your thyroid problem. What is the link between the adrenals and the thyroid? If the adrenals become overactive during chronic stress, the thyroid slows down to try to calm the system. If the adrenals are diverted (by chronic stress) from their job of regulating the immune system, thyroiditis can result. In thyroiditis, the thyroid becomes inflamed. This inflammation can scar and, eventually, destroy your thyroid gland. Your own best anti-inflammatory is the natural cortisone your adrenals would make if they weren't otherwise occupied. The adrenals are energizing partners of the thyroid. If the thyroid fails, the adrenals get overworked and run down. The result is a stressed—tired, but wired—sensation that won't go away. If you have adverse reactions to thyroid medication, because adrenal malfunction often causes low thyroid, it is crucial to test your adrenals as well as your thyroid. For information on how to do this see pages 49 and 51 in chapter 3.

Drug Use. Do you use lots of caffeine, or NutraSweet and caffeine (for example, diet sodas), or diet pills like Dexatrim or Ephedra? Do you use even stronger stimulants such as cocaine or methamphetamine? If you really need these substances for a lift, to get things done, to focus and concentrate, or to keep your weight from increasing, then your natural energy system is weakened. A likely cause is low thyroid.

When people who are addicted to stimulants come to us, we can't help them without considering why their bodies need "speed." Low thyroid is sometimes the reason. When we restore the gland's function, these clients no longer need their drugs. You won't either.

Prescription drugs can inhibit the thyroid. Estrogen (including the estrogen in birth control pills) and lithium are the most well known thyroid-inhibiting drugs. Sulfa drugs and antidiabetic drugs also slow thyroid function.[2] But there are many more thyroid inhibitors. Review any drugs you are taking with a pharmacist and your physician. Study the information on the enclosure that comes with the package, or ask the pharmacist to give you a copy.

Chemicals in Water. Chlorine and fluoride can also suppress thyroid function. Perhaps this is why so many people seem to have low thyroid symptoms nowadays; most water supplies are treated with both these chemicals. There are also harmful hydrocarbons in unfiltered water that have been shown to suppress the thyroid. (See the resources section for chapter 12 for information on unadulterated water.)

TESTING YOUR THYROID FUNCTION

Once you are certain about your symptoms and clear on whether you or anyone in your family has experienced symptoms of low thyroid, it's time to gather more information to determine once and for all if, indeed, you do have low thyroid function. Armed with this information, you can work with your health care professional to determine whether you need thyroid medication (which I will discuss in detail in chapter 12).

Test Results That Lie

The most common test for thyroid function is the TSH (thyroid-stimulating hormone) test. The TSH measures a chemical sent by the pituitary gland in the brain, which relays orders to the thyroid gland about how much thyroid hormone the body needs at a given time.[3] However, in my experience, TSH is not the most accurate indicator of a thyroid problem. Christine, a 50-year-old financial adviser, was a prime example of a person with a thyroid problem that went undiagnosed because of the unreliability of the TSH test. Christine, chubby as a child, had become quite heavy as an adolescent after she began to get unusually profuse and painful periods at 11 years old. She slimmed down briefly as a teenager and met her husband-to-be. Before her wedding a few years later, because her weight had started to go up again, she used diet pills for the first and only time. As soon as she quit the pills, her weight really surged, and she was on the dieting roller coaster for life.

A sensitive and lovely woman, Christine had been beaten raw by the contempt she had encountered everywhere. Most particularly she had been hurt by her husband (who was one of the wiry, eats-anything body types), who had never stopped complaining about her weight and berating her for "not trying harder." He tended to blame her weight for all of the problems in their marriage—this despite the years of self-torture he had witnessed as she struggled through one diet after another.

Christine said she had never been a sweets lover, though she enjoyed wine several evenings a week. Since menopause, she had developed a taste for fatty foods for the first time. But she had never been a binger.

After menopause began, she stopped being able to lose any weight at all even with her most austere and punishing diet standbys—like liquid fasting. She finally just gave up and let the weight come on until she heard about our program. As she and I reviewed her symptoms and history, a textbook case of hypothyroidism took shape. I kept exclaiming, "Not that symptom, too?!" In addition to all the classic ones, she had some symptoms that I had only seen listed in books—never in a person—such as excessive ear wax and an enlarged heart. Christine told me that she had always felt that she might have a thyroid problem. She said that she had mentioned this to every doctor that she had ever seen, and they had all shrugged and said, "Sorry, we've checked it, and your thyroid is doing fine." TSH tests confirmed that she was in the "normal" range. She never thought to ask any further questions. If she had, she would really have been "fine" years before.

More extensive lab testing, as well as ankle reflex tests, confirmed that both her adrenals and her thyroid were malfunctioning. As a result, her doctor started her on a dual treatment protocol, which solved the problem. We have heard this same story at our clinic countless times: The TSH test failed to reflect the true state of thyroid affairs. If the TSH test does not show abnormality, most medical doctors refuse to proceed further. They insist that their patient is lying about how much she or he eats, and then give lectures about how only increased self-discipline will achieve weight loss. Yet time after time I have seen a more complete work-up (with up to eight blood tests included) show results that correspond with the actual experience of the person tested.

Two Thyroid Tests

There are a couple of simple tests that are quite accurate at detecting a thyroid problem: the basal temperature, which you can do at home, and the ankle reflex test, which your doctor can do in his or her office.

Measuring Your Basal (Underarm) Temperature. This home-testing method has been demonstrated to be 77 percent accurate and has been used for many years by physicians. A study confirming its accuracy, conducted by Dr. Broda Barnes on one thousand patients, was first published in the *Journal of the American Medical Association* in 1942.[4]

1. Buy a mercury thermometer (a basal thermometer, if you can find it, is easier to read than a regular oral one). Do *not* use a digital thermometer, which is not as accurate.
2. Place the thermometer under your armpit 30 minutes after awakening but before you get out of bed or turn the light on and keep your eyes open.
3. Leave it there for ten minutes.
4. Do this for three mornings, or more, to get an average temperature. If you are menstruating, basal temperature is most accurate during your period. Ovulation causes the temperature to rise, which is why women can use the basal temperature for pregnancy planning as well as measuring thyroid function. Even if you are having hot flashes, your basal temperature will not be distorted. If the axial (underarm) temperature is consistently subnormal (under 97.8 degrees), your thyroid function is probably low.

Testing Your Ankle (Achilles Tendon) Reflex. Here is another way to test thyroid function. Does your foot bounce when someone taps the tendon at the back of your ankle? This is a good indication that you do not have a sluggish thyroid.[5] If your reflex is slow, keep testing it throughout therapy. It should begin to bounce nicely.

Thyroid Blood Tests

Because the TSH is not a reliable blood test, and because you won't be able to get thyroid medication easily unless blood tests reveal a problem, you can—and should—insist that the following tests be performed: TSH; T_4; T_3; RIA; T_3 Uptake; Reverse T_3; antithyroglobulin and antimicrosomal antibodies; and FTI.

T_4. This is the second most common thyroid test. T_4 (short for the amino acid tyrosine and four iodine molecules) is the primary hormone manufactured by the thyroid gland. Although T_4 is the most plentiful thyroid hormone, it is not the most potent. Sixteen percent of T_4 is used directly by the cells. The rest is converted by them into its sister hormone, T_3, which is ten times more active. T_3 is the thyroid hormone that has the greatest effect on the body.

RIA (radioimmune assay). RIA may be the most accurate method for testing T_3 levels.

T₃ Uptake. This test measures how much T_3 is actually reaching the body's cells once it has been converted from T_4.

Note: none of these tests measures what happens inside the cell, which is where the real action takes place—or doesn't.

Reverse T₃ (RT₃). This test measures a substance called RT_3 that plugs into the same outlets as T_3 on the cells and blocks it. You may have quite a bit of it blocking your T_3, which is usually adrenal related.

Thyroid Antibody Tests. These two tests measure the number of immune system terminators created specifically to do battle against the thyroid. There are two types of these well-named antibodies, therefore two tests are needed: antithyroglobulin and antimicrosomol. This is the test that helps identify whether you have thyroiditis, an allergy to your own thyroid. This autoimmune condition is becoming quite common.

FTI. Free Thyroid Index is the T_4 test result number multiplied by the T_3 Uptake number. Your FTI will reveal approximately how much thyroid hormone is available for use by your cells.

Test Results: Low, Low-Normal, or Normal

In addition to all the people who get false-negative results on their thyroid tests, particularly on TSH, there are lots of people who score in the low-normal range. They almost always have plenty of symptoms to indicate some kind of foul-up involving their thyroids. But sure enough, their doctors don't attend seriously to their symptoms and refuse to give thyroid medication a try. The patient gets worse, but again is admonished and sent away with a low-calorie diet. (I hope that you know by now that low-calorie diets make things even worse.) Yet a standard medical textbook advises that "patients with subclinical hypothyroidism [low-normal test results] may benefit from therapy even though their symptoms are not obvious.[6]

Fortunately, there are doctors who interpret the test scores differently. According to their interpretations, your low-normal score is likely to be considered *sub*normal. These practitioners will usually be glad to give you a monitored trial on thyroid medication, if you don't respond to simple nutritional strategies. (See chapter 21, pages 350–354 for assistance finding these doctors.) Remember that blood tests for thyroid function are relatively recent. Up until the 1940s, doctors treated thyroid by looking carefully for certain symptoms rather than relying solely on a blood-test number!

If your test results are outside of the normal range, or if they indicate low-normal thyroid function, your physician will have recommendations to make. Bring this book with you to the visit in which you review the test results that have come in and the treatment options described in chapter 12.

If your first results are negative—in other words, no thyroid (or adrenal) problems are reflected by them—you and your physician will have to look carefully at your symptoms and history again, and then decide whether a trial of medication is in order if you have already tried the nutritional strategies in chapter 12.

Most of my clients with many symptoms of low thyroid have found that test results have confirmed a problem. But almost 25 percent have had no confirming blood-test results. In most of those cases, a trial of thyroid medication has been very successful.

ARE YOU ALLERGIC TO YOUR OWN THYROID?

It may sound strange, but another common cause of low thyroid symptoms is thyroiditis, which means that you are actually "allergic" to your own thyroid. If your body's immune system is mistakenly trying to destroy your thyroid gland and its hormones, you will, at some point, suffer many of the symptoms in the questionnaire. Some thyroid experts now believe that *most* low thyroid symptoms are caused by thyroiditis.

Our clinic's experience is that about 25 percent of our clients with thyroid problems have had thyroiditis identified by blood antibody tests and by certain unique symptoms. They have all improved from various treatments that are described in chapter 12, but recovery is usually a complex and lengthy process.

Stephen Langer, M.D., in his *How To Win at Weight Loss*, gives this excellent summary of thyroiditis symptoms:

In descending order of frequency [they] are: (1) profound fatigue, (2) memory loss, (3) depression, (4) nervousness, (5) allergies, (6) heartbeat irregularity, (7) muscle and joint pain, (8) sleep disturbances, (9) reduced sex drive, (10) menstrual problems, (11) suicidal tendencies, (12) digestive disorders, (13) headaches and ear pain, (14) lump in the throat, and (15) problems swallowing.

Nervousness ranges from mild anxiety to full-blown panic attacks, of which some are true psychiatric emergencies. These are as puzzling to the patients as to their physicians, who, in desperation, recommend psychotherapy and powerful tranquilizers.

As with anxiety and panic attacks, patients tell me, "I feel so depressed, but I have no reason to feel that way. I have a loving husband, a good job, and caring friends."

. . . deep fatigue and psychological problems are the most prevalent complaints of patients with HAIT [Hashimoto's Auto-Immune Thyroiditis].[7]

When your thyroid is under attack from your own immune system, you may experience the flat, low thyroid depression, plus an agitated, distraught, even panicky, depression. One of our nutritionists who suffered (and conquered) this difficult condition calls it "tired and wired." You may not have a weight problem, or even a low body temperature with thyroiditis. Quite often malfunctioning adrenals are a big part of the problem.

No matter whether you have simple low thyroid (hypothyroidism) or thyroid allergy (thyroiditis), you will find that changing your diet and adding nutritional supplements can help. Some of you, however, will have to get further help from thyroid medicine. In chapter 12, you will learn all about the many tests for evaluating thyroid function and how to maximize your thyroid's health.

FIVE

Food Addictions and Allergic Reactions

The Three Culprits

What are the foods that you really love the best—the foods you can't stop eating once you've started? Cookies, ice cream, frozen yogurt, or sweet, cold cereal with milk at bedtime? Pastries and creamy pie? Are you a bread junkie or crazy for pizza and pasta? There are lots of people who live for hard candies, licorice, and caramel. Do you?

In this chapter, you'll discover whether or not you are actually allergic to these foods you are absolutely crazy about, even addicted to. You say you can't live without your bagels or your ice cream? Don't worry—if you are addicted and allergic, you can use amino acids and other supplements to get you over your cravings until you are ready to give these trouble foods up, on your own, for life. Any withdrawal symptoms will be minimal. And you will be happy to know that there are plenty of yummy substitutes for the foods you may need to give up.

HOW DOES ALLERGY-ADDICTION WORK?

Your immune system produces aggressive Pac-Man–like antibodies to protect you from hostile foreign substances known as antigens. These antibodies kill things such as viruses, which are dangerous to you. They also attack food fragments that they perceive as foreign or toxic. The antibodies in action signal the release of a chemical called histamine. Histamine produces many of the symptoms that you probably associate with allergies, such as runny nose, swelling of the throat, sinus headache, wheezing, and stomachaches—the things you relieve with *anti*histamines.

But we aren't going to be talking much here about these strong, obvious kinds of allergic reactions to foods. After all, no one gets addicted to foods that close his throat or cause rashes, like strawberries, shellfish, and peanuts, et cetera. We're talking about food reactions that you are so used to that you may just consider them normal, like bloating, stomachaches, gas, constipation, low energy, joint pain, headaches, earaches, runny noses, postnasal drip, and even ADHD (attention deficit hyperactive disorder). These are some of the most common symptoms of food intolerance or allergy. Ironically, the most "intolerable" foods, the ones most likely to cause these annoying and chronic symptoms, are often your very *favorite* foods.

It is possible to have allergic reactions to any number of foods, but there are commonly only three foods that cause allergy-addiction. They are a small family of grains that includes wheat, rye, oats, and barley; cow's milk; sugar. Unfortunately, these are the three most popular foods in America.

HAVE YOU EVER BEEN ON AN ALLERGY-FREE DIET, BUT DIDN'T KNOW IT?

Think back to your "best" diets. When did you feel good (if ever) on a diet? I don't mean feeling good because you were losing weight—try to remember how you felt physically and what your mood was like as you were losing it. Of course, starvation eventually kicked in and you had to quit every diet you ever tried. But before you reached that point, did you ever feel really good while you dieted?

The diets that reduce carbohydrates and emphasize proteins and vegetables are usually the ones our clients have felt the best on. The Atkins Diet is a diet that people often remember feeling good on; so are The Zone and the Diet Center plan. But if these diets worked so well, why did you, and most other dieters, continue to have weight problems? Why were you unable to "stay on maintenance"? Many of my clients felt that Dr. Robert Atkins's diet was too fatty and low in vegetable and other healthy carbohydrates for a permanent plan. The Zone was far too low in calories,* as

---

* *The Zone* claims to be the diet plan that made the Stanford swim team national champions. But it turns out that only a few team members actually followed The Zone diet exactly. What most of the team members did do was to adjust their diets to include more protein and vegetables and less starch. They certainly did not restrict their calories to 1,600 per day, as author Dr. Barry Sears says he does, yet they benefited hugely. Dr. Sears has a very good idea, but it does not need to be low cal to work.

was the Diet Center plan. Fasting programs can make some people feel great. But fasting is not a permanent "maintenance" possibility! Low-cal dieters can't maintain their sense of well-being or their weight loss for long, because the low calories trigger the starvation response: a rebound increase in food cravings and a decrease in ability to burn calories.

If only the diet despots understood better. Some of them almost have it right. They have diets that initially pretty much eliminate the most addictive foods we know of, the big-three allergy-addictors. It isn't the calories, it is the *kind* of calories that they eliminate that make certain weight loss diets more "successful" than others.

The Zone and the Diet Center provide an insurmountable obstacle to long-term success, besides being too low-cal, as does Dr. Atkins's maintenance plan. *None exclude all three allergy-addictors entirely*—the grains wheat, rye, oats, or barley; cow's milk products; and sugar—or even suggest it as an option. To maintain weight loss, Dr. Atkins advises against most refined sweets and starches, but allows wheat and dairy products. The Zone's Dr. Barry Sears puts sugar and chocolate in his Balance Bars, and he is adamant about the importance of oats and cottage cheese. He also allows moderate amounts of pasta, bread, and the other gluten-containing grains. Both Sears and Atkins do suggest that sugar and flour be kept at low levels, but do not realize that any amount of an allergy food can overcome the most Herculean willpower in many people by triggering allergy-addiction.

What about the other leading diet plans, like Weight Watchers and Jenny Craig? Besides being too low cal, they also recommend small or moderate amounts of all the allergy-addictive three. At least in the maintenance phase, *all* diets that I know of allow at least two of the three prime allergy-addictors.

When you are allergy-addicted, following these diets is like attending Alcoholics Anonymous meetings and being served small glasses of beer. The low-fat vegetarian diets may be the worst. They allow too little fat, escalating fat cravings by starving us of good fats, and they promote excessive consumption of starchy carbos, including the most irritating foods we know: wheat and its cousins rye, oats, and barley.

GRAINS, COW'S MILK PRODUCTS, AND SUGAR

It is obvious to the food industry that so many people crave wheat products, milk products, and sugar, so not surprisingly the three can be found everywhere, "conveniently" combined as cheesecake, milk chocolate brownies, and cookie dough ice cream. The three allergy-addictors have a unique effect on your brain that can make them impossible to resist. As with alcohol and drugs, the first taste can lead to trouble every time—if you are sensitive to these foods.

We know now that the body tries to calm the irritation caused by allergy foods by releasing powerful, soothing chemicals. Candy bars and hard candy loaded with sugar, cottage cheese and sour cream made from milk, and grain-based foods like bagels and noodles can set off powerful drug reactions in your brain, if you are sensitive to them. Sugar consumption can trigger a brain release of the powerful painkillers, the endorphins.[1] Casein, the protein in cow's milk, and gluten, a protein found mostly in the grains wheat, rye, oats, and barley, stimulate the production of exorphins, opiate chemicals very similar to endorphins.[2] Over time, these pleasurable brain chemicals can become heavily addicting. If you don't have your bagel and cream cheese with your sweet latte, you won't get that feeling of comfort that you like so much.

In fact, going without one or more of the big-three allergy foods could land you in an unbearable withdrawal state, causing your body to start screaming like any addict's body does without its drugs. You probably already know how hard it can be to "withdraw," especially if you are addicted to more than one of these three allergy foods. Even one allergy-addiction can easily become a nightmare of cravings, overeating, weight gain, mood swings, and guilt.

Reba is a good example of someone who had troubles caused by allergy-addictors. A graduate student in psychology, Reba came from a large Italian family and loved pasta, bread, and sweets. For years she'd had frequent digestive trouble: bloating, constipation, and gas. Over the prior six years she had gained twenty extra pounds that she could not shed. She had been aware that her heavy consumption of sugar was certainly part of the reason she was gaining weight, but she also suspected that wheat was a problem. Bread and pasta made her feel blocked and drowsy, with a heavy feeling, but she ate them anyway because they tasted so good to her.

I suggested that she try going off of wheat and sugar and recommended some supplements that would stop her sweet-dough craving and improve her mood. Reba suffered no withdrawal discomfort. Just a few days later, Reba said she had begun to feel "lighter," physically and mentally. After a week, her clothes became loose, her energy increased, and she needed less sleep. Although she was eating plenty of food, in one month she had dropped fifteen pounds.

Moreover, Reba found it easier to concentrate and produce at school, yet she felt calm and peaceful, which amazed her. And best of all, she said, was that she "didn't miss the pasta and bread that, being Italian, I never thought I would be able to go without." She found she enjoyed the rice pasta and loved her polenta crust pizza.

Because food allergies often have a genetic basis, they may have caused problems from birth for you as well as for other family members. Allergy-addiction can impair your digestion and the absorption of anything you eat, creating general malnutrition. Food allergies can also seriously affect your immune system by diverting it from its other jobs, such as protecting you from viruses, bacteria, and airborne irritants like pollen. As a rule, allergy-food addicts usually feel low and run down. They have often had inhalant allergies, to pollens and other plants, for years—*allergies that disappear when their allergy foods are withdrawn.* This is because by eliminating allergy foods, they free up their immune system to take care of all their other health needs, and it begins to do a much better job.

Allergy Addictor 1: A Family of Grains

The family of grains that is made up of wheat, rye, barley, and oats is actually a family of hybridized grasses. Grasses are high on the list of the most common causes of inhalant allergies. It makes sense that eating grasses is apt to cause problems as well. The proteins in these four grassy grains contain a substance called gluten (think "glue") that is very hard to digest. Gluten can actually inflame and even damage your digestive lining rather easily. It can, and has, killed infants by damaging their tiny digestive tracts (many of our gluten-intolerant clients report having been colicky, formula-fed infants).

The most severe kind of reaction to gluten-containing grains has a special name: celiac disease (CD). One in every four persons is genetically vulnerable to CD, especially if they have northern European ancestors.[3] CD is closely associated with both diabetes and colon cancer, as well as mental conditions such as depression and mania. Anemia and a blistery skin disease called dermatitis herpetiformis (also known as Duhring's disease) are also associated with celiac disease.

Your body might have this most severe celiac reaction to the four gluten-containing grains, but you are much more likely to have a somewhat milder form of the problem: gluten intolerance. Because these grains are universally so hard to digest, I don't recommend that anyone eat them often, even if there are no obvious adverse reactions to them. Not only are they hard to digest, but they also contain phytic acid, which blocks the absorption of calcium.

In general, wheat is far and away the most problematic of all these gluten-containing grains. Many people can actually digest gluten in small amounts, as it appears in oats, barley, rye, and in spelt and kamut (because these old forms of wheat have less gluten than the hybridized form that we eat today). After you have carefully investigated all of the possible gluten-containing grains, you may find that wheat is your only problem.

Eating foods made from these four grassy grains, particularly wheat, may have many surprising consequences. Routinely I read the food diaries that my incoming clients have written. Many people who love bread and pasta describe feeling heavy and tired after eating them. Others say, "I want a nap right after I have a sandwich every day at lunch." Low energy is a very common symptom of gluten intolerance, and it can lead to excessive need for caffeine, nicotine, and other stimulants. Some of my clients also often complain that they continue to feel hungry even after eating big meals and just keep on eating. They never feel full because their gluten-damaged intestines aren't absorbing food very well. Often they crave and eat sweets soon after they eat a meal that contains bread or pasta, because sugar *will* get into their systems, like a drug, no matter how damaged their digestive tract is, and give them a lift.

After eating even small meals that contain wheat or gluten, many people complain of bloating and gas, or say "I feel too full after I eat." Some even want to, or do, throw up after their heavy gluten-containing meals. When they bring in their initial food diaries, it is clear that after meals in which the only carbos are rice, corn, or potatoes, these same people feel light and energetic. They tend not to crave, or to binge on, these carbos the way they do on bread and baked goods, like croissants, pretzels, and crackers. Yet all these foods are equally starchy carbos with identical calorie contents. The crucial difference turns out to be what kind of carbos they are—whether they contain gluten or are gluten free.

Another reason for weight gain besides overeating baked goods and sweets is that the allergy causes them to retain so much water. Doctors tend to mistakenly rule out gluten intolerance as a problem for weight-gainers because a classic symptom of celiac disease is to be too thin, despite normal eating.

Because gluten-containing foods interfere so much with digestion, they set some people up to have problems with other foods that also tend to be hard to digest, like dairy and soy products, and the grains buckwheat, millet, amaranth, and quinoa. Only a first-class small intestine can handle these foods well. Because of intestinal inflammation caused by wheat, the digestive tube can eventually have trouble digesting anything at all. Many of my clients avoid food all day, then eat a lot at night and just sleep off their allergic reactions, sometimes waking up feeling hung over. If you tend to get through the morning with a cup of coffee and juice, and keep going on coffee or diet sodas and some candy, it may be because common foods like cereal and sandwiches don't agree with you.

The wife of one of my colleagues suspected she was gluten intolerant, so we told her to eliminate the suspicious grains for a week, then try eating some wheat to see how she felt. She felt less bloated and more energetic right away. But on her test day, as we'd suggested, she took a nice big piece of homemade bread to work with her. She had her bread with a cup of tea at her ten A.M. break. Fifteen minutes later she woke up, startled by her unexpected nap. Her experience was the most extreme we've seen, but drowsiness is the most common symptom we hear about from gluten "testers." Bloating, gas, bowel trouble, and general tiredness are common, too. Another grain-allergy clue is not being "regular." As soon as I see a dough junky who tends to have bowel problems (constipation, diarrhea, or both), low energy after eating, and a distended abdomen, I propose seven to fourteen days off of gluten-containing grains. Of course, I also propose amino acids and other nutrients to stop grain cravings and make it easy to give up the dough. Typically the characteristic problems, often lifelong, disappear for good in the first few days off these grains.

One of the problems with having a wheat allergy is that wheat can show up in lots of unusual places, from gravies and sauces to catsup. (See pages 189–190 in chapter 13 for a list of hidden sources of gluten.)

Allergy Addictor 2: Cow's Milk Products

Unlike women's breast milk, and even goat's or sheep's milk (which are usually fairly easily digested by human beings), cow's milk can cause big problems. One of the least known of them is addiction. Do you drink lots of milk, or overeat cheese, ice cream, or frozen yogurt? If you crave foods full of milk, you are likely to be intolerant to them. More understandably, if you hate (or ever hated) any of these foods, you are also likely to be intolerant of them. Did you need special formula as a baby because you couldn't tolerate milk? Ask your family if you or anyone else in the family has ever had problems with any dairy products. Do you have respiratory problems? Many of our clients have had everything from runny noses to asthma and chronic earaches since they were children, due to a milk allergy. Respiratory congestion is a classic symptom of intolerance to milk products, though it can be symptomatic of other food or inhalant allergies, too. (Antibiotic and cortisone treatment for childhood milk-allergy symptoms, like earaches and asthma, often sets off major addictions to sweets and starches by encouraging yeast overgrowth, as I discuss in chapter 7.)

The other part of your body that cow's milk products can typically affect is your digestive tract. Stomachaches, gas, bloating, belching, cramping, and diarrhea or chronic constipation are typical allergic reactions to cow's milk products. The good news is that even the most severe symptoms can be cured overnight by eliminating milk, cheese, ice cream, and other culprits from your diet. If you are addicted to milk-based foods, you are probably having an allergic reaction not only to milk sugar (lactose) but to milk protein, or casein. It can trigger the release of powerful pleasure chemicals in the brain, keeping you uncomfortable but hooked. According to allergist Doris Rapp, digestive problems are most likely caused by a reaction to lactose, while respiratory problems (and constipation) are most likely to be caused by other ingredients in milk, such as casein.[4]

If you can't digest milk sugar (lactose), you can use lactose-free milk and take a supplemental enzyme that helps you break down the lactose: lactase (brand name Lactaid). Thirty to ninety percent of us are not naturally equipped with our own lactase, depending on our genetic background. In fact, according to the National Institute of Diabetes and Digestive and Kidney Disease of the National Institutes of Health, 12 percent of American Caucasians, 75 percent of African Americans, and 90 percent of Asian Americans and Native Americans are lactose intolerant.[5]

Lydia, a dynamic Middle Eastern mother, had been having food problems all her life. She'd been a picky eater as a child (a red flag for food allergy) and had been force-fed by her nanny. By 20 she'd developed an ulcer and was living on Tagamet, a liquid antacid. Whenever she got upset, she would vomit. By 34 she was having alternating constipation and diarrhea, constantly taking Zantac, another potent antacid, and sometimes having stomach cramps after meals. At 44 she came to the clinic and reluctantly agreed to try going off all foods made from cow's milk, including milk chocolate, which she loved.

Lydia used amino acid supplements to stop her chocolate cravings and fish oil caps to help with her milk and cheese cravings, but she only needed them for six weeks. After that, she was able to stay away from her old dairy favorites with no struggle, although she found that taking Lactaid enabled her to eat them occasionally. Some people who have problems with wheat (or other gluten-containing grains) *and* milk can tolerate milk products more easily after cutting wheat and other gluten-containing grains out of their diets for a while. Grains can damage the digestive lining and make many foods difficult to digest, especially foods like milk products that are already troublesome. So after you've been off of wheat, rye, oats, and barley for three months, you could try milk, yogurt, or cheese again to see if you can better tolerate them. Cute milk-mustache ads aside, worldwide research increasingly indicates that milk consumption, especially in childhood, can lead to very serious problems: diabetes, heart disease, infant anemia, Crohn's disease, multiple sclerosis, infertility, and asthma. There are several good reasons for all of us to minimize the use of milk products, whether we can "stomach" them or not. Unless they are organic, milk products are laced with the antibiotics and hormones that are regularly used to treat dairy herds. In any case, because they are so hard to digest, milk products are *not* the best source of calcium, which is one reason why osteoporosis is still so common among milk-drinking women. But you will need your basic calcium supplements even more than the rest of us.

Allergy Addictor 3: Sugar

Dr. Ellen Cutler, author of *Winning the War Against Asthma and Allergies*, reports that 80 percent of her patients have significant allergic reactions to sugar. That doesn't surprise me. Sugar can cause standard allergic reactions like joint pain, headaches, and hyperactivity. Other symptoms are very much like the ones that sugar's cousin alcohol can produce: mood and energy swings, hangovers, headaches, agitation, and irritability. A sugar addiction might be caused by any of the imbalances that are described in this book, but if sweets literally make you feel high and then sick (with a headachy, groggy, heavy feeling), you are probably having an allergic reaction.

Sugar is a drug that can be extracted from many foods—corn, barley, sugar beets, sugarcane—and it is called by many names. It's important that you recognize sugar on food labels because it is often a hidden ingredient going by a different name (such as fructose or malto dextrin). A list of "sugar" words to help when you're reading labels is included in chapter 13, on pages 191–192.

Many studies have confirmed that pediatric allergist Dr. Benjamin Feingold's sugar-free (and food-additive-free) diet could quickly cure hyperactivity in children. It has similar benefits for adults who are sensitive to sugar and other foods. Mood and attention problems can clear up

---

The Blood Type Clues to Possible Allergies

Your blood type may give you a clue about food allergies. Two generations of naturopathic physicians and authors, John and Peter D'Adamo, have researched this possibility. Son Peter's best-selling *Eat Right for Your Type*, asserts that all the four blood types—O, A, B, and AB,—have trouble with the gluten-containing grains, especially in terms of weight gain, but that B and AB blood types can tolerate milk products. (More on this in chapter 20.)

---

overnight when allergy foods like sugar are removed from the menus of sensitive people. Amino acids and other supplements can make avoiding sugar easy, but any experimental return to sugar use will usually trigger a return to the original allergy symptoms. Doris Rapp, M.D., a pediatric allergist, has produced fascinating videos of children before and after exposure to sugar. Their allergic reactions of restlessness, tears, rage, violence, or exhaustion are immediate and obvious. So is the relief when the reactions are reversed with a neutralizing treatment.

Though I don't recommend it, because sugar is hard on everyone's body whether they are allergic or not, some can tolerate being "recreational sugar users." But if you are allergic to sugar, you'll have to say goodbye to your sweet drug. You may experience a few days of druglike detox, but you've probably been through that many times before. This can be your last farewell to sugar, partly because you understand more about why you can't tolerate it, mostly because your supplements and new way of eating will silence your sweet cravings—*permanently.*

TESTING FOR FOOD INTOLERANCES

Allergist Theron Randolph paved the way in the 1970s for a broader definition of allergy by describing case after case of patients with severe physical and mental reactions that could be turned off overnight by removing a single food, then turned back on instantly by reintroducing that food.[6] Psychiatrists like William Philpott, author of *Brain Allergies*, and pioneering biochemists like Carl Pfeiffer, author of *Nutrition and Mental Illness*, developed exciting nutritional techniques to clear up unbalanced emotional states by identifying and removing allergy foods.[7] Though many haven't heard of allergy-addiction, it's a phenomenon that has been recognized and studied by wholistic physicians for many years.

But most doctors still insist that food allergies are very rare. This may have a lot to do with the unreliability of the testing methods available. Neither the conventional blood test for allergies (RAST) nor the skin-prick testing picks up food allergies anywhere near as reliably as it does inhalant allergies. Perhaps because of this, many doctors refuse to test for food allergies at all. Saliva testing does a good job of identifying allergies to gluten and casein milk (protein), but not lactose. At Recovery Systems, there are two methods that we will try if our clients' symptoms continue even after they eliminate the big-three allergens: a special form of skin-prick testing and a new blood test. Both are described in chapter 13 along with other allergy-indicating methods. But *always* consider your symptoms first and foremost. Home testing is quite accurate, so you may decide to skip the lab tests altogether.

The Home Test for Hidden Allergies

Home testing for food intolerance is called "elimination and challenge" and is the most commonly accepted and accurate way of identifying problem foods. When you are ready, eliminate the suspected allergens— gluten-containing grains, milk, or sugar for seven days, then reintroduce them for one day. (See chapter 13 for specific instructions on how to perform a home test for allergies.)

Please note that there are special problems with testing for severe gluten-intolerance (i.e., celiac disease). If you have extensive intestinal damage from gluten, you have CD. Once you start religiously avoiding gluten, this damage will heal. If you "test try" gluten after a few months of healing, you may not get the old symptoms right away. It may take a few weeks of redamaging your gut before you notice them again.

There is also the problem of delayed reaction. Some people get arthritic or muscular pains days after the allergy food is eaten, making it extremely difficult to connect the symptoms to the food eaten two or three days before. But if you retest and these symptoms go away, you have your answer.

As for determining whether you are allergic to sugar, I feel it's not worth testing. Do you think you might be allergic to the poison strychnine? You could try it and see . . . that's the way I feel about suggesting that you try sugar once you've gotten off of it. After fifteen years of seeing how much damage sugar can do, I would much rather that *everyone* stay off it. But if you want to find out for sure whether your addiction to sugar stems from an allergic reaction, you'll get a quick answer after you've been off of

---

Saliva, Blood, Skin-Prick, or Biopsy for
Severe Gluten Intolerances (Celiac Disease)

Saliva testing, the gold standard for hormone testing according to the World Health Organization, seems to reliably identify gluten problems, from mild to severe. So far, I have been impressed by the results because they correspond with real symptoms. Like blood tests, they measure antibodies, but the blood test seems to identify only the most severe celiac types. Specialized skin-prick testing is another reliable allergy test, but a biopsy of the small intestine is the most accurate way of diagnosing celiac disease. (See chapter 13 for specifics on these test procedures.)

---

it for seven to fourteen days by reintroducing sugar on *one* day at both breakfast and lunch.

Don't just suddenly decide to test, because you're at someone's birthday party and getting pressure to try the cake. Do it in a situation where you can watch your reactions carefully, not in any social situation where it might be hard to keep close track of any emerging symptoms. If you are allergic to sugar, your old adverse symptoms should return within forty-eight hours.

From the special skin-prick tests we describe in chapter 13, you might be able to find out which types of sugar are worse for you. For instance, you may be allergic to corn syrup, but not to beet sugar. This might give you more freedom in your food choices, but, again, freedom to use sugar is not a goal that I would encourage. Sugar in any form will cause problems, even if they aren't allergic problems.

As for milk allergies, if you eliminate milk products from your diet for a week or two, then reintroduce them and find your nasal congestion or stomach problems come back along with your cravings, try eating only lactose-free milk products or taking lactase supplements, like Lactaid. If you still have bad reactions, it's time to move on to milk products derived from goats or sheep instead of cows. If you react to those foods, then forget about trying to consume milk products. However, you may find that cottage cheese, aged cheese, buttermilk, and yogurt are easier to digest because they are already partially digested by being cultured.

ARE YOU AFRAID OF FEELING RESTRICTED OR DEPRIVED?

If giving up bread, milk, and sugar makes you feel like you're being deprived, I sympathize. You've probably been tortured by food restricting—i.e., dieting—much too often already. Believe me, I would not propose these restrictions if I knew any guaranteed way around them.

Remember, though, that this time you will *not* be restricting *calories.* I know, too, that many of you will feel socially awkward having to refuse foods that you are allergic to. But I also know from years of experience that if you are very upset about giving up these foods, this in itself is a strong clue that you are allergy-addicted. Would you have the same feelings if I suggested that you might need to give up celery or cabbage for life?

What you probably won't believe, until you experience it, is that the amino acids and other supplements that you'll be taking from day one will stop the cravings that are causing you to panic. They will minimize your withdrawal symptoms, too. So this will be totally unlike any food eliminating you've ever done before! I promise. And the outcome will be thrilling: your energy will rise, your digestion and bowels will normalize, your mood will elevate, your extra weight will fall, and your health prospects for the future will be greatly improved, too.

Now that you have an idea of whether or not you are addicted to wheat, milk, or sugar, it's time to test to see if you truly are and to learn how to avoid these all-too-common foods. Turn to chapter 13 for details on testing and on what tasty substitutes you can use.

SIX

Hormonal Havoc

PMS, Menopause, and the Food-Mood Connection

The "Male" Box—for Men Only

If you are male, rather than read this whole chapter, please just read the information on hormonal imbalances here and on page 89.

Men should be aware that two common things can eventually result in consistently lowered testosterone levels (that is, male menopause):

1. Eating too many high carbohydrate foods (sweets and starches) for too long
2. Too much stress, which wears out the adrenals, major testosterone-producing glands.

If you are past age 40 and are gaining weight and becoming moody, check the symptoms of low testosterone on page 89 of this chapter. If you then feel it is indicated, test for any stress-caused depletions by getting saliva tests for your testosterone, DHEA, and cortisol levels. (See page 352.)

If these three hormones are low, you can use DHEA (an over-the-counter supplement), which converts to testosterone and also shores up your adrenal stress response.* Natural testosterone is available only

---

*Note: DHEA can also convert to estrogen, so watch your reaction carefully and don't overdose.

by prescription. Don't get synthetic methyltestosterone, which may cause cancer and is very hard on the liver.

The nutrient solutions to excessive stress can be found on pages 159–164, chapter 11.

Eating more protein and low-carbohydrate vegetables and less sugar and starch and repairing adrenal stress will naturally raise your DHEA/testosterone levels. To eliminate carbohydrate cravings, identify which imbalances are causing them and follow the recommendations in the pertinent chapters.

After more than fifteen years of helping people with food addictions of all kinds, I know that nothing matches the ferocity of hormone-driven food cravings. Premenstrual chocolate cravings have brought more women to Recovery Systems' door than any other single problem. Fortunately, it's an easy problem to correct. If you erupt in premenstrual sweet cravings every month, or have developed permanent cravings and unnecessary weight gain (among other woes) in menopause, you will find solid answers here. Most of my clients lose all of their hormonal cravings and other, more debilitating symptoms of PMS, such as irritability and cramps, within two months. The same is true of menopausal women, who suffer from hot flashes, night sweats, and insomnia. Relief from these symptoms is a result of a significant improvement in their diets combined with supplements that lift their brain's mood chemistry and balance their hormones.

ESTROGEN AND PROGESTERONE IN PMS AND MENOPAUSE

Normally, your estrogen level should peak when you ovulate in the middle of your menstrual cycle. Then it should subside until after menstruation, gradually rising again to its ovulation peak. Once you have peaked, your estrogen levels deflate, but your progesterone levels quickly begin to swell dramatically. Progesterone supports pregnancy (think "progestation"), and your levels of it will remain elevated for nine months if you become pregnant. When your body is sure you aren't pregnant, your progesterone levels deflate. Then around menstruation its levels become as low as estrogen's, the only time in the month that the two hormones are at equal levels.

Estrogen stimulates many of your brain's mood sites, leading to the production of serotonin (your natural Prozac) as well as norepinephrine (your natural caffeine) and endorphin (your natural painkiller and plea-sure enhancer). If estrogen levels drop too low, in PMS or menopause, your moods can drop with it. This is one way that hormonal food cravings get triggered: sweets and fats lift your mood by indirectly increasing the amount of serotonin and other pleasure enhancers in your brain.

Here is another way that mood and eating are affected: Progesterone increases your levels of GABA, a brain chemical similar to Valium. If pro-gesterone levels don't rise high enough, you might be tense, wired, and sleepless. If progesterone levels are very high, they can either de-stress and relax you, or make you tired, or both. They can also make you want to eat more yet keep your metabolism high enough, usually, to burn off the ex-cess calories (as in PMS). If you, like so many of us, are already deficient in any of your four key mood-enhancing chemicals (see chapters 1 and 9), you are likely to have even more mood and craving problems if you have the wrong amounts of estrogen or progesterone, or both, or they are out of balance with each other.

Signs and Symptoms of Premenstrual Syndrome

+ Craving for sweets
+ Nervous tension
+ Increased appetite
+ Mood swings
+ Irritability
+ Mild to severe personality change
+ Fatigue, lethargy
+ Forgetfulness
+ Confusion
+ Weight gain
+ Uterine cramping
+ Diarrhea and/or constipation
+ Abdominal bloating
+ Heart pounding
+ Oily skin
+ Anxiety
+ Heightened or lessened sex drive
+ Depression
+ Crying
+ Insomnia
+ Swelling fingers and ankles

+ Backache
+ Breast tenderness and swelling
+ Headache
+ Dizziness or fainting
+ Acne[1]

After 35 your ovaries gradually make less of both estrogen and pro-gesterone, until they run so low that your adrenals have to start extra pro-duction to compensate. Menstrual cramping can become more painful and bleeding heavier.

These are among the most common signs that premenopausal changes (perimenopause) are underway. If you are in perimenopause or have already reached menopause, think back to what your periods were like before age 30, and if they changed over time. Are you having any of the clearly menopausal symptoms, such as hot flashes, night sweats, memory loss, or intense food cravings?

Perimenopausal and Menopausal Symptoms

+ Menstrual irregularity
+ Hot flashes and/or flushes; night sweats
+ Dry vagina
+ Memory problems
+ Insomnia and/or weird dreams
+ Sudden, intense food cravings
+ Sensory disturbances (vision, smell, alterations to taste)
+ Waking in the early hours of the morning
+ "Funny" sensations in the head
+ Lower back pain (crushing of vertebrae)
+ Fluctuations in sexual desire and sexual response
+ Onset of new allergies or sensitivities
+ Sudden bouts of bloat (waistline increases by two to three inches for an hour or two)
+ Annoying itching of the vulva (area around the vagina)
+ Indigestion, flatulence, gas pains
+ Chills or periods of extreme warmth
+ Overnight appearance of long, fine facial hairs
+ Rogue chin whiskers
+ Crying for no reason
+ Bouts of rapid heartbeat

+ Waking up with sore heels
+ Graying scalp and pubic hair
+ Aching ankles, knees, wrists, or shoulders
+ Thinning scalp and underarm hair
+ Frequent urination
+ Mysterious appearance of bruises
+ Prickly or tingly hands with swollen veins
+ Nausea
+ Lightheadedness, dizzy spells, or vertigo
+ Urinary leakage (when coughing or sneezing, or during orgasm)
+ Weight gain, especially in unusual parts of the body
+ Sudden and inappropriate bursts of anger
+ Sensitivity to being touched by others
+ Inexplicable panic attacks
+ Tendency to cystitis (inflammation of the bladder)
+ Vaginal or urethral infections
+ Anxiety and loss of self-confidence
+ Depression that cannot be shaken off
+ Painful intercourse
+ Migraine headaches
+ Easily wounded feelings
+ Crawly skin[2]

A Woman Who Had It All

Farrell was a redhead with a big laugh. She was a clothing artist who came to Recovery Systems originally at age 40 because she had food cravings that were completely out of control during the ten days before her period. She put a quick stop to her PMS cravings with a good multi–amino acid supplement, a multivitamin/mineral, a low-carbohydrate diet that daily included eight cups of vegetables and eighteen ounces of animal protein (she was a meat-eating, O-blood type); she ate no refined carbohydrates. She also began to attend Overeaters Anonymous meetings. Her weight normalized as her cravings disappeared, and Farrell quit bingeing and vomiting. All of her PMS symptoms, including chocolate cravings, were gone in two months.

Eight years later, at 48, Farrell's cravings for carbohydrates suddenly came back, even though she had continued to eat very well, take her supplements, spend years in therapy, and attend O.A. Her problem? Menopause. It had sent her into exhaustion and deep depression as well as back into compulsive overeating, night sweats, weeping, nausea, and insomnia. Before returning to see us, she had checked with her doctor. He had tried her on the hormonal drugs Premarin and Provera. Her energy had improved, but her cravings worsened, her weight gain sped up, and she became bloated, depressed, and full of rage. Finally, Farrell quit both drugs and came back to see us and our wholistic medical consultant, hoping for a more natural, and effective, solution to her hormonal imbalance. She got it: we gave her L-glutamine, 5-HTP, and DL-phenylalanine. Her cravings disappeared and she began to eat well again, increasing her protein and vegetable intake. Her new wholistic M.D. evaluated her thyroid function, which had always been borderline. Indeed, her thyroid test results showed that she needed thyroid hormone medication. Her energy increased and her sleep improved. To rebalance her estrogen and progesterone, she was given natural progesterone pellets and a Climera skin patch that administered 17 beta-estradiol (which is exactly like human estradiol and not implicated in the adverse effects found in studies that used Premarin). This combination eliminated her night sweats, nausea, and rages. Why did Farrell have so many hormonal problems in the first place? Her biggest problem was that she lived in the U.S.A.

WHAT IS HORMONALLY HAZARDOUS ABOUT THE U.S.A.?

It is unnatural and unnecessary to have uncomfortable hormonal symptoms. Women in healthier, less developed countries, like Indonesia, don't experience hot flashes (they don't even have a word for them!). They often love menopause because they're so happy to stop dealing with their periods and pregnancies. PMS is not a common problem for them, either. Many believe that the American diet is responsible for the PMS that so many American women suffer. It was mentioned in chapter 3 about how diabetes isn't a common problem among Mexican Pima Indians, but that among the Pima of the United States diabetes is epidemic. Very similar things can be said about "female problems" inside and outside of the U.S. For example, Japanese women have much lower breast cancer rates than do women in the U.S. As with diabetes, though, genetics are not protective. Once Japanese women start eating an "American" diet, their breast cancer rates shoot up.

A new study shows that America's poorest immigrants are healthier than most other Americans are, but that after they've been on our diet for a few years, their health deteriorates dramatically. This is why the nutritional suggestions that you will find in this book are so vital. They can help you back to a "primitive" nutritional state that can protect you from some of the discomforts and the dangers of hormonal imbalances.

Poor countries tend to be much richer nutritionally because they don't have as much junk food. It seems the more supermarkets and fast-food outlets a country has, the more its women suffer from PMS and menopausal troubles. Caffeine can be a big contributor to PMS, too. Too many sweets, junk fats (such as margarine and fried foods), chocolate, alcohol (the supercarbo), and refined starches raise estrogen levels too high. Too much estrogen relative to progesterone levels seems to be a common cause of PMS and menopausal discomfort as well as more serious hormone-related problems, such as cancer.

YOUR HORMONAL HISTORY
Unbalanced by Genetic Factors

What are the hormonal patterns and trends among the women in your family? When did each of you begin menstruating? Did you develop breasts and hips quickly or slowly? Has pregnancy, miscarriage, or childbirth affected your appetite, mood, or weight long-term? Do you all crave and craze premenstrually? Have you had more difficult periods as you've moved into your forties? Have you all gone into menopause at a particular age?

Does low thyroid function run in your family? Chapter 3 explained about the thyroid's tendency to falter at hormonal milestones like the start of menstruation and menopause, or after a pregnancy, slowing down metabolism, thereby reducing the ability to maintain comfortable energy or weight. Be sure to review the symptoms of low thyroid on page 54 as you consider your own and your family's hormonal history: unusually early or late onset of menstruation (13 is the average age), heavy menstrual bleeding, permanent weight gain after childbirth, and infertility can all be examples of thyroid-related problems. If your thyroid is a culprit, chapter 12 will help you check it out and get it functioning properly again, helping your thyroid-related PMS and menopause symptoms to disappear.

How Else Can You Upset Your Estrogen/Progesterone Balance?

Undereating. The foods we *don't* eat can cause even more problems. Do you avoid fresh vegetables and fruits and high-protein foods like fish, eggs, and tofu, because you want to cut your calories to make up for eating junk food? Do you eat breakfast? Do you try to subsist on coffee, cigarettes, and diet sodas, instead of food, as much as possible? If so, your hormones can be stressed and starved into imbalance and depletion. Have your periods become irregular or stopped as a result of undereating? Are you bulimic or anorectic?

Too little body fat can also reduce your sex hormones. Fat is hormonally vital. In fact, all of your reproductive and stress-fighting hormones are made from the much maligned fatlike substance called cholesterol! Especially in menopause, the fat on your abdomen can actually produce estrogen when you run low, as your ovaries start making less estrogen (usually sometime after age 35). Because dieting encourages slowed metabolism and weight gain, it hampers your ability to maintain a good weight in menopause, when your metabolism is already naturally slower, from lower thyroid and progesterone, too.[3]

Alcohol, Drugs, and Drug Foods. I already cautioned that the druglike foods—chocolate, sugar, refined starches, and fried foods—can alter estrogen/progesterone balance. Tobacco, with its high sugar content (up to 90 percent!) can interfere, too. So can alcohol, the supercarbo that increases the risk of breast cancer. Another way that alcohol and drugs can distort hormone levels is by impairing your liver function. Your liver removes hormonal excesses if it is functioning well.

Chemical Hormones. The pesticide residues in nonorganic meats, dairy products, and produce supply fake estrogens that can raise your estrogen levels too high. Also, drug estrogens like DES are fed to cattle and poultry to fatten them; then, when we eat their fat, we ingest the estrogen. That's why you should eat organic meat and poultry, and leaner meats.

Petrochemical products like plastic containers (and, sorry, even water bottles) are now known to emit estrogen impostors as well, particularly when exposed to heat. These are all major factors in what may be a growing epidemic of estrogen-related problems, such as PMS, breast cancer, and low sperm counts in men.[4]

Another cause of hormonal imbalances is the birth control pill, which can cause hormone levels to drop. Sixteen-year-old Maria had a steady boyfriend and an allergic reaction to condoms, so she decided to start the pill. She stayed on it for eight years and loved the regular, light periods and sense of safety. But she gained twenty pounds, and when she quit the pill, developed a huge fibroid tumor in the lining of her uterus, and suffered miserable PMS and heavy periods. She also put herself at risk for breast cancer. Why? Because the pill, with its estradiol (synthetic estrogen) and progestins (artificial progesterone) had kept her low in both her natural estrogen and the other important female hormone, progesterone, which can protect against fibroid tumor growth.

Taking the birth control pill can add to or create a hormonal imbalance—even years after going off the pill. (Staying on the pill for more than ten years can raise your risk of breast cancer, too.)

HORMONE IMBALANCES

The following are lists of adverse symptoms associated with either too much or too little estrogen, progesterone, and testosterone. If you experience any of these symptoms, you should test your hormone levels. Then compare your test results with your symptoms. For example, if your test results say you're too low in testosterone, and you begin taking testosterone, you should see the symptoms in that list go away.

Symptoms of Possible Progesterone Imbalance

+ Sweet cravings
+ Tiredness
+ Bloating
+ Sleeplessness
+ Bone loss
+ Constipation
+ Depression
+ Lower sex drive[5]
+ Breast tenderness
+ Acne[6]

Symptoms Indicating Possible Estrogen Imbalance

+ Irritability, negativity
+ Bone loss

✦ Increased blood pressure[7]
✦ Breast tenderness
✦ Sleeplessness
✦ Diarrhea
✦ More sensitive to pain
✦ Tension, anxiety
✦ Increased weight around the abdomen
✦ Hot flashes
✦ Headaches[8]
✦ Racing heart
✦ Increased cholesterol
✦ Reduced memory, concentration[9]
✦ Tearfulness
✦ Inability to tolerate the pill
✦ Gallstones

Symptoms of Testosterone Imbalance in Women

Too Little	*Too Much*
✦ Low energy	✦ Hyper feelings
✦ Loss of sex drive	✦ Increased libido
✦ Slowed down	✦ "Scattered" thoughts
✦ Mildly depressed	✦ Irritable, anxious
✦ Thin, fine hair	✦ Facial hair
✦ Dry, thin skin	✦ Acne
✦ Fewer dreams	✦ Intense dreaming
	✦ Aggressive dreams
	✦ Violent dreams[10]

How Adrenal Stress Affects Your Hormonal Balance

The adrenal glands and the ovaries make your reproductive hormones. The adrenals actually govern the ovarian hormone production and produce all of the same reproductive hormones themselves as well as other hormones that are designed to protect you from every kind of stress. The primary stress-coping hormones—adrenaline, cortisone, and DHEA—are deployed at the first sign of emotional upset or physical danger. Levels of cortisone and DHEA continue to be high during a prolonged stress, such as illness, and can remain on the job for years helping you to cope. The adrenal glands

Male Box

Symptoms of low testosterone in males

✦ reduced sense of well-being
✦ reduced energy, vitality
✦ reduced sex drive, muscle
✦ apathy; reduced purpose, courage, direction
✦ increased insulin and blood glucose
✦ increased abdominal fat
✦ coronary clogging
✦ increased total and LDL (bad) cholesterol
✦ bone loss, hip fractures[11]

are also forced into overdrive by dieting. Their mission, there, is to organize the cannibalizing of muscles and bones to salvage the proteins and minerals that the body must have while it's not getting the nutrients it needs. And if you are overexercising to keep the weight off, as so many Americans do, your adrenals regard that as stressful, too, and march out more troops.

All of this keeps the attention of your adrenals firmly off your reproductive needs. Your levels of estrogen, progesterone, and testosterone can all begin to falter as a result. In fact, adrenal exhaustion from too much stress of various kinds may be a major factor in all hormone imbalances. See chapters 3 and 11 for more on adrenal exhaustion and how to treat it. It is particularly implicated in perimenopause and menopause, where accumulated stress can accelerate naturally, diminishing hormone levels to cause severe hormonal deficiencies and imbalances.

MENOPAUSE AND HORMONE REPLACEMENT THERAPY

Are you perimenopausal or menopausal, or for any other reasons do you take synthetic hormones, such as Provera (nonexact, laboratory-made copy of human progesterone) or Premarin (made with estrogen derived from pregnant mare's urine), as hormone replacement therapy (HRT)? Sometimes we see someone who is really happy and satisfied with these hormonelike drugs, but more often my clients, like Farrell, have found that they have not only not eliminated all the problem symptoms but they have

---

The Shocking Results of a Study of 122,000 Nurses

Their Increased Risk of Breast Cancer:

Estrogen (Premarin alone)	36%
Premarin plus Provera (progestin) together	50%
Estrogen (Premarin) and synthetic testosterone	78%
Provera (progestin) alone	240%

Plus a doubled risk of gallbladder disease and lupus from hormone therapy (mainly Premarin).[12]

---

also caused new problems. The most common adverse symptoms they report to me are mood swings and food cravings. But much more serious, even life-threatening, changes may be set in motion by these drugs— changes that you might not be aware of until you begin to see signs of breast cancer, or cancer of the uterine lining (endometrial cancer). Although these problems can occur because your own hormonal levels are unbalanced to begin with, using hormonal drugs can further disrupt your hormone balance and increase your risk of developing these cancers by 50 to 75 percent or more, depending on which drug or combination of pharmaceuticals you use.

Unwanted Effects of Conventional "Estrogen" Replacement

+ Breast tenderness
+ Blood clots
+ High blood pressure
+ Nausea and vomiting
+ Fluid retention
+ Impaired glucose tolerance
+ Headaches
+ Leg cramps
+ Gallstones
+ Worsened uterine fibroids and endometriosis
+ Vaginal bleeding
+ Increased risk of endometrial cancer and breast cancer[13]

Unwanted Effects of Conventional Progestin (e.g., Provera) Replacement

✦ Can help cancers to become more invasive[14]
✦ Depression
✦ Bloating
✦ Bleeding resumes
✦ May increase the risk of breast cancer

In chapter 14, you'll learn about how to nourish your hormones back to balance, using hormone-balancing supplements, herbs, and acupuncture. Finally, you'll learn how to test for hormonal imbalances, and I'll tell you about some excellent alternatives to traditional hormone replacement therapy.

SEVEN

Yeast Overgrowth

A Hidden Cause of
Food Cravings

Years ago at Recovery Systems, although we were having lots of spectacular successes eliminating food cravings, we were troubled by the occasional client that did not respond as expected. Typically we'd hear that cravings had subsided considerably, but were erupting again every three or four days. Often we would hear, "It doesn't even feel like it's me wanting this junk food." It turned out that our clients were right. It *wasn't* them, it was organisms called yeasts.

These yeasts are exactly like the yeast that bread is made with. Yeast is great for bread making because it gobbles up the sugar or honey that is added to it, making a big, puffy, gassy mess that gets bigger as flour is added in. And that's essentially the way our yeast-afflicted clients usually feel: bloated, puffy, gurgly, and distended, especially after sweets, starchy foods, and alcohol. They also tend to get yeast infections, which is a real tip-off that something beyond depleted brain chemistry or allergies is at work. Other common symptoms are sinus infections, mental fog or "spaciness," and nail fungus.

Check your own symptoms on the following questionnaire to see if yeasts could be a problem for you. If your questionnaire score is high, you should confirm it with the saliva or stool test that I describe later in the chapter.

There is a lot of skepticism in the medical community about just how common yeast overgrowth really is. Actually, we used to be skeptical, too.

Identifying Yeast Symptoms

Section A. Major Symptoms
Choose the score that fits your symptom best and circle it. Scoring:
Don't Have Symptom = 0; Mild = 4; Moderate = 8; Severe = 12

Energy/Toxicity
0 4 8 12   Fatigue or lethargy
0 4 8 12   Irritable or uncomfortable when hungry
0 4 8 12   Headache

Mental/Emotional Functioning
0 4 8 12   Anxiety, sometimes without apparent cause
0 4 8 12   Depression
0 4 8 12   Feel spacey, light-headed, or disoriented
0 4 8 12   Poor memory
0 4 8 12   Inability to make decisions and to concentrate

Digestive Symptoms
0 4 8 12   Bloating or gas
0 4 8 12   Chronic diarrhea
0 4 8 12   Chronic constipation
0 4 8 12   Abdominal pain

Reproductive System
0 4 8 12   Loss of sexual interest or ability
0 4 8 12   Troublesome vaginal burning, itching, or discharge
0 4 8 12   Premenstrual tension or cramps

Muscles and Joints
0 4 8 12   Muscle aches and weakness
0 4 8 12   Cold hands or feet or physical chilliness
0 4 8 12   Pain or swelling in joints

Section B. Other Symptoms
Scoring: Don't Have Symptom = 0; Mild = 3; Moderate = 6; Severe = 9
0 3 6 9   Chronic eczema, rashes, or itching
0 3 6 9   Body odor or bad breath not relieved by washing
0 3 6 9   Chronic sore throat, laryngitis, cough, or tender glands
0 3 6 9   Urinary frequency, burning, or urgency
0 3 6 9   Pain or tightness in chest, wheezing, or shortness of
                  breath
0 3 6 9   Recurrent ear infections, fluid in ears, or nasal congestion
0 3 6 9   Tendency to bruise easily

0 3 6 9   Insomnia
0 3 6 9   Lack of coordination, dizziness, or poor balance
0 3 6 9   Food sensitivity or intolerance

_____ Total—Sections A and B

Section C. Major Influences—Personal History
Scoring: Yes = Number Indicated; No = 0

Antibiotics and Drugs as Factors
35 Have you taken tetracycline or other antibiotics for one month or longer?
35 Taken frequent short courses of other broad-spectrum antibiotics?
15 Taken prednisone or other cortisone-type drugs for one month or more?
10 Taken birth control pills for more than a year?

Symptoms and Sensitivities
25 Have you had persistent yeast infections, prostatitis, vaginitis, or other reproductive problems?
20 Been frequently exposed to high mold environments and seem to have a sensitivity to mold?
20 Severe athlete's foot, nail or skin fungus, ringworm, or other chronic fungus?
10 Have you been treated for internal parasites?
20 Does exposure to perfumes, insecticides, or other chemicals provoke noticeable symptoms?
10 Does tobacco smoke _really_ bother you?

Cravings
10 Do you crave or consume lots of sweets?
10 Do you crave or eat lots of starches, such as pastas or breads?
10 Do you crave or consume lots of alcoholic beverages?

_____ Total—Section C

_____ Grand Total—Sections A, B, and C

Scores over 100 suggest the possibility of a yeast overgrowth; over 175 indicates a high probability.

From _Inner Health_ © 1997, J. Anderson, N. Faass, T. Kuss, J. Ross, and J. Stine.

But now we're believers, having seen hundreds of clients who finally lost their bloat and their cravings only after their yeast problem was addressed.

WHAT IS CANDIDA?

Candida, also known as *Candida albicans* and Monilia, is the most well known of the problematic yeasts, but it is just one of many different types of yeasts commonly found in human bodies, in bread, and even in the air. From the time we are born, we have had some candida and other yeasts living in our intestinal tracts. Normally, candida and other yeasts live in harmony with us, their hosts. It is only when they overgrow their normal boundaries that yeasts like candida pose a problem.

When you have too much yeast in your system, it's called a "yeast infection," or yeast overgrowth. Since yeasts love warm, wet places, yeast infections show up in places like your intestines, vagina, or your mouth (where it is called "thrush"). When enough of these yeasts overgrow in your body, they can become quite troublesome. They also have the chameleonlike ability to change to fungi as they overgrow, producing long rootlike structures that are invasive and can penetrate the lining of your intestine. A fungus can release toxins and incompletely digested food and fecal matter into your bloodstream. This damages the digestive tract and causes food sensitivities, allergies, and other problems.

THE EMERGENCE OF YEAST AS A MAJOR CAUSE OF FOOD CRAVINGS

Yeast infections are fairly common. Researchers estimate that 25 to 35 percent of the population suffers from yeast and related fungal conditions. Many more women than men are affected.[1]

Yeast infections have become a much greater health risk in the second half of the twentieth century than ever before. Modern medicine's introduction of the wonder drugs known as antibiotics started yeast on its rise to prominence. Antibiotics kill all bacteria, regardless of type. But this means that antibiotics also destroy good bacteria, mainstays of our immune defenses. The "friendly" bacteria—such as lactobacilli acidophilus and bifidus—are killed off by antibiotic therapy. Opportunistic yeasts quickly overgrow, stepping in to fill the void left behind after antibiotic therapy kills off the helpful bacteria that used to line our intestinal tract. Birth control pills and steroids also directly contribute to yeast overgrowth.

When you swallow sweets and starchy carbos, you feed the yeasts, which starts a fermentation process, hence the gurgle and bloat. Of all the food groups, undigested and unabsorbed carbohydrates (sweets, starches, and alcohol) most directly feed the growth of these intestinal microbes. Good digestion absorbs the carbs that you eat quickly into your body, but if you have been eating too many sweets and starches, you may have overwhelmed your gut's ability to digest and absorb them. As the yeast feeds on excess carbs, it multiplies and spreads, and its feeding frenzy is felt as the overwhelming cravings for carbohydrates that so many people now suffer from.

Who Gets Yeast Infections

Many women are afflicted with vaginal yeast infections. They may be rare or all too recurrent. The most typical symptoms are a white vaginal discharge and itching of the genital area. You may also experience irritation, swelling, and redness, discomfort during sex, and painful urination. Recurrent yeast infections are an indication that a yeast overgrowth may be affecting your whole system, though many of our yeast-ridden clients don't get them. (Males with yeast infections rarely have obvious genital symptoms, but can infect their partners if not tested and treated along with them.)

How Do Yeasts Multiply and Take Over?

Antibiotics. These wonder drugs kill the good off along with the bad, wiping out lots of beneficial bacteria that normally keep yeasts in check.

The Pill. The hormones in birth control pills encourage yeast growth. They also increase levels of glycogen (sugar) present in vaginal secretions, promoting further yeast infections.

Spermicidal Creams and Foams. The active ingredient in these creams, nonoxynol 9 fosters the growth of both candida and E. coli (a bacteria that causes cystitis). Nonoxynol 9 also destroys vaginal friendly lactobaccilli bacteria, which are part of the body's natural defense system.[2]

Cortisone, Prednisone, and Similar Steroids. Use of these medicines encourages yeast growth as they suppress the immune system.

Nutritional Deficiencies. Deficiencies of lactobacillus acidophilus (bacteria) and the B vitamins (such as biotin) allow opportunistic yeasts to spread.

Poor Digestion. Poor digestion and malabsorption set the stage for yeast overgrowth. If you don't have enough digestive juices (hydrochloric acid) in your stomach, yeast is more likely to overgrow. If you have enough, the yeast gets burned up in the digestive fire. Eating foods you are allergic to, such as dairy and gluten-containing grains (especially wheat), can slow down, irritate, and damage your gastrointestinal tract, allowing yeasts more feeding time and defenseless tissue to invade.

Poor Diet. The lack of nutrients in fast food and junk food directly lowers immunity, allowing yeasts an easy takeover.

Excessive Carbohydrate and Sugar Intake. Of all the food groups, these foods most directly fuel yeast overgrowth.[3]

Antibiotic Residues in Commercial Meat. Most commercial meats contain small amounts of residual antibiotics. Eat antibiotic- and hormone-free meats instead (see chapter 20).

Weakened Immune Function. Are you highly stressed? Do you have frequent colds and flus? Yeasts thrive when your immune response is impaired or debilitated. AIDS patients are typically killed by yeast that has taken over as they have grown weaker.

Use of Recreational Drugs. Alcohol, marijuana, tobacco, and other recreational drugs stress the liver, adrenals, and the immune system, further depleting the body and its resistance to yeasts.

Operations, Catheterization, Radiation, Anti-Cancer Drugs. Opportunistic yeast thrives after these traumas to the body.

Preventing Yeast Overgrowth

When the following three conditions are met, the yeast in your body usually remains harmless:

1. You have a stable population of "friendly, beneficial" bacteria in your intestines.
2. Your immune system is strong and intact.
3. Your diet is balanced with adequate protein, vegetables, and essential fats, and you're not overeating carbohydrates (particularly sugar, refined carbohydrates, and grains).

How Yeast Spreads

When yeast spreads in the GI tract, you'll know it's there from the gas, bloating, indigestion, heartburn, nausea, and constipation and/or diarrhea that develop. You'll also get major cravings for sugar, starches, and alcohol—the foods that yeasts prefer. The more you feed the yeast, the more it proliferates, releasing toxins and interfering with your digestion as it expands.

Eventually the yeast may enter your bloodstream and spread through your body. At this point, your immune system really can begin to be overwhelmed and to falter. A frail, sluggish immune response is an open invitation for yeast to overgrow, as yeasts are far more aggressive even than viruses.[4]

As the yeast spreads, your symptoms may grow more diffuse and convoluted: depression, lethargy, mental fog, mood swings, PMS, confused thyroid function, susceptibility to infections (sinus, respiratory, bladder, gums, et cetera), sensitivity to pollutants and fumes (which can become full-blown "environmental" illness), achy muscles and/or joints, and skin and nail fungus.

TESTING FOR YEAST INFECTIONS

If you believe you might have a yeast infection, given the symptoms listed in the Quick Symptom Questionnaire and the more complete questionnaire here, you can get saliva and/or stool testing to be sure. If your self-diagnosis is confirmed, you can start a three-month, anti-yeast food-and-supplement plan, which usually stops yeast-related symptoms very quickly, even in the first week.

Many have been trying to eliminate yeast overgrowth for years without success. It can be easily wiped out using the methods developed at Recovery Systems.

A diagnostic stool analysis at a specialty lab (see chapter 21, page 353 for listings) is one good method of diagnosis. Any health professional can order this analysis, and some testing labs will let you order it yourself.

The Problem of Parasites

Like yeasts, microscopic parasites are aggressive organisms that can cause cravings, bloating, and many other problems. Some people with parasitic infections may have no noticeable symptoms, but others will manifest severe symptoms. Parasites usually affect already weakened systems. For example, if you have a predisposition to weakness in the lungs because you are asthmatic or have had pneumonia in the past, you might develop wheezing, shortness of breath, or respiratory symptoms.

Parasites are suprisingly common due to world travel, which spreads them around, so that even nontravelers get them. They can be extremely difficult to kill off, and they can be quite destructive, so if you suspect you have parasites, please work with a health professional to test for and eradicate them. You can have your health professional send for the protocol that we use at our clinic. Send $2 and a self-addressed, stamped business envelope to Recovery Systems, Suite 402, 775 E. Blithedale Avenue, Mill Valley CA 94941.

The presence of yeast progressively suppresses immune function, which may lead to a parasite invasion, and vice versa. If it turns out that you have both a yeast infection and a parasite infection, you should start an antiparasite program first, *before* tackling the yeast. At Recovery Systems, we tried to do it the other way around and failed a number of times before we learned this valuable lesson. Fortunately this dual infestation has not been a common problem.

Parasite Questionnaire

Please circle the appropriate number next to each question.

A = Symptom never occurs/never exhibit this behavior
B = Symptom/behavior occurs occasionally
C = Symptom/behavior occurs often
D = Symptom/behavior occurs most of the time

	A	B	C	D
1. Chronic fatigue for no apparent reason	0	1	2	3
2. Swollen or achy joints	0	1	2	3
3. Increased appetite, hungry after meals	0	1	2	3
4. Eat out at restaurants	0	1	2	3
5. Nervous or irritable	0	1	2	3
6. Restless sleep/teeth grinding while asleep	0	1	2	3
7. Night sweats	0	1	2	3
8. Blurry, unclear vision	0	1	2	3

	A	B	C	D
9. Fevers of unknown origin	0	1	2	3
10. Frequent colds, flu, sore throats	0	1	2	3
11. Recurrent feelings of unwellness	0	1	2	3
12. Constipation	0	1	2	3
13. Diarrhea alternating with constipation	0	1	2	3
14. Thinning or loss of hair	0	1	2	3
15. Allergies, food sensitivities	0	2	4	6
16. Irritable bowel, irregular bowel	0	2	4	6
17. Rectal, anal itching	0	2	4	6
18. Bloating or gas	0	2	4	6
19. Abdominal or liver pain/cramps	0	2	4	6
20. Mucus in nose that is moist or encrusted	0	2	3	4
21. Dark circles under the eyes	0	2	3	4
22. Bowel urgency	0	2	3	4
23. Skin problems, rashes, hives, itchy skin	0	2	3	4
24. Vertical wrinkles around mouth	0	2	3	4
25. Kiss pets, allow pets to lick your face	0	2	3	4
26. Go barefoot outside the home	0	2	3	4
27. Travel in Third World countries	0	2	3	4
28. Eat lightly cooked pork/salmon products	0	2	3	4
29. Eat sushi, sashimi	0	2	3	4
30. Swim in creeks, rivers, lakes	0	2	3	4
31. History of parasitic infection	0	2	3	4
32. Loose stools or diarrhea	0	2	3	4
33. Pale, anemic, or yellowish skin	0	2	3	4
34. Foul-smelling stools	0	2	3	4
35. Low-back or kidney pain	0	2	3	4
36. Indigestion, malabsorption	0	2	3	4

Total _____

Scoring Index:

0–19	Possible parasitic presence
20–29	Likely parasitic infection
30–39	A stronger possibility
40 or more	Odds are quite strong that parasites are present

Note: If your score is 15 or higher, there is some likelihood that parasites may be affecting your health. Consult your health care practitioner for further discussion and laboratory testing. Questionnaire was mutually developed by Timothy Kuss and Dr. Jack Tips of Apple-A-Day Clinic in Austin, Texas. © 1996 Timothy Kuss, Infinity Health, 1519 Contra Costa Blvd., Pleasant Hill, CA 94523 (925) 676-8982.

Another possible step would be to take a yeast-antibody blood test. If your yeast-antibody presence is above 100 you probably have a yeast overgrowth. A saliva antibody test may be the best way of all to test for yeast overgrowth; it certainly is the easiest. You can order this test yourself or get it through any health practitioner. We often recommend that our clients take a saliva test first, then a stool test to confirm (blood tests have not been as useful). See chapters 15 and 21 for more testing information.

Yeasts are a much more common problem among our clients than parasites. In chapter 15, you'll learn about how to effectively kill off these unwelcome diners and start feeling better and eating better than you've been able to for quite a while.

EIGHT

Fatty Acid Deficiency

Why You Can't Stop Eating
Chips, Cheese, and Fries

A re you someone who doesn't care much about bread or potatoes—
unless they are drenched in butter or cheese, or deep fried? If you
like sweets at all, do you only like Reese's peanut butter cups (peanuts and
chocolate are both high in fat) or ice cream, not hard candy? Do you love
potato or corn chips, but not the baked kind? Would you lose interest in a
chicken breast if it was served with no crispy skin? If this all sounds like
you, you're probably addicted to fat.

I meet several true fat addicts every month. But usually fat cravers are
also carbohydrate addicts, who are stuck with serious cravings for both
carbos and fats. In this chapter, you'll discover what causes fat cravings,
and I'll lay out painless ways for you to extract your "fat tooth" easily and
quickly.

Maybe you are like 32-year-old Bronnie, a typical fat-and-carbohydrate
addict. She had a fascinating, high-energy lifestyle, working as a producer
of dance exhibitions all over the country. She had lots of friends that
she loved to entertain with lovely, lingering, candlelight dinners. But those
dinners, and all of the other food that she ate, tended to be overly rich.
Bronnie had always craved cheese, chips, olives, salami, ice cream, popcorn
with lots of butter, and rich, creamy, sweet coffee. By age 18, she was 100
pounds overweight, and she weighed 285 pounds when she came to our
clinic for help. We started out by eliminating her sweet cravings with
chromium and L-glutamine. Then we went after her fat cravings.

Bronnie had mixed northern European ancestry that included some
Scandinavian forebears. Her family history also contained depression,

anxiety, alcoholism, irritable bowel syndrome, PMS, and winter depression, all signs of a simple nutrient deficiency. With the right nutrient supplements to treat her cravings, she could begin the changes in eating habits that had been so impossible for her to adopt before.

In fact, most of the fat cravers that we work with lose their interest in fats in a few days. The secret? Supplements that contain . . . fat! These nutritious oils also help burn off unneeded body fat, so I hope you won't be afraid to try them. I want to help you dispel the fear, even horror, of fat that all of us in the United States have been feeling unnecessarily for years.

The fact is, human beings need plenty of good fat in their diets and on their bodies, for the production of all hormones, to protect their internal organs, to insulate them from cold, to burn for fuel when food is scarce, to cover every single body and brain cell, to make hair and skin lustrous, to keep sex drive from waning, to maintain mental stability and concentration, to avoid carbohydrate cravings, and to keep our bowels regular. Without enough body fat, women experience fertility problems.

FAT IS NOT THE ENEMY

Many people fear consuming fat not so much because they perceive it as a health risk but because they think it will make them fat and therefore ugly. As humans, our ideas of beauty have often been grotesque: The Chinese at one time thought that the ideal woman should have feet the size of teacups. In Africa, Ubangie women still stretch their lips to the size of saucers. But never in all of human existence has the complete absence of body fat looked beautiful to people until now.

It's time to let go of your fat fears and be sure you're getting *enough* fat.

(See the list of some of the degenerative diseases that occur when you are too low in essential fatty acids, later in this chapter on page 111).

HOW MUCH FAT SHOULD YOU BE EATING?

Too much of the nonessential fats, especially the hydrogenated (fried) fats like margarine and shortening, can cause heart disease. So can too many carbos. But just as with the ideal number of calories, the ideal percentage of fat keeps eluding us. Is it 10 percent; 20 percent; 30 percent (the RDA); 35 percent (what we are actually eating in the U.S. and also the percentage that Crete's healthiest-men-in-the-world eat); 40 percent (the healthy Italians' average); or 75 percent (the Eskimo ideal)? We do know

---

Fat Facts

✦ Every cell of our body is made up of a fat (lipid) coating. The fat acts as a barrier to keep out harmful microbes.

✦ Our endocrine glands require fat in order to construct hormones like estrogen and testosterone.

✦ The human brain, the most complex organization of matter we know, is 60 percent fat.

✦ Fat maintains the integrity of neuron connections—the brain's vital communication system.

✦ Nerve, brain, eye, heart, and adrenal and thyroid cells must have essential fats to function.

✦ Essential fats are necessary for normal reproduction and growth. They are converted into prostaglandins, which regulate all body functions at the cellular level. Prostaglandins control blood pressure, clotting, inflammation, allergies, sodium, and water excretion, tumor growth, among other functions.

✦ Fat is required for the production of serotonin, which elevates mood and promotes good sleep.

---

that all people need to get enough of the essential omega-3 and omega-6 fats. As long as you eat well, and your cholesterol is normal, you can eat as much *healthy* fat as your particular genetic programming requires. *Try not to count fat grams.* If you crave fats, ask yourself, "Am I eating enough food in general, and good fat in particular? Did my fat cravings start when I quit taking my fish oil capsules or cut back on the amount of fish I was eating?" You are the only expert on your best fat percentage. If you are from a culture that's been heart healthy (most any culture but American), eating along traditional lines is your safest bet.

THE NUMBER ONE CAUSE
OF FAT CRAVINGS

Many people who are overeating fatty foods are deficient in certain fats. If you are a fat addict, your real problem probably isn't that you are eating too much fat, it's that you aren't eating enough of the right type. You are probably so deficient in certain essential, healthful fats that your body continually calls for oily, creamy foods, hoping that you will eventually swallow the particular kind of fat that it really needs. And you are not alone. According to Artemis Simopoulos, M.D., distinguished researcher and author of *The Omega Plan*, we are getting one tenth of the fats that we really need, and 20 percent of us have levels so low "as to be undetectable."[1]

People who do overeat fat may develop health problems. I don't advocate excessive fat consumption, but as Americans, we've won that battle. The problem associated with excessive weight gain today—dieting, high blood pressure, and heart disease—are caused by too many carbos, *not* too much fat. Nationally, on average, we take in about 35 percent of our calories from fat, so most of us are doing fine in the fat department!

Fat Is Rich in Many Ways

Craving and overeating fatty foods, especially when you are trying not to, is a signal that something is wrong. The solution is not to cut out all fats, but to find the *right* fats.

It turns out that fats are fascinating and complex as well as essential to your health and well-being. There are many kinds of fats, each fulfilling a special need in your body. Butter, for example, contains at least five hundred different elements; none are "bad," some are healthy, while others neutral (not harmful). If you don't eat enough of the more essential fats (such as fish oil from salmon), you can develop fat cravings and overeat greasy foods. Your health can suffer quite seriously, not so much from the fats that you are eating as from the fats that you aren't eating. And you're not going to get the good fats by downing a bag of potato chips or a bacon cheeseburger.

Instead of taking in oils from the vegetables, nuts, or fish that are high in most essential fats, you may be eating fats from fried foods or chemically fried fats like margarine, which prevent the absorption of the "good" fats. Eating butter, cheese, and fatty meats could be quite harmless because these foods do not contain the damaging trans-fatty acids that margarine does, but they do not give you enough of the essential fats that your body requires, so too many can throw off your fat balance.

There are certain fats that have tremendous health benefits. The omega-3 fats are sometimes called vitamin F_2, because, like all the vitamins, they are essential to life. (*Vita* means "life.") The other equally essential fat vitamin is called omega-6. Both of these fatty vitamins must be consumed regularly in our food. Otherwise, we cannot protect ourselves from hormonal imbalances, dry skin and hair, immune system weakness, adverse effects on the brain (which is 60 percent fat), the eyes, the adrenals and the thyroid, as well as gallstones, heart and cholesterol problems, and many other health troubles. Hundreds of studies have confirmed the extraordinary benefits of the two omega oils in preserving our health.

Of course, we've already mentioned another benefit of increasing intake of these essential fats—it will stop fatty food cravings that can lead to unneeded weight gain.

The Omegas and Weight

Are you afraid that fats will make you fat? Studies have shown that adding fish oil to the diets of lab animals causes their weights to drop, even when they continue to eat the lard and vegetable fats that had originally caused them to gain weight.[2] Our clients, too, experience a drop in weight when they add fish or flax oil to their menus, even though they also eat nuts, seeds, and other kinds of fats, and eat a full-calorie diet (averaging 2,800 for men; 2,500 for women). Why? One reason is that omega-3 fats raise our metabolic rate so that we burn calories briskly, not sluggishly. They also act as diuretics, helping the kidneys to flush out excess water from our tissues. Omega-3 fats energize us, allowing us to exercise more easily. Getting these benefits will require that one third to half of your essential fat calories come from omega-3 fats. The other half to two thirds would come from omega-6 fats. Together they should total 4 to 8 percent of your calories for the day (or at least 125 calories a day).[3]

One breakdown product of omega-6 fats offers benefits similar to those of omega-3. It is called GLA. Like fish oil supplements, GLA supplements have been shown to reduce weight by stimulating the more active burning of fat by the body, and by stimulating the thyroid gland to raise metabolic rates. The best source of GLA is oil from black currant seeds and the evening primrose plant. My clients sometimes use it along with the fish oil capsules, but at half the dose (that is, one GLA per two fish oil capsules).

Do You Have Fat-Loving Genes?

The answer to this is yes. We all do! Originally we had only healthy, beneficial fats to choose from, and our attraction to fats helped preserve our health. We ate the fats in vegetables, fish, and wild game. The animals we ate (deer, birds, and others) fed on nutritiously varied and rich wild food, not the feed-lot grains our meat and poultry consume now. For example, wild fowl eggs, or eggs from chickens that feed off of weeds and worms, are much richer in all the essential fats than commercial eggs from animals that are fed on fat-deficient grains.

There are certain peoples, from specific genetic stock, that we know have very special needs for essential fats. They need a continual ration of the fatty nutrients found only in fish like salmon, tuna, and sardines. Did you descend from them? Even a distant ancestor could have passed the genetic need for fish fat to you, though you are most likely to have the problem if your ancestry includes 25 percent from one of these specific genetic stocks.

✦ Scandinavians
✦ North American coastal Native people
✦ Celtic Irish (native to Ireland, not England; these people are or were usually Catholic, not Protestant), Scottish, or Welsh

If you are descended from any of these genetic groups, or possibly other island or coastal people, you may crave fats because your ancestors relied heavily on fish, for as long as twenty thousand years.[4] Your genetic code adapted itself to a fish-based diet. Your body design may still require lots of fish fat, and it may not be able to substitute the fats from other animals or vegetables.

What's so special about the fat found in fish? It is a particularly rich kind of fat. For example, fatty nutrients in fish provide one of the most activating brain foods known (DHA). Those of us who do not come from this coastal stock have bodies that can make these special fatty nutrients out of flax seeds, walnuts, canola oil, leafy greens, or any other food that contains omega-3 fatty acids. But the decendents of fish-dependent peoples cannot. They need to eat fish frequently and take fish oil supplements (algae oil may work for vegetarians).

Many of our clients come from alcoholic families that are Scandinavian, Irish, or Native American and suffer alcoholism and depression at unusually high rates. Depression and cravings for alcohol, as well as fat, can usually be relieved by the use of fish oil. Without the omega-3 fats in their food, these genetic types suffer depression as a brain fat (DHA)–deficiency symptom. They may be unable to use any other kinds of fats to make DHA, as other people can. So they use alcohol to numb the depression, and overeat all kinds of fat, blindly searching for the right one—omega-3, which is hard to find.

One research gave fish oil or GLA-rich evening primrose supplements to chronic alcoholics and found that their interest in alcohol disappeared. The depression that their alcohol use had relieved was eliminated by the supplements. (These supplements also helped them to detox comfortably after they quit drinking, by preventing seizures, which can be quite dangerous as well as frightening.)[5]

If you tend to abuse alcohol, or feel that it affects you differently from others, or if you are an alcoholic, these could be signs that you have essential-fatty-acid deficiency. Alcohol can relieve the depression caused by EFA deficiency, so if you are deficient you may be drawn toward drinking. Other problems with alcohol that could be symptoms of or risk factors for essential-fatty-acid deficiency are:

+ Anxiety or depression during hangovers
+ Suicide, schizophrenia or other mental illness, religious fanaticism, or fanatical teetotalling among close relatives
+ Being a dry alcoholic who still experiences depression

THE OTHER CAUSES OF FAT CRAVINGS

Even if you do not have (or don't know if you have) the ancestry that I just described, essential-fatty-acid deficiency could easily be your problem. How?

Low-Fat Diets, Which Deplete You of Healthy Fats

Like so many of us, you are probably shocked by the idea that fat can be good, let alone essential for your health. The antifat movement has been very successful, though misguided, since the 1970s, when the Pritikin Institute's now famous low-fat, heart disease diet hit the headlines. What never got into print was important information from the institute's own former head nutritionist, Ann Louise Gittleman. As noted previously, in her book *Beyond Pritikin*, Gittleman reported that Pritikin clients, who went very low-fat (10 percent) for more than three months, developed new health problems and regained unneeded weight. A big part of their new problems stemmed from the fact that they had lost the healthy fats along with the unhealthy ones! Gittleman helped us to see how vital some fats could be. She found that adding certain essential fats back into the diet quickly helped return unneeded weight to ideal levels. Why? Because certain fats control how much fat is burned by our bodies and how fast it is burned. At our clinic we, too, have found that fatty acid supplements can help with weight loss. In fact, eating approximately 8 percent of your diet as balanced essential fatty acids (1:1 to 2:1, omega-6 to omega-3) will keep your fat-burning capacity at its peak.[6] That's because the omega fats are *activating* fats.

As you can see, although you want to quit *over*eating fat, you can't do it by cutting fat out of your life. Please stop trying to eat a super-low-fat diet (10 percent or 20 percent) unless you have cardiovascular disease, and even then you may have to beware of other problems that such a low-fat diet can cause. Even if you have been able to lose pounds on very low-fat regimens like McDougall's, Pritikin's, or Ornish's, you have probably rebounded out of them eventually and into the opposite extreme, overeating fats more than ever.

Another major problem with low-fat, high-carb diets is that they don't give you enough protein. You may already know how important it is to eat enough protein along with your carbohydrates. We talk a lot more about that in chapters 20, 21, and 22. What you may not know is that without good fats, your body can't use the protein. Protein and fat are a team. The fat doesn't get utilized without the protein, either—it just gets stored. Many foods that are high in protein also contain fat: chicken, eggs, tofu, meat, fish, nuts, and seeds. So don't be afraid of fat. It will help you build muscle and brain power by helping you utilize protein, and protein will activate the fat.

Too Many "Karbo-Fats"

If you've been fighting your fat cravings and eating too little fat for too long, you may have noticed that you've been eating too many carbohydrates because you've had a hard time feeling satisfied. In all of us it takes a certain amount of fat in meals to trigger this satisfaction sensation: "I've had enough to eat now." If you can't stop eating your low-fat foods, you may find that adding in more fats, expecially the omega fats, will make you feel satisfied and "full" more quickly. Here is the other crucial problem with low-fat diets: the high carbohydrate contents of these diets convert directly to poor quality stored fat. This is because low-fat diets usually abound in sweets and starchy carbohydrates that your body just gets overwhelmed by and slaps onto your body for quick storage. This is true even when you're eating those carbohydrates as whole grains and vegetables. This body fat that originates from carbos, I call "karbo-fat."

Only a small amount of sweets and starches (that is, low-fat carbos) can be burned for energy. The rest is stored as fat. This low-fat karbo-fat, called palmitic acid, accounts for much more unneeded weight gain than high-fat foods. And karbo-fats are considered among the most damaging fats of all for the heart and entire cardiovascular system. Yet they are made from foods that we've been taught are very healthy precisely because they're so low in fat! One of the reasons that karbo-fats cause problems is that they are very sluggish. They form the bulk of the excess triglycerides that clog the arteries, and they block the benefits of the active omega fats.

Sugar, Alcohol, and Fat

Too much of the super-karbo twins, sugar and alcohol, can block our utilization of the omega fats. Sugar and alcohol convert to excess cholesterol. They trigger excess insulin, a magic potion that converts them instantly from glucose into stored karbo-fat and triglycerides. All of the fats derived from excess sugar and alcohol keep us from benefiting from the omega fats that we take in. So we keep on needing and craving fats.

Too Much of a Good Thing: Excess Omega-6

Too much omega-6 in relation to omega-3 can cause fat cravings. Where do you get omega-6? You can find it in seeds, nuts, vegetables, beans, grains, and most salad or cooking oils. It is much harder to get the omega-3 oils, which is why you're probably deficient, and why you'll be using omega-3 supplements.

The cholesterol scare in the 1960s prompted a rush away from butter and fatty meats and toward vegetable oils. Most vegetable oils (such as corn, safflower, and peanut oil) are high in omega-6. Unfortunately, too much omega-6, without balanced omega-3, now seem to be causing some of our most common and serious health problems in addition to fat cravings. We do need omega-6 fats, but we need almost as many omega-3, which are much harder to find. The ideal ratio is somewhere between 1:1 and 2:1, omega-6 to omega-3. In the typical U.S. diet, the ratio of omega-6 to omega-3 fats is 20:1. Canola is the only oil that contains both omega-3 and omega-6 in a decent balance. Flax, hemp, and fish oil contain high levels of omega-3 and little omega-6.

Some of the serious consequences of too much omega-6 are that by unbalancing omega-3 oils, it contributes to inflammatory and auto-immune problems, such a rheumatoid arthritis, asthma, Crohn's disease, osteoporosis, cancer, and Alzheimer's disease.

If you're been eating mostly junk food, you probably aren't getting enough of either omega-6 or omega-3 oils. But if you have been trying to be healthy, you have been getting plenty of omega-6—so just add some omega-3 now to balance it out.

FACTS ABOUT SOME FAT SOURCES

Cholesterol, Butter, and the Other Saturated Fats: Surprise!

Cholesterol is a word, like fat, that we have learned to fear. But guess what is made from the cholesterol in our bodies? Estrogen, testosterone, adrenaline, and all of our other sex and stress-coping hormones. Fats like butter, cheese, coconut, and the fats in shellfish, meat, and poultry are high in cholesterol, but 70 percent of us are not affected by them. Our bodies know how to dispose of unneeded cholesterol.

About 30 percent of us are born with a tendency to make too much cholesterol.[7] But a low-cholesterol (low saturated fat) diet does not usually help much. We do better to increase our vitamin and mineral intake from vegetables and fruit, and take special supplements, including *essential* fats.

Coconut, palm kernel, butter, and cocoa are types of saturated fats. If they are not hydrogenated (to prolong shelf life), they don't cause harm and can help lower tryglycerides. But they are very low in the essential fats. If we eat fats like these in excess, these oils will block the benefits of the essential omega-3 and -6 oils that we take in.

What About Meat, Poultry, and Milk Fat?

These, too, are saturated (firmer) fats. Saturated fats are rather inert compared to the liquid omegas. They keep our cell walls firm while the omegas make them flexible. We need both kinds of fat to stay in balance. But red meats actually include some beneficial fats, as well as important minerals (iron and zinc). Lamb, even, contains some omega-3 fat. But trimming extra fat off of meat, as well as poultry, is a good idea. Too much saturated fat interferes with essential fat absorption. Another problem is that animal and dairy fat also harbor pesticides and antibiotics. Buy the organically produced versions whenever you can. Remember: animal fat is only junk fat if you consume it in excess. But you will not be doing that, because you'll be eating special foods and taking supplements that will stop your excess-fat cravings.

Many people, particularly those who have type O blood, seem to digest animal fat quite well.[8] They seem to need meat, poultry, and eggs, as well as fish (though they do not seem to do as well as those with other blood types do with cow's milk products). A blood types may not be able to utilize saturated animal fats as well, because they may be best adapted genetically to a vegetarian diet based on legumes, corn, rice, nuts and seeds, and leafy green sources of fat. Both blood types need to get enough omega-3 oil. Vegetarians can get too much omega-6 and meat eaters can be deficient in both omega-3 and omega-6.

DO YOU DIGEST FAT WELL?

You may be eating plenty of healthy fats, but if you aren't an efficient fat processor, you may not get the benefits from them. You may not be making enough of the enzymes that do your fat digesting, or your liver and gallbladder, key players in fat digestion, may be in some kind of trouble. If so, the benefits of your anti-fat-craving program will be reduced. How do you know if you're digesting fat poorly? If you are, you will feel overly full, heavy, or nauseous after a high-fat meal, have oily skin, or experience burping or belching after eating fatty foods. In this case, lipase, a fat-digesting enzyme, can help.

Your Fat-Digesting Enzymes

Lipase is part of the digestive brigade that breaks fats down so that your body can use them most beneficially. Lipase (*lipid* is another word for "fat") meets up with your fat soon after you swallow it. So does bile—a powerful acid made by the liver and stored in the gallbladder. Bile breaks fat into little pieces so that lipase can easily dissolve it for your body to utilize, rather than just store.

If you are having trouble digesting fats, you should take extra lipase supplements to help you break down the fats you eat. Lipase supplements are exactly like your own digestive enzymes. You have many kinds of enzymes in your digestive track, each one only capable of digesting one particular kind of carbohydrate, protein, or fat. If you don't have enough lipase, your body can't get the full nutritional value of the fats you eat.

Once you've improved your general eating and health over the next few months, you'll be making lots of your own lipase and you won't need lipase supplements any more. That's because your pancreas, which produces digestive enzymes like lipase, will no longer be stressed by a high-carbohydrate diet. Now it will be able to manufacture enough of the enzymes you need instead of working overtime to produce insulin to handle all those extra carbs.

Fat and the Liver and Gallbladder

The liver and its intimate partner, the gallbladder, process all of our incoming fats. If either is unable to do its job, our bodies may not receive the fats that they need, and they will put out the call for more fat. This can turn into a vicious cycle, as the liver gets more inefficient because of an overload of fats to process, on top of whatever problems it had to begin with (for example, from drug or alcohol use, parasites, chemicals, or pesticides).

Your liver is the gallbladder's boss in processing the fats that come into your body. It can get overworked and congested. It can even become diseased, especially now with various forms of hepatitis becoming more and more common. Symptoms of liver problems include yellowing of the skin and eyes, intolerance of greasy foods, and unusual bowel movements.

There are a number of nutritional supplements that can help your liver function better. You'll see in chapter 16 why an herb called milk thistle (or silymarin) is our favorite as a liver regenerator.

MICROBIAL PARASITES AND FAT

Tiny intestinal invaders can increase your appetite for fatty foods. The parasite blastocystis hominis ("blasto") actually feeds on the fat that you eat until it literally explodes. These and other parasites can invade the liver and affect the gallbladder, too. If you increase your omega-3 fats and improve your liver and gallbladder function, and you still have strong cravings for fats, then take the parasite questionnaire in chapter 7 and check with your doctor about testing and treatment.

Whatever the cause of your fat cravings, you don't have to be enslaved by it anymore. Nor do you have to cling to fat addiction because when you get the essential fats your body so needs, you won't miss the ones you don't need. Turn to chapter 16 for liberating nutritional solutions.

Part II

Correcting Your Imbalances

NINE

Refueling Your Brain Chemistry with Amino Acids

This may be the most exciting chapter in *The Diet Cure* because it will teach you how to use amino acid supplements to correct your brain chemistry deficiencies. Soon you'll be free of food cravings, depression, irritability, anxiety, obsessiveness, and mental dullness. You'll use the Amino Acid Therapy Chart on page 118 to carefully check off your brain deficiency symptoms in each of the four key areas. Then you'll learn which aminos you'll need, at what dosages, and when to take them. You'll also learn some other ways to boost your brain's chemistry.

As part of your master plan, you'll of course be taking basic supplements as well. The basic vitamins, minerals, and others are detailed in chapter 17 on page 241. And while amino acids and other nutritional supplements will do wonders for your brain chemistry, certain foods are important, too. Protein-rich foods are essential for replenishing your body's supply of all twenty-two amino acids. So once you have chosen your amino acid supplements, you can read the chapters in part 3 to ensure that you get all the most beneficial foods for your brain-refurnishing project.

You may want to test your amino acid levels for confirmation that you are indeed low in certain ones before you begin to use them, so I've provided information on testing at the end of this chapter. Finally, I'll give you some guidance here on when you can stop taking your amino acid supplements and simply continue with your basic supplements and master eating plan.

> **Warning:** Not all amino acids and supplements are safe for all people. See "Are Your Supplements Safe" in chapter 17, page 251. If you have doubts, talk to your health care practitioner.

USING THE AMINO ACID THERAPY CHART: RESTORING YOUR DEPLETED BRAIN CHEMICALS

The following chart will help you determine what amino acids you should take, in what amounts, and when, to address the imbalances in your moods. Let's start by examining the columns at the top of the chart.

Column A, Deficiency Symptoms. This tells you how you might feel if you did not have enough of each natural mood booster. Check off the symptoms that apply to you.

Column B, Addictive Substances Used. Here is a list of the drugs or drug-foods you will be drawn to if you don't have enough natural mood boosters. Check off each one that applies to you.

Column C, Natural Solution: Amino Acids. This lists the amino acids that correct the deficiencies. Look first at the boxes you checked off in columns A and B. These are the areas of your brain chemistry that need the most mood-food (amino acids). Column C then tells you which specific aminos you will need.

Column D, Neurotransmitter or Brain Fuel/Promotes. These are the natural brain boosters, or neurotransmitters, that are made from the amino acids you will be taking. This column indicates what benefits will result from building up these neurotransmitters.

Now let's look at each of the five horizontal sections, starting at the top of the chart.

Section I, Relieving Cravings for Sweets, Starches, and Alcohol. If your cravings are triggered by a drop in blood sugar (hypoglycemia), the L-glutamine should alleviate them in just a day. Two 500-milligram capsules three times a day between meals is usually sufficient. For fast, emergency relief of carbohydrates and/or alcohol cravings, take 500 milligrams of L-glutamine sublingually. As L-glutamine stabilizes your brain's blood sugar level, your mood tends to stabilize as well.

Section II, Curing a Lack of Energy and Focus. For low energy, depression, and poor concentration, take 500 to 2,000 milligrams of L-tyrosine three times per day (before breakfast, midmorning, and midafternoon). L-tyrosine is an energizing and stimulating amino acid. If it is too stimulating (for example, if it interferes with sleep), eliminate it or reduce the dose, particularly the midafternoon dose.

If you look for a "lift" or better concentration from foods or drugs like nicotine, NutraSweet, and caffeine, you probably need to overhaul your brain's natural energy system. I usually recommend L-tyrosine first. Then, if you still feel draggy, or if the tyrosine makes you feel wired or jittery, try a similar amino acid, L-phenylalanine. Work with these two aminos until you get your own natural energy and concentration back. If they don't do the job, your master energy glands—the adrenals and the thyroid— probably need help. Tyrosine is a primary food that their hormones are made from, but if these glands are too dysfunctional, they may need special medical attention.

Section III, Enhancing Your Ability to Relax. If you have checked off several of the symptoms and substances in this section in columns A and B, try adding 100 to 500 milligrams of GABA (gamma amino butyric acid) to your daily regimen of amino acids whenever you need extra help relaxing. Taking GABA for the first time early in the day is not a good idea because you might get too relaxed to drive or to begin work. Several popular formulas combine GABA with two other relaxing amino acids, taurine and glycine, 300 to 500 milligrams each. This combination can be even more calming for some people than GABA alone. Several popular formulas combine all three aminos: GABA Calm, by Source Naturals, meant to be taken sublingually, contains 100 milligrams of GABA plus 50 milligrams glycene and 40 milligrams of magnesium taurenate (both of which relax muscles, and magnesium taurenate relaxes the brain as well), plus 25 milligrams of tyrosine (to prevent getting too drowsy). Another, Amino Relaxer, by Country Life, has 100 milligrams of GABA and higher doses of taurine and glycene. Try 500 milligrams of GABA if you need more relaxation. If these aminos do not relieve your stress, you may be suffering from adrenal exhaustion. (See chapter 3.)

Amino Acid Therapy Chart

Sec. No.	A. Deficiency Symptoms	B. Addictive Substances Used	C. Natural Solution: Amino Acids	D. Neurotransmitter or Brain Fuel/Promotes
I	❑ cravings for sugar, starch, or alcohol ❑ reduced mental stability	❑ sweets ❑ starches ❑ alcohol	L-glutamine	**Emergency fuel source for entire brain** stable, calm, alert brain function
II	❑ depression ❑ lack of energy ❑ lack of drive ❑ lack of focus, concentration ❑ attention deficit disorder	❑ sweets ❑ starch ❑ chocolate ❑ aspartame ❑ alcohol ❑ marijuana ❑ caffeine ❑ cocaine ❑ speed ❑ tobacco	L-tyrosine L-phenylalanine	**Dopamine/ Norepinephrine** arousal energy mental focus drive
III	❑ stiff and tense muscles ❑ stressed and burned out ❑ unable to relax/loosen up	❑ sweets ❑ starch ❑ tobacco ❑ marijuana ❑ Valium ❑ alcohol	GABA (with relaxing aminos taurine and glycine, if needed)	**GABA** calmness relaxation

Sec. No.	A. Deficiency Symptoms	B. Addictive Substances Used	C. Natural Solution: Amino Acids	D. Neurotransmitter or Brain Fuel/Promotes
IV	☐ very sensitive to emotional or physical pain ☐ cry easily ☐ crave comfort, reward, or numbing treats ☐ "Love" certain foods or drugs	☐ sweets ☐ starch ☐ chocolate ☐ tobacco ☐ heroin ☐ marijuana ☐ alcohol	DL-phenylalanine D-phenylalanine	**Endorphin** psychological and physical pain relief pleasure reward loving feelings numbness
V	☐ negativity, depression ☐ worry, anxiety ☐ low self-esteem ☐ obsessive thoughts/behaviors ☐ winter blues ☐ PMS ☐ irritability, rage ☐ heat intolerance ☐ panic, phobias ☐ afternoon or evening cravings ☐ fibromyalgia, TMJ ☐ night-owl, hard to get to sleep ☐ insomnia, disturbed sleep ☐ suicidal thoughts	☐ sweets ☐ starch ☐ tobacco ☐ chocolate ☐ Ecstasy ☐ marijuana	L-tryptophan 5-HTP Melatonin for sleep at bedtime	**Serotonin** emotional stability self-confidence **Melatonin** good sleep (made from serotonin)

Taking Your Aminos

Taking an amino acid (or any other nutrient) sublingually—opening the capsule and pouring the contents under your tongue—speeds its effect because it is absorbed by the large blood vessels there, but only L-glutamine tastes good. Try to take your aminos at least twenty minutes before or ninety minutes after a meal in which you eat protein; otherwise, the protein in your food will compete with the amino acid and some of the amino will not get into your brain. If you have no negative reactions, such as headaches, but you are still feeling cravings or other deficiency symptoms an hour after taking a 500-milligram capsule (the smallest dose usually available), try using 1,000 to 2,000 milligrams, gradually increasing 500 milligrams at a time. *Stop if you have any adverse reactions.*

Section IV, Eliminating the Need for Comfort Foods. Which amino acids can free a food junky? D-phenylalanine seems to be the single most helpful amino acid for building up optimal amounts of our natural "painkillers or opiate." Many studies have confirmed its usefulness in increasing pain tolerance by keeping endorphin levels high.

Most supplement formulations combine D-phenylalanine with equal amounts of L-phenylalanine, its more stimulating twin. Since the L form is also needed to create the pain relievers called enkephalins, this combination usually works well, especially if energy is needed. When it doesn't and you feel too stimulated, the D form can be taken alone. (See page 9.) Try a combination of DLPA (DL-phenylalanine) with L-glutamine three times per day (on arising, midmorning, and midafternoon) if you overeat to help you deal with emotional pain. You will also need to consume plenty of high-protein foods and perhaps add a complete blend of amino acids, because endorphin building requires more amino acids than are needed to build any of the other three neurotransmitters. (Note: If you take DLPA, you won't need to take L-phenylalanine for energy, because DLPA contains L-phenylalanine. Try L-tyrosine if you need more energy than you get from DLPA alone.)

Section V, Raising Serotonin, Our Natural Prozac. The deficiency symptoms in column A of the last section of the Amino Acid Therapy Chart make it clear that depleted brain serotonin can cause some of the most extensive suffering of all.

If you have low serotonin levels, take a 250- to 1,000-milligram dose of L-tryptophan midmorning, midafternoon, and two hours after dinner (or at bedtime, if sleep is a problem, because, as explained in chapter 1, L-tryptophan creates serotonin, which creates melatonin, which helps you sleep).

Since L-tryptophan is available only by prescription, another supplement you can take to boost serotonin is 5-HTP (hydroxytryptophan), which is a chemical halfway between tryptophan and serotonin. It is widely available in health food stores and some drugstores as well as Wal-Mart. My clients find that they often need only 50 to 100 milligrams or less, two to three times a day.

Tryptophan in either form, as L-tryptophan or as 5-HTP, usually works best when it is taken thirty minutes or longer before rival amino acids (tyrosine or phenylalanine), caffeine, or protein foods are consumed. Too much tryptophan can make some people sleepy, even when it's taken in the daytime. If you have this problem, eliminate morning doses, experiment with smaller amounts, or take tryptophan along with meals. You may need to vary your dose according to your response to tryptophan quite a bit, as different individuals respond differently to this amino acid (more so than with any of the other aminos). Occasionally, very low doses (e.g., 10 milligrams of 5-HTP) work best.

Be sure to take the multiple vitamin-mineral in your basic supplement plan while you are taking either form of tryptophan, as you should with any amino acids. The B vitamins and zinc are particularly important because they help the brain to manufacture its neurochemicals out of the amino acids. Vitamin B_3 (niacin) is particularly important because your body makes it out of tryptophan, and you want your limited store of tryptophan making serotonin, not niacin.

To increase serotonin, emphasize the following protein sources of tryptophan and serotonin, along with moderate amounts of carbohydrate at meals, and get plenty of exercise and light.

Eat foods containing tryptophan. Most foods that are high in protein contain much less tryptophan than they do the other amino acids. Here are some foods that have higher amounts of tryptophan or, for reasons not entirely clear, seem to raise serotonin levels:

✦ Seeds (pumpkin, sunflower, and sesame)
✦ Filberts and almonds
✦ Pork
✦ Beef

+ Wild game
+ Shrimp
+ Chicken
+ Turkey
+ Tempe
+ Tofu
+ Kelp
+ Bananas
+ Milk (if you are not dairy intolerant)

Try St. John's Wort. Wort means "herb," and this one increases serotonin activity. Studies from Europe and the United States find that it is as effective as Prozac, without as many of the side effects. Some people do best taking St. John's in combination with L-tryptophan or 5-HTP; some do better on St. John's Wort alone. Try taking 300 milligrams of St. John's Wort (which includes 0.3 percent of the active ingredient hypericin) three times a day. Start with the tryptophan or 5-HTP, and then add St. John's Wort (which is the more likely to create a negative side effect, such as sensitivity to sunlight) if you need it, with professional supervision.

Be sure to get enough exercise. Moderate levels of exercise can temporarily raise serotonin levels. That's why many of us feel so good after physical activity. The exercising muscles pull all of the competing amino acids out of the bloodstream, allowing L-tryptophan to pass freely through to the brain. Caution: When exercise is the only tool used to raise serotonin, exercise addiction can result. (See chapter 21.)

Expose yourself to enough light. If you tend to get depressed and/or overeat in winter or in the evening, it is probably because you are not getting enough light or enough serotonin. In the late summer, your brain registers a decrease in light levels and begins to reduce serotonin levels in favor of melatonin—your "hibernation" or sleep chemical. As fall and winter set in, your serotonin levels can drop too low. This is called SAD, or seasonal affective disorder. Increasing your exposure to light sources to over two thousand lux helps trick your brain into raising serotonin to summer levels. Two thousand lux is about ten times brighter than normal office lighting (one lux represents the brightness of one candle; ten thousand lux is as bright as a sunny day at noon); to get that intensity with regular lightbulbs you would expose yourself to far too much infrared light, which would hurt your retinas, so the key is either sunlight or cool fluorescent lighting. When you use the light to encourage your brain to take in extra tryptophan to make more serotonin you can build in permanent immunity from the winter blues. Also, plenty of full-spectrum lighting, which mimics natural outdoor light, has other benefits, including activating the synthesis of vitamin D, which helps absorption of vitamin C. Emergency visits to tanning booths in winter have also lifted the moods of many of our clients suffering from winter depression. (For sources of high-lux lamps and full-spectrum bulbs, see Resources.)

Consider taking SSRIs (selective serotonin reuptake inhibitors). As I mentioned at the beginning of chapter 1 raising serotonin can make the difference between life and death if you are severely depressed, anorectic, or bulimic. SSRI drugs such as Prozac, Paxil, Zoloft, and Effexor can be crucial for making that difference. Since the effects of tryptophan and 5-HTP can be felt in a day or two, you may want to try one of them first. If it doesn't make a vast improvement in how you feel, I suggest you consult a medical doctor, preferably a psychiatrist, and ask about possibly taking an SSRI or similar drug. Unfortunately, these drugs improve, but do not eliminate, all symptoms of low serotonin. Even worse, you may experience mild or severe side effects such as suicidal depression, inability to achieve orgasm, insomnia, jitteriness, and more. Lastly, SSRIs can be safely taken only short-term, and their benefits are not usually sustained after discontinuation. Fortunately, my clients almost never need SSRIs long-term. Why? Because I direct them to physicians who help them with their low thyroid function, which is the most common reason we've found for tryptophan not working as well as SSRIs.

Consider combining tryptophan with SSRIs. Do this in consultation with a physician who can prescribe and monitor medications. Amino acid therapy expert Eric Braverman, M.D., who recommends the use of tyrosine along with Ritalin, Phentermine, or similar drugs for attention deficit disorder (ADD), cites many studies documenting L-tryptophan's successful coadministration with SSRIs. Though most had no problems, a few patients in initial studies on Prozac experienced agitation, restlessness, and mild digestive distress when they took Prozac and L-tryptophan together. Many of the psychiatrists that I work with are happy to combine the two, and the results have been excellent. (The *Physicians' Desk Reference* doesn't note any problems with combining Paxil or Zoloft with L-tryptophan.) As to whether St. John's Wort can be taken with even low doses of SSRIs, the jury is still out.

If the combination of medication and tryptophan is successful, you might (in the late spring or summer only) try reducing your medication. At our clinic, we have often collaborated with M.D.s or D.O.s to get clients off of their Prozac and similar medications for a trial of L-tryptophan or 5-HTP—which often worked better than SSRIs right away.

Melatonin: The Natural Sleeping Pill for Nighttime Eaters

Your brain begins to make its own sleeping pill, melatonin, out of serotonin as the sun gets lower in the sky each afternoon. If it can't produce enough, you don't sleep well. The food that your brain needs as raw material to manufacture melatonin is the amino acid tryptophan. In the afternoon and evening, you need extra supplies of serotonin because your brain begins to convert it into melatonin. As serotonin levels decline in this daily cycle, if you are low in serotonin to begin with, you will start to crave carbohydrates, which can give you a temporary lift of serotonin (especially if they are simple carbohydrates, like sugar). Your midafternoon cravings may get worse as the evening wears on. Unable to sleep, you eat more sweets and starches, usually along with milk products. Ice cream and cereal are common favorites.

Because melatonin can cause grogginess and troubling dreams, as well as add to depression for someone already depressed, I recommend melatonin for relieving late-night cravings only when L-tryptophan, 5-HTP, and/or St. John's Wort do not normalize sleep. Taking 500 to 1,500 milligrams of L-tryptophan (or 100 to 150 milligrams of 5-HTP) at bedtime is usually effective for insomnia, interrupted sleep, and night-owl syndrome. If you still wake up after two A.M. and can't get back to sleep, try a 2-milligram time-release capsule of melatonin at eight P.M. and an oral or sublingual tablet at bedtime (0.5 to 3 milligrams). This latter is also a good dosage range if you are trying to adjust to a change in time zones because of traveling; melatonin is famous for its effectiveness in relieving jet lag.

If you need to take L-tyrosine or DLPA and tryptophan: Remember that L-tyrosine and DL-phenylalanine compete with tryptophan, so either take them at different times of the day or take a form of L-tryptophan thirty minutes or more before either of the other two amino acids. If you take them together they will still help, but not as effectively. We often recommend L-tyrosine and DLPA for early morning (AM) and midmorning (MM) use, and L-tryptophan or 5-HTP for midafternoon (MA), evening (predinner) and bedtime (BT) use.

Finding DPA: Only one company that I know of, Amino Health, carries D-phenylalanine (DPA) by itself. If emotional or physical pain is a real problem for you, it can be worth the trouble of ordering it. See Resources.

Amino Acid Supplements

With a pencil, check off the amino acids and other supplements listed below that you should be taking, as indicated by your responses on the Amino Acid Therapy Chart and the other information in this chapter. You should photocopy this chart to make clean copies for future use, because your amino plan is likely to change as you begin using the aminos and by your reactions to them you find that you need more or fewer. Where a range of doses is listed, start with the lower amount to see how it affects you. It is important that you also take the vitamins, minerals, and other nutrients in the basic supplement plan in chapter 17 to optimize the effects of your amino acids.

	AM	B	MM	L	MA	D	BT*
❏ L-glutamine, 500 mg (to stop sweet, starch, and alcohol cravings, and enhance relaxation)	1–3	__	1–3	__	1–3	__	__
❏ GABA, 100–500 mg; or GABA w/taurine and glycine, 100–300 mg of each as needed† (to destress and relax muscles)	__	__	1	__	1	__	1
❏ L-tyrosine, 500 mg (to energize and focus)	1–4	__	1–4	__	1–4	__	__
❏ DLPA, 500 mg; or DPA 500 mg (to enhance feelings of comfort and pleasure and to reduce pain)	1–2	__	1–2	__	1–2	__	__
❏ L-tryptophan, by prescription, 500 mg (to improve mood, sleep, and PM cravings) or	__	__	1–2	__	1–2	__	2
❏ 5-HTP, 50 mg (to improve mood, sleep, and PM cravings)	__	__	1–2	__	1–2	__	2
❏ St. John's Wort, 300 mg, with 900 mcg (0.3%) hypericin (to help raise serotonin levels)	__	__	1	__	1	__	1

*AM=on arising; B=with breakfast; MM=midmorning; L=lunch; MA=midafternoon; D=with dinner; BT=at bedtime.
†Note: GABA Calm by Source Naturals and Amino Relaxer by Country Life combine GABA, taurine, and glycine.

	AM	B	MM	L	MA	D	BT
❏ Complete essential amino acids, 500 mg	1–2	—	1–2	—	1–2	—	2

Note: Add the complete amino acid blend, if:

1) You are unable to eat enough protein-containing foods, at first.
2) You have been severely malnourished; e.g., after anorexia, alcoholism, or too many low-calorie diets
3) Your endorphins seem to be very depleted. (See section IV of the Amino Acid Therapy Chart.)
4) If you tend to have blood sugar drops (or hypoglycemia)

Caution: Find an amino blend that contains at least the eight essential amino acids, particularly tryptophan. The eight essential aminos are:

lysine
phenylalanine
leucine
threonine
isoleucine
tryptophan
methionine histidine
valine

AMINO FOODS

Protein is the only food source of amino acids. Mature adults should be sure to have at least 20 grams of protein at each of their three meals. You must build protein into your diet in order to be able to stop using the amino acid supplements in three to twelve months. Chapter 18, "The Best Foods for Your Special Biochemistry," will help you determine how much protein you will need and detail more about your complete eating plan, including what kinds of carbohydrates and fats will work best with your protein. But don't forget, muscle and brain power can be built *only* from protein.

TESTING FOR AMINO ACID LEVELS

If you would feel more comfortable getting tested to confirm your need for amino acids, you can ask your doctor for a urine or blood plasma test for amino acid levels, before and three months after you start taking amino acids. Remember that the test may show you have plenty of amino acids, but your symptoms might indicate that you need more. Some individuals simply need more of specific amino acids and other nutrients than others do. The proof is in how the aminos make you feel. A test can help you to decide when to try eliminating your aminos or point you to aminos that are not on the chart, but that, if deficient, may be adding to your discomfort.

TAPERING OFF AMINOS

Unlike the basic supplements, your amino acid supplements will be needed only temporarily. But how will you know when you no longer need them?

+ You get adverse symptoms, like headaches, tiredness, or jitteryness.
+ You stop taking them to see if your cravings or mood symptoms return, and they don't.

When should you start tapering off your aminos to see whether they are still needed? After one to three months, start consciously skipping your amino doses to see what happens. Experiment with one amino at a time; don't drop all of them at once. If you still need your aminos, try eliminating them again monthly until you are ready to do without them. But keep them on hand for short-term use during any future brain slumps.

ACTION STEPS

1. Study the deficiency symptoms on the amino acid therapy chart in this chapter.
2. Try the supplements indicated by your symptoms as directed, along with your basic supplements, detailed in chapter 17.
3. Eat plenty of protein as suggested in chapter 18.
4. If you continue to have symptoms of low serotonin:
   + try using a full-spectrum lamp
   + exercise regularly.
   + consult your doctor about using SSRI drugs
5. Consider with an M.D. or D.O. whether to test your amino acid levels before and three months after you start taking aminos.
6. Cut down, then eliminate, your amino acids over the next three to twelve months, as you no longer need them.

Reading

Braverman, Eric R., M.D., with Carl C. Pfeiffer, M.D., Ph.D., et al. *The Healing Nutrients Within.* (New Canaan, CT: Keats, 1997).

Erdmann, Robert, and Meiri Jones. *The Amino Revolution.* (New York: Fireside, 1989).

Larson, Joan Mathews, Ph.D. *Seven Weeks to Sobriety.* (New York: Fawcett Books, 1997).

Norden, Michael J., M.D. *Beyond Prozac: Brain-Toxic Lifestyles, Natural Antidotes and New Generation Antidepressants* (New York: HarperCollins, 1995).

Sahley, Billie Jay. *Healing with Amino Acids.* This book (and other materials) can be ordered by calling (800) 669-CALM.

Slagle, Priscilla. *The Way Up from Down* (New York: St. Martin's Press, 1994).

Resources

For compounding pharmacies where your M.D. or D.O. can order L-tryptophan, see Resources in Chapter 21, page 353.

Most amino acids can be purchased from any health food or drug store, supplement catalogue, or our clinic's order line. Three exceptions:

1) DPA (D-phenylalanine) is available only through a few private practitioners, our clinic order line, or Amino Health
   (800) 293-1683.

2) L-tryptophan must be ordered from a compounding pharmacy by your physician's prescription. It's easy. See page 353.

3) Ott Biolight Systems, Inc.
   28 Parker Way
   Santa Barbara, CA 93101
   (800) 234-3724
   <www.ottbiolight.com>

   Founded by Dr. John Ott, who pioneered the concept of light for wellness, Ott Biolight sells full-spectrum and extra-bright lighting.

   Ott's full spectrum and extra-bright lighting is also available through our clinic's order line (800-733-9293.) Also, check your local Office Depot for bargain Ott lights.

TEN

Nutritional Rehab for the Ex-Dieter

W henever I see someone with signs of any of the eight physical imbalances discussed in this book, I always look at the role of low-calorie dieting, because it can set off several of the other imbalances, in addition to all the damage it can do by itself.

Some dieters can recover on their own by making a decision to stop dieting forever. But many others need more education and support to return to normal, nondiet eating, which can then restore normal appetite and mood, often very quickly. With the help of better foods, simple nutritional supplementation, and supportive education, you can reduce your fears about weight gain and eliminate your food cravings quickly. Then you will be able to start enjoying healthy eating, your weight and mood will stabilize, and you will no longer have to deal with the many side effects of poor nutrition that have, until now, interfered with your quality of life. But first, you've got to reeducate yourself about dieting.

In this chapter, you'll get some suggestions about how to break out of the dieting mentality and develop a more realistic sense of how much food you should be eating—and what kind. I'll provide nutritional supplement protocols for ex-dieters, including anorectics and bulimics. Finally, I'll give some pointers on finding books, videos, magazines, and supportive organizations and professionals that can help keep you safe from dieting.

DEFECTING FROM THE DIET CULT

One young woman came to Recovery Systems after years of intermittent dieting and ten- to twenty-pound weight shifts. She was eating candy bars in the afternoons and too often lots of ice cream after dinner. When I went over her diet diary with her, I immediately pinpointed the culprit: she was always skipping breakfast. This particular client did not even seem to need any special nutrient supplements to help get her back on track. As soon as she began to eat a protein-rich breakfast daily, her afternoon and evening junk food cravings just disappeared. Soon she was eating three well-balanced meals per day and finding her weight stable for the first time in years.

By returning to three-meals-a-day eating you too may be able to eliminate overeating and weight gain. Unfortunately, many of you are too afraid of putting on pounds to try eating normal amounts of food again, but you don't have to be, as you will learn in this chapter.

YOUR "IDEAL" WEIGHT

Where do we get our perception that we are "fat"? Most of us rely on standard height and weight charts, but as we saw in chapter 2, these are misleading. Body fat percentages are not accurate measures of health, either. Perfectly healthy people can have high percentages of body fat. (Think of Eskimos, with 75 percent body fat!) Excessive deep abdominal fat stores may cause health problems, but not the fat in hips and thighs that women so despise.

Unfortunately, too many of us look to the media to get a sense of what we "should" look like. Entire books have been written on the effect of the media's distorted images of women's bodies (and let's not forget that our visually oriented media are now presenting unattainable "ideal" bodies for men as well). Try some of the following exercises to reeducate your eye, and your mind, about what a healthy body should like.

1. Stop weighing yourself. Toss out your bathroom scale. Even at the doctor's office, do not allow yourself to be weighed (unless you are underweight) or insulted about your weight.
2. Pick one day a week where you totally avoid any conversation about anyone's weight, especially yours! Expand this to seven days a week as soon as possible.
3. Check the body shapes of people on your family tree. If you didn't know your grandparents or great-grandparents, or great-aunts or -uncles,

when they were young, before they ever dieted, get photos and study them. Go as far back into pre-dieting (pre-1970) family history as you can. You'll probably find your genetic double, who will be the healthy ideal weight that you should be. Remember the further back you go, the healthier the diet, and the more realistic the weight standards. I found that my body was almost identical to my paternal grandmother's, and to no one else's on either side of my family.

You may wish that you had your aunt's green eyes or your uncle's long eyelashes, but you know it's impossible. Remember, the rest of your body is inherited, too.

4. Question your family messages about weight. Did you grow up hearing things like, "I hope you don't get my thighs," or "Don't eat so much or you'll end up looking like your uncle Benjamin"? It's sad to think that these inherited body types are held up as something you should, or even could, try to avoid developing. If only we all grew up hearing messages like, "I think you'll be built just like your wonderful aunt Jane," with no negative baggage attached to any particular body type.

5. Look at old photographs and great artwork of the past. Take a trip to the flea market, a store that sells old magazines or prints, a museum or art reproduction shop, or view some old movies. Look at the bodies of models, actors and actresses, and ordinary people of the past. You may be astonished to see the beefy thighs and arms on 1940s pin-ups or on women in paintings (such as those of Rubens, Michelangelo, or Botticelli), or the fleshy legs on 1920s bathing beauties. Notice the thick middles of some of the most dashing male movie stars of the past. Remember, Marilyn Monroe was a size 12 and above, and the full-figured Mae West was considered quite the sex symbol. You may want to get copies of these old photographs or artworks to hang on your wall as a reminder that the "ideal" body has changed drastically over time for no good reason.

6. Stop reading fashion magazines and watching soaps and sitcoms with emaciated actresses and superbuffed actors. Women and gay men will have an especially hard time avoiding unrealistic body images in magazines and media aimed at them. Keep in mind that television, magazines, movies, and even newspapers rarely show images of average-shaped bodies. Moreover, print images are often drastically altered by computer to "fix" every possible flaw. You can try reading magazines that feature larger-size models and realistic body shapes, but if they still make you hate your body they will have to go, too. Self-body hate, like any hate or other strong negative emotion, contributes to unneeded weight gain by triggering junk-food binges.

7. Keep in mind the following eye-opening facts:

✦ Only 5 percent of us have "skinny" genes.

✦ In healthy 20- to 50-year old women worldwide, 28 percent body fat is average.

✦ The average American woman is a size 14.

✦ If Barbie were a real person, she would have so little body fat that she would be unable to menstruate.

✦ *No* study has convincingly shown that overweight is an independent *cause* of health problems.

✦ Premenopausal women who are medically "obese" have a 40 percent lower risk of breast cancer.

✦ Among elderly women, the thinnest have a death rate 50 percent higher than average-weight women.

✦ In a study of seventeen thousand Harvard alumni published in the *New England Journal of Medicine,* the men who had the best chance of living the longest were those who gained the most weight (twenty-five pounds or more) but stayed physically active.[1]

While it's true that with very serious obesity we can have health problems, very modest weight loss will get rid of them. Weight loss, even in those extreme and rare cases where excess weight is causing real health problems, has to be approached very, very cautiously. Many studies worldwide have confirmed that weight loss in both men and women correlates with a shortened lifespan. For example, the famous forty-year Framingham Study found that those whose weight fluctuated frequently, or by many pounds, had a 50 percent higher risk of heart disease.[2]

Sadly, many of my clients look back at the weight that prompted their first diets and tell me, "That was a great weight. I'd love to be that weight again, even though I wasn't skinny." Quite often that was their "ideal" weight and they never needed to diet in the first place. They were strong, full of energy, and emotionally positive. It was dieting that sapped their energy, disturbed their moods and their appetites, and caused them to lose their true balanced weight point. If you have dieted, you've probably been yo-yoing above and below your true weight for years. Sometimes illness, injury, or imbalances, like inherited low thyroid function, prevent you from finding your true weight. (Dieting, of course, just slows your thyroid even more.)

Fortunately, whatever the reason you lost track of it, your body can find its own natural weight again, if it is allowed to. Just as your natural voice reappears after a bad cold, your natural weight can reappear after a bad period of underfeeding or misfeeding.

THE "IDEAL" MEAL

In chapters 18, 19, and 20, you'll find lots of ideas for creating healthy meals that will enhance your particular biochemistry and get you on the road to health. To eat healthfully, you will have to reeducate yourself about what a meal should look like.

To start, try to forget about counting calories or fat grams. Focus on new ways of viewing food. What do you consider a healthy portion of chicken? Six ounces? Three ounces? What constitutes a "balanced" meal? After reading chapter 20, you will, I hope, have a different idea of what you should be eating.

I typically eat 3,000 calories or more a day. I'm almost five feet ten inches, I don't know what I weigh, but I do know that I feel good most of the time. My neighbor and I compared calories one day, because, though he is a daily runner, he is overweight. I exercise moderately three or four times a week. My neighbor considers my weight to be ideal and was astounded when I told him my calorie intake. When we calculated his daily menus, we came up with just under 1,600 calories. He fills up with diet Cokes all day. He undereats whenever he can. The food that he does eat is poor quality: sweetened hot or cold cereal for breakfast; chips and half a sandwich for lunch; and for dinner an iceberg lettuce salad with some carrot and tomato and kidney beans, and thousand island dressing. He decided to add in more protein, vegetables, and fruit, and cut out the diet drinks, bringing his calorie count up and his weight down. He lost even more when he replaced his wheat cereal and bread with rice and beans, even though his caloric intake went up to more than 3,000 a day.

My 3,000 calories:

+ Breakfast: Usually I eat 2 servings of fruit with 1/4 cup of nuts and seeds, protein powder, and nutritional yeast, blended into a smoothie; or, 3 eggs scrambled with veggies, avocado, and black beans, and a corn tortilla or two.
+ Lunch: I often eat a very large raw vegetable salad with 4 ounces of salmon and a bowl of split pea soup or a side of roasted potatoes.

◆ Dinner: 2 to 4 cups of sautéed veggies with tofu or sheep's feta cheese and 1 cup wild rice pilaf with brown basmati rice.

◆ Plus snacks of trail mix or fruit with cheese or nuts.

VEGETARIANISM

Are you a strong, vigorous, healthy vegetarian with rosy cheeks? Or are you tired a lot and a bit pale? Are you in between? Vegetarian dieters can be extra deficient in certain nutrients, because they not only cut calories, they eliminate whole groups of foods from the diet, such as protein. The other nutrients that are most commonly deficient in vegetarian diets are the minerals iron and zinc, vitamin B_{12}, and the amino acid L-carnitine. These are all easy to find in red meats. For guidance on how to construct a vegetarian, or vegan, version of the Diet Cure, turn to chapter 18. Supplements for vegetarians can be found in chapter 17, "Laying Out Your Master Plan." If you are a vegetarian, get your iron and ferritin levels tested, and check your blood count (CBC) for signs of anemia. Get medical suggestions for B_{12}, iron, and/or folic acid supplements if you are anemic. Monitor your levels by retesting regularly.

GOOD-BYE TO DIET SWEETENERS

Many dieters have become dependent on aspartame, also known as NutraSweet or Equal. You may find it surprisingly hard to do without your sweetened diet drinks and foods and your pink packets. Rather than search for another sweetener (I don't know of any that are problem-free) I'd like you to eliminate the drinks and foods that you've felt the need to "sweeten." Think instead about why you crave those beverages. Do some nutritional investigation and repair work. If you like diet sodas only with caffeine, take some tyrosine (500 to 1,500 milligrams) at the times you'd usually drink your caffeine (before or between meals is best). You should lose your interest in caffeine very quickly. Ditto decaf coffees or lattes, which still contain some caffeine. If you like only (or mostly) noncaffeinated beverages sweetened with aspartame, try DL-phenylalanine (500 to 1,000 milligrams) when you'd usually have your diet drink. You should not miss it. If you decide that you miss both caffeinated and NutraSweetened foods, you can try L-tyrosine (500 milligrams) and DL-phenylalanine (500 milligrams) together first thing in the morning and between meals.

You won't need these extra amino acid supplements for long. If they begin to make you a little jittery, or if you've been free of cravings for two weeks, go off of them. If your yen for aspartame or caffeine comes back, take a smaller dose for another week or so, then try going off again. Repeat until you're permanently free of cravings. You might think about your old drug favorites, but if you don't actually crave them, you're fine.

What should you drink instead? Warm beverages are a good idea, especially in the morning when you're at your coldest after eight hours of inactivity and no food, especially in cold weather.

Pure water with a squeeze of lemon or lime is delicious, but keep your bubbly drinks to a minimum because the phosphorus added through the carbonation process strips you of calcium. Herbal teas without caffeine or matte (another stimulant) can also be satisfying and tasty.

Respect Your Red Flags

If, at any point after you start the Diet Cure, you find yourself regularly wanting a cup of coffee, a diet soda, or some chocolate, that is an important red flag that can alert you to nutritional problems that need attention. Keep a food-mood log (see chapter 22, page 362) so that if you experience cravings you can spot any problems that might account for it. You'll usually find that you've skipped meals or supplements, or eaten foods that make you tired, or not eaten enough for your unique nutritional needs. The red flags of craving can alert you to important nutritional problems that need attention.

You might also discover that you'll need to review the Quick Symptom Questionnaire again. Even if your total score was not very high, a few significant symptoms might indicate a real imbalance. For example, if you tend to have cold hands and feet, and you've never taken your temperature in the morning but assume it's normal, take your morning temperature as instructed in chapter 12, and generally explore the possibility that you have a sluggish thyroid.

HOW TO UNDIET

1. **Do not skip meals.** Eat three substantial, balanced meals (containing protein, fat, and carbohydrates) per day. Skipping breakfast automatically slows metabolism and induces evening food cravings and overeating.

2. **Eat at least 25 percent of the day's calories at breakfast.**

Breakfast is the only meal that speeds up calorie burning. You may be able to stop all compulsive eating simply by adding a solid breakfast that emphasizes protein (at least 20 grams).

3. **Do not undereat.** Dr. Wayne Calloway, an expert in Third World malnutrition as well as eating disorders, describes patients who had dieted so often that they were gaining weight on 700 calories per day. When he raised their intake above 1,500 calories (with 25 percent taken in at breakfast), they finally began to lose weight and gain energy. My clients thrive on 2,500 or more calories per day.

4. **Start your meals with plenty of protein** (fish, chicken, beef, tofu, turkey, eggs, among others). Twenty grams or more of protein will reduce your interest in empty carbohydrates and make you alert and strong.

5. **Eat unlimited amounts of green vegetables with your protein. Eat some red and yellow ones, too.**

6. **For snacking, eat fruit or vegetables with proteins** (for examples, nuts, seeds, or cheese), not sweets or starches (like bagels or pretzels).

7. **Be sure to include some good fats in each meal** for optimal health and to trigger your appetite to turn off. Eat nuts, seeds, salad oil, olives, and avocados.

8. **Stop counting calories and fat grams.** If you are eating according to the guidelines of *The Diet Cure*, you don't have to worry about crunching numbers to be healthy.

9. **Turn to chapters 18, 19, and 20 for detailed guidance on using food to recover from dieting,** including a list (on page 307) of how much protein common foods contain.

Supplements for Antidieting

You will need to take the basic vitamin, mineral, and other nutrient supplements recommended in chapter 17. If, however, you have an eating disorder, you will need to take some extra nutritional supplements.

BULIMIA AND ANOREXIA

Please combine the following nutritional suggestions with visits to expert counselors and health professionals. I urge you to work with a physician who can monitor your progress and your health. I'm particularly concerned that you get your heart and electrolyte levels checked regularly.

You must also confer with a doctor about adding the serotonin-raising nutrient 5-HTP along with whatever prescribed SSRI (such as Prozac or Paxil) you may be taking. Taking them together is often necessary in the first few months of recovery to effectively relieve you of your compulsion and your mood swings. If you are vomiting, your doctor may need to provide the stomach-activating medicine propulsid for you for a while so that your food will stay down.

If you've been bulimic for less than ten years, you should respond immediately to this program; hundreds have. If you have a severe problem that has gone on for many more years, please be patient. It may take a while to get you totally stabilized, but you are on the right track.

Supplements for Bulimia

The supplements that will stop food cravings and binge eating and heal the digestive track for most bulimics include aloe vera juice (to repair your damaged gut lining and get your digestion and bowels moving); chromium (to decrease your sugar cravings and stabilize your blood sugar); and calcium, magnesium, and potassium to support your heart (plus extra magnesium if you have constipation). Vitamin C, B complex, and pantothenic acid lower stress and restore energy. L-tyrosine will decrease your depression and increase your energy. L-glutamine eliminates sugar cravings and has a calming effect (or use GABA, which has a more calming effect). Fish oil capsules will stop any fat cravings and help with PMS symptoms. 5-HTP and St. John's Wort, or L-tryptophan (by prescription), will raise your serotonin levels, eliminating obsessive thinking, negativity, irritability, and insomnia. (Check with your doctor, if you are taking antidepressants, and see page 253 on mixing these supplements with your medication.)

Eating soft or pureed food for a while and taking digestive enzymes and aloe juice should help enormously in getting rid of that awful "too full" feeling that makes you want to throw up even when you've "been good." If not, get a prescription for propulsid to use until your stomach begins emptying into your intestines normally, on its own. Delayed gastric (stomach) emptying is a double problem. Because it takes hours for you to get the benefit of the foods you eat, it can trigger severe low blood sugar cravings in addition to the perpetual bloated feeling that makes you want to throw up. Bulimics share this problem with many diabetics; you'll find great advice on exercises and medicines that can help get your stomach moving in the right direction in *Dr. Bernstein's Diabetes Solution* by Richard Bernstein, M.D.

Relieving the Special Stresses of Bulimia

Bingeing, purging by vomiting or with laxatives or diuretics, and over-exercising are extremely stressful to your adrenal glands, which have to take care of all your ordinary stresses, too. The adrenals can malfunction badly after a while. That knocks your other hormones (like estrogen, progesterone, and testosterone) out of balance and contributes to the particularly vicious PMS that many female bulimics suffer. It also makes you feel too stressed and easily overwhelmed.

I strongly recommend that you have your adrenal hormone levels checked with saliva testing, an easy and accurate way of testing now available. (See list of labs, page 352.) Many bulimics continue to have elevated levels of the harsh adrenal hormone cortisol, even after they stop bingeing and purging. This makes them anxious and stressed even in recovery. (See chapters 3 and 11.)

Saliva testing for your reproductive hormone levels is also a must if you have severe PMS. Otherwise, you'll be thrown off every month, back into demoralizing bursts of bulimia. Once you know how your reproductive hormones—estrogen and progesterone—are out of balance, you can act more effectively to get them balanced. (See chapters 6 and 14.)

Zinc for Bulimics and Anorectics

If you are bulimic or anorectic, along with your basic supplements, start drinking a bottle a day of Ethical Nutrients' Zinc Tally (a third of the bottle with each meal). Do this until it begins to taste awful. Then taste it once a week to be sure that it still tastes awful, signifying that you have enough zinc to keep your appetite and brain function normal.* Keep taking extra zinc in your multivitamin/mineral. Retest yourself with your liquid zinc every month to be sure that it still tastes awful. If not, take extra zinc again until it does.

Recovery from the Special Stresses of Anorexia

Note: If you are recovering from anorexia, you must work with a medical specialist. Do not try to follow the Diet Cure suggestions alone.

Starvation is one of the techniques that researchers use to study stress

---

*This technique was described by Alex Schauss, Ph.D., an eating disorder specialist and pioneering nutritional researcher, in his monograph on zinc therapy (see Resources).

reactions in lab animals. Exposure to cold is another. You've probably been suffering from both if you are anorectic. Please see that you get your adrenal stress function tested (see page 353 for special saliva testing information and subsequent treatment recommendations). Taking the nutrients that will start to restore your overworked adrenal glands will renew your ability to handle stress. Vitamin B1 along with your B complex and vitamin C with electrolytes will help. Typically, if you are anorectic, your adrenals are hyperactive and you have high cortisol levels. You must bring down the levels of this harsh adrenal hormone that is breaking down your muscles, bones, and brain cells during the emergency of your starvation in a desperate effort to keep you nourished. Otherwise it can continue to do its destructive work even after you begin to recover. (See chapter 3 and 11 on adrenal repair.)

Supplements for Anorexia

In addition to zinc, you'll need to take a multivitamin/multimineral, extra B complex, and vitamin C (Emergen-C, which includes electrolytes to protect your heart, is a good choice). If you are constipated, drinking aloe vera juice and/or taking extra magnesium will help. GABA will ease any anxiety; L-tyrosine will bring back your energy and sparkle by restoring your thyroid function. L-tryptophan or 5-HTP (especially with St. John's Wort) will help stop your mood swings and mental obsessing, and help you to sleep. Fish oil will help your dry skin and hair and your hormone function. DL-phenylalanine (DLPA) will help you wean yourself from NutraSweet, if you're addicted to diet gum or soda, as well as caffeine, and will restore your natural pleasure in life along with raising your vitality level. If it is too stimulating, then use just D-phenylalanine (DPA, without the L form). Because anorexia (starvation) stimulates endorphin release, you need to build up your endorphin levels quickly with DLPA or DPA (it's the D form that raises endorphin levels; the L form is energizing), so that you won't need to starve to feel "high." A complete "free form" amino acid blend will help quickly restore all of the most essential aminos to their muscle, brain, and other vital functions. Take for at least three months, early morning, midmorning, and midafternoon.

Aloe vera juice is wonderful for anorectics who are constipated or who vomit or use laxatives. It heals and stimulates the digestive tract. And complete digestive enzymes will help you to break down and utilize your food efficiently. This is particularly important if you have been vomiting. Take one or two with each meal.

Supplements Used in Recovery from Bulimia or Anorexia

Chose the nutrients you'll need and try them, along with the basic nutrients covered in chapter 17, under the supervision of a good nutritionist.

	AM	B	MM	L	MA	D	BT*
❏ Liquid Zinc, 40 mg (Ethical Nutrients' Zinc Status, or Metagenics Zinc Tally)	1	—	1	—	1	—	—
(later, Country Life Zinc Target Mins, 50 mg)	—	1	—	—	—	—	—
❏ George's Aloe Juice, 8 oz.	—	1	—	—	—	1	—
❏ L-glutamine, 500 mg (to reduce early cravings)	—	—	—	—	—	—	—
❏ Vitamin B complex	1	—	1	—	1	—	—
❏ Vitamin B₁ (thiamin), 200 mg	—	1	—	—	—	1	—
❏ Emergen-C Lite packets (1,000 mg vitamin C with extra electrolytes)	1	—	1	—	1	—	1
❏ 5-HTP, 50 mg	—	—	—	—	1–3	—	1–3
❏ St. John's Wort, 300 mg (if not on SSRIs)	—	1	—	1	—	1	—
❏ DLPA, 500 mg (or DPA 200–500 mg) (to restore pleasure and energy, help stay away from aspartame and caffeine)	1–2	—	1–2	—	—	—	—
❏ GABA† 100–500 mg (for relaxation at bedtime and as needed during the day)	—	—	—	—	—	—	1
❏ Tyrosine, 500 mg (for low energy and caffeine cravings)	1–2	—	1–2	—	—	—	—
❏ Complete Digestive Enzymes with HCl	1–2	—	—	1–2	1–2	—	—

*AM=on arising; B=with breakfast; MM=midmorning; L=with lunch; MA=midafternoon; D=with dinner; BT=at bedtime.

Note: If you continue to experience constipation, add magnesium 200 mg. If your bowels become too loose, stop magnesium. If loose bowels continue, stop vitamin C and aloe juice.

†GABA Calm by Source Naturals or Amino Relaxers by Country Life are good 100–mg. GABA formulae, but stronger (500 mg) versions are also available. Watch for low blood pressure, especially with any alcohol use. Available through the Vitamin Shoppe or our clinic order line if you can't find it in stores.

HEALTH PROFESSIONAL SUPPORT

When working with a health professional, keep in mind the following tips:

1. Do not allow yourself to be weighed (unless you are underweight) or insulted about your weight by any health professionals.
2. If you'd like more support, find a wholistic health professional who can advise you about supplements and help you to find healthy foods that work for you without restricting calories.
3. Do not allow health professionals to prescribe fasts, low-calorie diets, or extended, low-fat diets unless you are very ill and the natural techniques in this book do not help.
4. Join support groups that are antidieting, or take a course in women's issues to help you get in touch with yourself and an appreciation for your other qualities beyond your weight. (Check your local adult education or community college courses.)
5. Before committing to a counselor, check his or her stance on weight, body image, and diet issues. For some women, a women's issues specialist might be your best bet.
6. *For men:* A men's support group might be helpful, but interview the group leader about his knowledge and attitudes first. If you have an eating disorder, you may be able to find a men's group, but they are not as plentiful as they should be, even here in the San Francisco Bay Area.
7. Remember, all health professionals have their own biases. None of us has all the answers! See chapter 21 for guidance in finding any wholistic help that you might need.

ACTION STEPS

1. **Deprogram yourself about dieting.** Stop weighing yourself and counting fat grams and calories. Stop kidding yourself that low-calorie dieting will help you lose weight—it will make you gain.
2. **Reject unhealthy messages about body image and fat.** Use some of the suggestions in this chapter to remind yourself that there are many ideal body weights.
3. **Be sure to eat:**
   + 3 meals *minimum* per day.
   + 4 cups *or more* per day of colored low-carb veggies, mostly green. Eat as many of your vegetables raw as you can.

✦ 20 grams protein *or more* per meal.

✦ at least one quarter of your day's total calories at breakfast (600 calories or more).

✦ 2 servings of fruit or more per day.

✦ other whole-food carbos—beans, rice, corn—as needed after you've eaten your vegetables, protein, and fat.

✦ good oils, like olive and canola, in your salad dressings and sautéed dishes.

4. **Keep a food-mood log of what you eat (or don't eat) and how you feel (strong, energetic, free of cravings, or the opposite). See chapter 22 for information on how to set it up.**

5. **Use the basic supplements detailed in chapter 17 to eliminate food cravings and dieters' malnutrition.**

6. **Consult with a health professional and an individual counselor as needed (especially if you have an eating disorder).**

Reading

BOOKS

Check out these books on the dieting industry, dieting and your health, body image, and self-acceptance.

Berg, Frances M. "Health Risks of Weight Loss." (Hettinger, N.D.: *Healthy Weight Journal*, 1995).

Burke, Delta, with Alexis Lipsitz. *Delta Style: Eve Wasn't a Size 6 and Neither Am I.* (New York: St. Martin's Press, 1998).

Fraser, Laura. *Losing It, America's Obsession with Weight and the Industry That Feeds on It.* (New York: E. P. Dutton, 1997).

Gaesser, Glenn A. *Big Fat Lies: The Truth About Your Weight and Your Health* (New York: Ballantine Books, 1998).

Wolf, Naomi. *The Beauty Myth.* (New York: Anchor Books, 1992). (I especially recommend the chapter called "Hunger.")

MAGAZINES

Mode, which features larger-size models, is available at most newsstands.

Radiance: The Magazine for Large Women
P.O. Box 30246
Oakland, CA 94604
phone/fax: (510) 482-0680

VIDEOS

Body Trust: Undieting Your Way to Health and Happiness. 60 minutes, $24.95
Production West
2110 Overland Ave.
Suite 120,

Billings, MT 59102
(406) 656-9417
Other (more expensive) videos are available through Gurze and EDAP.

Resources

ONLINE SUPPORT
<www.about-face.org>
about-face was created by the inspired and delightful Kathy Bruin, who led the
    successful 1995 national campaign against emaciated models in Calvin Klein
    ads. Check out their directories of organizations, magazines and books, and
    a number of links to other Web sites.
<http://members.aol.com/edapinc/home.html>
EDAP is a national nonprofit organization dedicated to increasing the awareness
    and prevention of eating disorders.
<www.fatso.com/fatgirl/largesse/html>
Largesse, the Network for Size Esteem, is an internationally recognized resource
    center and clearinghouse for size-diversity empowerment, founded in 1983.
    It offers a computer database of up-to-date resources, an extensive library of
    archival and research materials, and connections to all areas of the growing
    nondiet and size-rights community worldwide.
<www.gurze.com>
Gurze publishes and sells books and other educational materials on body image
    and eating disorders. It provides a free catalog of books and videos and a di-
    rectory of treatment centers.
<www.something-fishy.org>
Loaded with information and support, this site is maintained by a very creative re-
    covering anorectic, but is not limited to anorexia and bulimia.
<www the-body-shop.com>
This international body-products company's Web site expresses its social, envi-
    ronmental, and animal protection values, offering a message of self-esteem
    honoring all sizes, shapes, and colors of selves.

OTHER RESOURCES
Gurze Books & Catalogs
Box 2238
Carlsbad, CA 92018
(800) 756-7533
Gurze publishes and sells books and other educational materials on body image
    and eating disorders and provides a free catalog of books and videos. Their
    Web site (listed above) has a directory of treatment centers. Gurze also pub-
    lishes a bimonthly newsletter, *Eating Disorders Review*, featuring summaries
    of relevant research for the professional treating of eating disorders.
<www.gurze.com>
EDAP (Eating Disorders Awareness and Prevention)

(800) 931-2237

Between the hours of 8:00 A.M. and 5:00 P.M. Pacific Standard Time, EDAP's staff will answer your questions regarding body image or eating disorders. They have a national database of eating-disorder counselors that they can refer you to by using your zip code. EDAP also has lists of curricula, videos, organizations, and an educational materials order form.

Resources Especially for Girls and Parents

MAGAZINES

New Moon Magazine
P.O. Box 3620
Duluth, MN 55803-3620
(218) 728-5507
<www.newmoon.org>
The magazine for girls and their dreams.

BOOKS

Cooke, Kaz. *Real Gorgeous: The Truth About Body and Beauty.* (New York: W. W. Norton, 1996.)

Jacobs, Joan. *The Body Project: An Intimate History of American Girls.* (New York: Random House, 1997.)

Mackoff, Barbara. *Growing a Girl: Seven Strategies for Raising a Strong, Spirited Daughter.* (New York: Bantam Doubleday Dell, 1996.)

Odean, Kathleen. *Great Books for Girls: More Than 600 Books to Inspire Today's Girls and Tomorrow's Women.* (New York: Ballantine, 1997.) Odean, a librarian, created this invaluable resource for parents. *Great Books for Girls* is a guide to hundreds of books with positive female characters

Waterhouse, Debra. *Like Mother, Like Daughter.* (New York: Hyperion, 1997.)

ELEVEN

Balancing Your Blood Sugar

I hope that you now really understand how dangerous to your health, mood, and weight excess sweets and starches can be. You may already have known this and been fighting a losing battle with carbos for years. Fear not, you are about to receive the secret weapons that will win the war for you, as they have for so many hundreds of my clients.

Some of you have chronic low blood sugar, also known as hypoglycemia, which may cause you to get dizzy when you stand up; to be irritable, headachy, and/or unable to concentrate when a meal is late or skipped; and to experience frequent and powerful cravings for sweets. Rather than rely on candy bars or coffee to perk you up in a pinch, you can learn to even out your blood sugar levels so that you don't fall prey to these blood sugar dips. Others of you may be diabetic or borderline diabetic and experiencing the classic symptoms of high blood sugar: excessive thirst and urination, fatigue, sugar cravings, and poor circulation, which causes any cuts or wounds to heal very slowly. You, too, can address these symptoms through key changes in your eating habits and through nutritional supplementation.

In this chapter, you'll learn how to get rid of your destructive sweet tooth and how to use certain minerals and amino acid supplements to keep your blood sugar stable. The supplements will make it much easier for you to stick to the healthy eating plan we recommend at Recovery Systems, which focuses on raising protein, lowering carbohydrates, and adding plenty of green vegetables.

Special Note to Diabetics

Before you even think about using any of the techniques laid out in this chapter, be aware that they will lower your blood sugars, so you must be ready to use your glucometer throughout the day to be sure you don't drop dangerously low. Also, consult with your doctor as soon as possible, so you will be ready with a medication-adjustment plan to keep you from getting into trouble as your diet and blood sugar improve.

One of our diabetic clients, addicted to both sugar and alcohol, really had not believed that she'd be able to quit both so easily. When suddenly she really did lose her interest in both, she found that she had not prepared for the consequences. The next thing she knew, she was being hauled out of her office on a stretcher by paramedics. She had gone into hypoglycemic shock. Now she measures her blood sugar frequently and has worked out an insulin-decrease plan with her M.D.

In addition, I highly recommend *Dr. Bernstein's Diabetes Solution,* because of his approach of high protein and low carbs; we've seen diabetics do exceptionally well on similar plans. In fact, at Recovery Systems we have seen many diabetics who have followed this type of plan and found that not only did their blood sugars level out, but that their cholesterol fell as well.

TESTING YOUR BLOOD SUGAR LEVELS

If you're experiencing the symptoms of low blood sugar, you really can rely on symptoms as your gauge. The standard three- to six-hour glucose-tolerance test is guaranteed to make you feel worse than you do already—dizzy, headachy, nervous—because you can have sugar water only during the test period. At the clinic, we have never regretted omitting this test, because it is also notoriously inaccurate at detecting hypoglycemia.

If you suspect you are diabetic, I refer you to your M.D. or D.O. for advice on testing your levels of insulin and blood sugar.

USING NUTRITIONAL SUPPLEMENTS TO HELP YOU KILL YOUR SWEET TOOTH

The following information will open the door that you've been banging on for years. It will allow you to freely choose what you are going to feed yourself and to really enjoy foods that are not overly sweet and starchy. You're going to be able to eliminate those foods containing sugar and white flour, which actually have *less than no* nutritional value, stripping you of whatever nutrients you take in from other, more nutritious foods. The B vitamins, vitamin C, and the mineral chromium are among the vital lost nutrients that you must replace immediately.

The Importance of Chromium

The United States is distinguished by being perhaps the most chromium-deficient country in the world. At least 90 percent of us don't have enough in our systems.[1] Chromium is crucial for keeping blood sugar stable, and it directly prevents carbohydrate cravings. Ironically, too much sugar, white flour, and alcohol block us from absorbing the chromium that would stop the yo-yo blood sugars and the carb cravings. One of the clients who tried chromium supplements had been eating 8 to 10 cups of vegetables a day, plenty of good fat in salad oils, and 4 to 8 ounces of protein at each meal. She avoided all grains and other high-carb foods. In most ways she felt and looked wonderful, but she still got low blood sugar spells that included daily headaches. The problem was that prior to getting on this food plan, she'd been a longtime junk-food binger, which had seriously depleted her of this key mineral. By taking 200 milligrams of chromium three times a day, she was able to bring her chromium level back up and was completely headache-free from the first day on.

If any of us becomes too deficient in a nutrient, food alone may not give us enough of that nutrient to restore adequate levels. But supplements can replenish our supplies and quickly make a dramatic difference in how we feel. Several of our other clients who elected to try chromium found that it helped stop their sugar cravings and all of their other low blood sugar symptoms as well. In fact, many studies have confirmed chromium's effectiveness in normalizing blood sugar levels in both hypoglycemics and Type II diabetics.[2] Chromium also helps build muscle, promotes the burning of unneeded body fat, and helps normalize our cholesterol levels.[3] All forms of chromium (picolinate, GTF, and others) seem to us to be equally effective. Chromium recommendations are included in the basic supplement plan in chapter 17.

Biotin and Your Blood Sugar

Several years ago we began recommending that our hypogycemic and diabetic clients use Glucobalance, by Biotics, a multiple vitamin with minerals designed specifically to stabilize blood sugar. It has turned out to be the

---

Diabetics and Biotin

The study of diabetics taking biotin used 9 to 16 milligrams per day, three to six times what we usually use.[4] High-dose biotin treatment for Type I and II diabetics drops blood sugars very fast, so if you take it be sure to work closely with your M.D.

---

single most useful multiple vitamin-mineral formula that we have ever found. Three mealtime doses (of two caps per meal) provide 1,000 micrograms of the mineral chromium and 3,000 micrograms of the B vitamin biotin. Research has shown that biotin helps stabilize blood sugar and eliminate carbohydrate cravings in people with both low and high blood sugar. One of our advisers, William Timmons, N.D., has found it more effective than chromium for some people with low blood sugar.

Thiamin (vitamin B1), like chromium, is easily depleted by high sugar (and caffeine) intake. It is another stellar nutrient crucial for cellular energy, blood sugar regulation, and protection from stress.

L-Glutamine: The Amino Answer

Our other key sugar fighter is an amino acid called L-glutamine, which can stop cravings for sweets, starches, and alcohol instantly. It works by preventing the brain from dropping into the low blood sugar, code-red, must-eat-candy-or-have-a-beer state. How? When the brain is low on glucose (blood sugar), it can burn glutamine instead. L-glutamine was first synthesized by a biochemist who quickly discovered how remarkable it was in eliminating alcoholics' cravings for alcohol (the most potent carb). It can have the same miraculous effect on cravings for sweets and starches as well. It works fastest when used sublingually.

The Other Nutrient Helpers

The following nutrients, vigorous sugar fighters as well, are included in your basic supplement plan, which will be laid out for you in chapter 17. Extra B complex has to be added to regulate blood sugar. Certain B vitamins, the mineral zinc, vitamin E, and omega-3 fatty acids help eliminate low blood sugar instability and cravings for carbohydrate, sweets, and alcohol. Zinc supplementation helps restore the appetite for real food and is

Supplement	AM	B	MM	L	MA	D	BT*
❑ Biotin 1000 mcg	—	1	—	1	—	1	—
❑ L-glutamine 500 mg	1–3	—	1–3	—	1–3	—	1–3
❑ Vitamin B₁, 100 mg	—	1	—	—	—	1	—

*AM=on arising; B=with breakfast; MM=midmorning; L=with lunch; MA=midafternoon; D=with dinner; BT=at bedtime.
†Take for one to three months.

Help in Detoxing from a High-Carb Diet

For the first three or four days off sweets and white flour products, you may feel tired and headachy. These detox symptoms are caused by your system's becoming too acidic. There are a few tricks to making it easier. Minerals in vegetables and fruits can neutralize that acidity and your supplemental minerals will help speed up the antiacid detox project, too. You can also use Alka-Seltzer Gold. Try warm baths with four cups of Epsom Salts each, too. (More on detox in chapter 22.)

involved in the entire blood sugar regulation process. Zinc is stripped by sugar use and is particularly low in diabetics. Like chromium, it is vital to blood sugar stabilization. Niacin (take it in the form of niacinamide to avoid sudden flushing and/or liver damage) and thiamin are two of the B vitamins that are essential for maintaining an even blood sugar state as well as lower cholesterol while vitamin B₅ (pantothenic acid) is famous for reviving adrenals exhausted by too much sugar. Vitamin E is important because it improves insulin's effectiveness. The mineral magnesium is notably deficient in diabetics (and is low in the general population, too). Healthy omega-3 fat (naturally found in dark green leafy vegetables and fish such as salmon) raises your metabolic rate, regulates fat burning, and supports your insulin function to keep your blood sugar stable. In a study of obese diabetics and prediabetics, just adding omega-3 fish oil as a supplement brought both weight and insulin levels down. (The group fed a low-fat, high-carbohydrate diet got worse!)[5]

THE FOOD SOLUTIONS

When special nutrients have freed you from your cravings for sweets and starches, you can start eating foods that will keep you craving-free permanently. By that I mean you'll eat delicious low-carbohydrate foods along with as many wholesome carbos as you need and can tolerate. For example, if you rush around in the morning and don't have time for breakfast, you can make high-protein breakfast smoothies or prepare cottage cheese and fruit. But you could also have eggs and healthy sausage (such as the kind made with turkey) with potatoes, or a feta cheese scramble with avocado, salsa, and beans. Lots of it! You won't even miss the donuts, I promise.

Diabetics Note: You may need to reduce or eliminate fruit and other whole food carbos along with the junk carbos because, for you, they may be equally destabilizing. At least for a while, concentrate pretty exclusively on lots of protein, low-carb veggies, and good fats.

I don't recommend that you try to eat according to the guidelines of the famous Food Pyramid. The nutritionists whom I hired in the early 1980s advocated that way of eating, emphasizing complex carbohydrates such as whole grain breads and brown rice. It worked better than sugar-based diets did. The pyramid diet consists of more than 60 percent carbohydrates. But within seconds after bread, pasta, potatoes, and other starchy carbs enter your body, these high-carbohydrate foods act just like sugar—your blood sugar spikes, then dives. If these foods make up the bulk of your meals, you will most likely continue to crave sweets and experience all the other consequences of blood sugar imbalance.

What has really made the difference for our clients is avoiding too many high-carb foods of any kinds. So what do they eat? Loads of salads and other low-carb vegetables, like asparagus, green beans, broccoli, red cabbage, and chard, topped by lemon and butter or oil and vinegar. (For a list of low carb vegetables, see chapter 20, page 305.) They do not restrict fats except deep-fried food and junk fats like margarine. And they eat generous portions of protein, like turkey and chicken, lamb chops, cracked crab, and salmon steaks and smaller portions of beans, fruit, and whole grains. They love these foods but don't overeat them, or anything else. They quickly lose interest in their old high-carbo standbys.

Over the years we learned that some people, after an initial detox period, need to add more carbohydrates, particularly if they are very active physically or are blood type A (A's tend to do better on vegetarian diets). We help monitor our clients as they introduce whole-food carbs like brown and wild rice, winter squash, and potatoes. If these starchy foods trigger a return of sweet cravings, we recommend that they limit them or cut them out altogether.

What Is Enough Protein in One Meal?

✦ 3 eggs (24 grams of protein)
✦ 1/2 to 1 can of tuna (about 22 to 45 grams of protein)
✦ at least 1/3 of a 16-ounce carton (2/3 cup or 5 ounces) of cottage cheese (20 grams of protein)
✦ 1 cup of beans (10 to 19 grams of protein) plus 2 to 4 tablespoons of seeds (5 to 10 grams of protein)
✦ 3 to 4 ounces of lean meat, fish, poultry, approximately the size of your palm; or a slightly larger 5-ounce piece of firm tofu (20 grams of protein)

Protein Helps Keep Blood Sugar Stable

I would like you, too, to experiment until you find the balance of foods that makes you feel the best. Gradually you will learn how to eat to protect your hard-won blood sugar balance. You will find that the food that keeps your blood sugar most stable always turns out to be protein.

Foods high in protein trigger the release of glucagon, a hormone that helps provide balance when excess carbos trigger excesses of insulin. Glucagon stimulates fat burning instead of fat storage, shuts down cholesterol overproduction, and discourages water retention, among other things. Protein alone, or together with fat (most high-protein foods, like meat, eggs, and fish, contain fat as well as protein), stimulates glucagon activity. (Fat alone has no effect either way.) Carbohydrate triggers the release of insulin, which results in their conversion to fat and low-blood sugar cravings. But don't get glucagon-fixated. What you want is *level* blood sugar. When your insulin and glucagon are both normalized, blood sugar stays level.

Fat Is Innocent

Fat by itself does not raise insulin. Only carbohydrates do. Fat really is innocent when it comes to most weight gain. Fats can be converted into blood sugar if necessary, but slowly, not in bursts that overstimulate insulin release. And fat actually keeps the carbos in your meals from hitting you too hard. It also makes you feel satisfied so that you know when to stop eating.

Convinced that a high-fat, low-carb diet will make you fat? Dr. Bernstein, the author of three books on the treatment of diabetes (and a fifty-year diabetic himself), describes a study published in the *Journal of the American Medical Association* in which two healthy men spent one year in a hospital eating 2,500 calories a day. Seventy-five percent of their calories came from fat, 25 percent from protein, none came from carbohydrates. By the end of the year, both men had lost six pounds and lowered their cholesterol. (One was a famous arctic explorer, who had volunteered for the experiment after seeing Eskimos fare well on no-carb, high-fat fare.)

Eat some fat at every meal. It helps stop carbohydrate cravings. The body yearns for fat and won't stop eating until the fat arrives. You don't have to eat gobs of it—on the Diet Cure plan you will probably consume approximately 30 to 35 percent of your calories as fat—but a dressing of oil and vinegar with lime juice for a salad, guacamole with your sautéed shrimp and rice, and butter or olive oil and lemon on your veggies will ensure that you enjoy your food and are satisfied by it.

So please relax and don't worry about good, sugar-free salad dressings, butter, and salad oils. If you crave fats and overeat them, turn to chapter 8.

Watch your own reactions as you make changes in your protein, fat, and carbohydrate ratio. You'll know when it's right. Unless you are diabetic, this kind of eating should work well for you right away. (Diabetics may need fewer carbos.)

Vegetables Are Vital

Along with protein and fat, vegetables are of primary importance. They should become your primary source of carbohydrates. Even low-carb, green veggies contain some slow-acting carbohydrates that won't spike insulin but will fill you up—*if you eat enough of them.* You'll need to make peace with vegetable preparation: washing, chopping, dressing, and cooking. Make vegetables your friends! Aim at 4 cups a day of colored veggies.

Veggies not only contain vitamins and fiber, they also contain crucial minerals and, particularly in the raw state, many digestive enzymes. If you've had low blood sugar for years, you are low—or even out of—all four kinds of nutrients.

Eating Ideas

✦ **Breakfast.** If you don't break the fast that has been going since you ate last night, your blood sugar will just keep dropping until you are so des-

---

What Is 4 Cups of Vegetables a Day?

✦ Enough to fill a one-quart milk carton

Remember, you have to eat twice as much salad greens per vegetable serving because they are so bulky. Imagine a half-gallon milk carton filled with lettuce, tomatoes, cucumbers, green onions, and red bell peppers. (See chapter 20 for information on how to visualize your vegetables for a meal.)

---

perate that you will grab the first Danish that floats by. Break your night-long fast with protein—eggs, healthy sausage, a tofu scramble, a high-protein shake. Eat plenty of food—at least 25 percent of your day's intake—within an hour after you wake up if you possibly can (it gets easier quickly).

✦ **Lunch.** If you can tolerate wheat, a sandwich loaded with protein (tuna, turkey, meat, egg salad, for example) can be okay. Otherwise, try a large salad with chicken, beans, veggies, avocado, and dressing. Or a burrito without the white flour tortilla wrap (ask for corn tortillas on the side), with meat or chicken, beans, lettuce, salsa, and guacamole. Or a big bowl of chili and a mixed vegetable salad with sliced hard boiled eggs.

✦ **Dinner.** Try fish, chicken, or tempeh with veggies and a baked potato with butter. Or have a shrimp and veggies stir-fry with rice, or cooked fish sushi and miso vegetable soup.

✦ **Snacks.** If your blood sugar has a great tendency to dip, you will need to shore yourself up with midmorning and midafternoon and maybe bedtime snacks that are strong on protein: peanut butter and celery, an apple with cheese or almonds, salmon or turkey jerky, a between-meal protein smoothie (no juice, just whole fresh fruit, protein powder, a few nuts, and water).

✦ **Legumes.** Try putting more legumes (beans, peas, lentils, and others) into your diet. If you can digest them easily (that is, without gas), I think you will like them as a carbohydrate source.* They are actually the highest-fiber food (which keeps your digestive track healthy), and fairly high in protein and other nutrients. Have them in salads, chili, bean and pea soups, tacos, burrito fillings, beans with rice, among others.

*See chapter 18, page 274 for hints on reducing the gas-causing properties in beans, and page 275 for a list of legumes you can try.

Diabetic Note: Beans may not work for severe diabetics because of their relatively high-carbohydrate content.

✦ **Fruit.** Because it is the only food that we tend to eat uncooked, fruit is loaded with fiber, vitamins, minerals, and vital enzymes. Remember, cooking destroys a good portion of the nutrients in your food (another reason to use supplements). But fruit is also loaded with fruit sugar (fructose). You may find that fruit is too sweet for you, causing you to have a blood sugar dive up to two hours afterward. Fructose does not tend to cause the immediate spike and dive of other sugars, but if you find yourself feeling tired and craving sweets after eating an apple as a snack, then next time be sure to eat it with nuts or cheese. Or avoid fruit for a while, until it does work for you. (For more meal and snack ideas, see chapters 19 and 20.)

✦ **Don't skip meals.** Ever. If you do, I guarantee your blood sugar will crash and spike. Then you'll eat cake.

✦ **Don't forget to take all of your supplements.** If you suddenly want a frozen yogurt, you can bet you have either forgotten a key supplement like glutamine, or a meal!

✦ **Liquids.** Sweet juices and sodas (including diet sodas of any kind) are sugar monsters. Drink filtered or spring water with a squeeze of fresh lemon, lime, or grapefruit. Try guava tea: in China, it is used to control and maintain proper blood sugar levels. Have carbonated water for occasional treats, but their phosphorus content makes them a calcium blocker.

I have already explained in chapter 3 that blood sugar problems are closely entwined with worn-out adrenal glands. We have just laid out the first steps in how to level blood sugar. In the final section of this chapter we will lay out what to do to repair exhausted adrenals.

TESTING AND RESTORING EXHAUSTED ADRENALS

If you suspect that your adrenals are exhausted, as indicated by the symptoms listed in chapter 3, I encourage you to get tested right away. If you suspect you have a thyroid problem, you should certainly test your adrenals immediately, as well as your thyroid, since the two are so closely linked. It's time to find out exactly how worn down you and your adrenals are. It will take a few weeks to get your results back. In the meantime, you'll be getting some relief from your new foods and supplements. The test results will let you know if you need extra help for your adrenals. I strongly recommend that you use the following suggestions for testing and treatment in collaboration with a health professional.

Blood Pressure Can Indicate Adrenal Exhaustion

Normally, systolic blood pressure (the first number in the measurement of blood pressure; for example, 120 in 120/80) is about 10 points higher when you are standing up than when you are lying down. If the adrenal glands are not functioning well, however, this may not be true.

Have your health professional take and compare two blood pressure readings—one while lying down and one while standing up. First, lie down quietly for five minutes and have your blood pressure taken. Then stand up and immediately have your blood pressure taken again. If your blood pressure reading is lower after you stand up, suspect reduced adrenal gland function. The degree to which the blood pressure drops upon standing is often proportionate to the degree of adrenal depletion.[6]

Saliva Testing

Arrange to get tested to measure your levels of cortisol and DHEA—the adrenal glands' primary stress-coping hormones. You can do this yourself or have a health professional do it for you.

Saliva testing is accurate and easy. We have been thrilled with the information it has given us, allowing us to help people at a whole new level. You'll collect saliva in little tubes four times: once in the early morning, once midmorning, once midafternoon, and once late at night. A lab will test your samples. If your test results show hormone levels that are overly high or overly low, you will know which kinds of repair strategies to implement. (This is important, because choosing the wrong strategy could make you worse.)*

We use a consulting service that provides the test kits and actively educates health professionals on how to understand test results and treat particular adrenal imbalances. Many health professionals, even wholistic ones, are not yet acquainted with this invaluable tool and effective remedies for restoring the adrenals to their optimal function. See chapter 21, page 352 for a list of saliva test providers and consultants.

---

*There are a number of labs in the United States and abroad that do saliva testing and have done it for twenty years. As for being an accurate measure of body chemistry, the World Health Organization has published a paper indicating that saliva testing is now the gold standard for hormone testing.

Test Results: Finding Yourself on the Stress Map

When your adrenal-stress saliva-test results come back, they will tell you some fascinating things about how stress is affecting you now, and about how long it has been beyond what you and your adrenals could handle.

Stage I of Adrenal Exhaustion. Here levels of your stress-coping king, cortisol, are abnormally high part or all of the day and night. You may still have energy, perhaps too much of it, because your emergency stress response is overamped. You may not be sleeping well or restfully if your cortisol levels are high at night (when they should be shutting down) or in the morning (when they should be just rising for the day, not left on all night). You may be very hungry and eating a lot, but losing weight. High cortisol lowers your mood-elevating serotonin, your sleep-inducing melatonin, and cannibalizes your own muscle and bone for emergency fuel. You may be getting sick a lot as your defense team drops its heavy immune-protective responsibilities, because it literally "can't cope" anymore. Your mood may be impatient and negative, with pronounced PMS. This stage is appropriately called hyper-adrenalism. While cortisol will be too high in this stage, DHEA, cortisol's backup, will have become worn down to subnormal levels.

Stage II of Adrenal Exhaustion. Your stress-fighting cortisol supplies have finally run low. But they haven't run out yet. For a year or so, at most, both cortisol and DHEA will hover in the low-normal range, leaving you tired and stressed, but functional.

Stage III of Adrenal Exhaustion. Now both your cortisol and DHEA levels are low most, or all, of the day. Your energy is low. You can tolerate very little stress. This situation is far more common than you might suspect.

One of our clients, Monique, was a highly skilled nurse who worked in a hospital that required all of its nurses to work twelve-hour shifts. She became alcoholic under the stress (she came from an alcoholic family that could not handle stress well). When she came to us, she was irritable, weepy, hopeless, and exhausted. She had a lovely family and she'd been going to A.A. for a year and loving it, but could not keep from drinking on her way home from her long work shifts. She felt better on the supplements right away and quit drinking for a month with no problem—until she went back to work. She took another medical leave while we waited for the results of her cortisol and DHEA levels to come back. When they did, all her scores were *very* low.

Now it has been three months and she is doing fine, even after she gets off from work. She takes her breaks regularly and has protein-carb snacks. She gets to sleep by ten o'clock most nights, exercises moderately, goes to her supportive A.A. meetings, meditates, and has fun with her little daughter. Without the testing and the special targeted supplements you're about to be introduced to, she would never have been able to stay sober.

Note: Since more than 90 percent of alcoholics are hypoglycemic, adrenal stress evaluation and treatment are crucial if you're an alcoholic.

RECOVERING FROM STRESS: RESTORING YOUR ADRENAL FUNCTION WITH SUPPLEMENTS

The cascade of hormones from your adrenals, ovaries, thyroid, and other glands rules your body's functional capacity. These hormones all "speak" to each other and all are affected by changes in any single hormone level.

The hormones the adrenals generate are powerful, as are some of the supplements used to balance them. For successful treatment, it is imperative to have a competent health care professional monitor treatment and progress.

The Supplements That Help at Any Stage of Adrenal Exhaustion

Among your basic supplements (see chapter 17) and your blood sugar stabilizing supplements are several supplements that will help restore your adrenal function. Vitamin C and the B vitamins are top helpers. In fact, 90 percent of the vitamin C you take in is used by your adrenals, and the vitamin B complex is at least as important.

Your basic multivitamin/mineral, taken with meals, and your basic vitamins B and C, taken between meals, will supply your body with adrenal support all day. C and B complex vitamins are water soluble and do not store in the body, unlike proteins, fats, minerals, and fat-soluble vitamins. The kidneys quickly excrete any excess. Because of the rapid turnover of these vitamins, a lower dose and more frequent intake assure a steady supply of stress-reducing, adrenal-supporting nutrients.

A Note on B Complex: The highly recommended coenzymatic B complex by Source Naturals that dissolves under your tongue contains the sweetener sorbitol and peppermint or orange oil flavoring to cover the unpleasant B vitamin taste. If you are diabetic or sensitive to any of these substances, use Country Life Coenzyme B-Complex capsules instead.

It is usually important to take extra amounts of vitamin B_5 (pantothenic acid) in the early repair process over the next few weeks or months. "Panto" allows the adrenals to make more of their antistress (and antiinflammatory) cortisone. It also burns away excessive cholesterol and triglycerides in your blood. Take 100 to 500 milligrams with meals, depending on the extent of your stress. Take one bottle and stop to see if you still need more than you get in your B complex and multi. If you notice an increase in the feeling of stress, continue to take it for another bottle's worth but probably not more.

Another key stress buster is GABA, an amino acid that works as your brain's natural Valium. It can be very relaxing, even at only 100 milligrams, because it helps deactivate the stress hormones. Try the 500-milligram size if you need more, especially at bedtime. A mildly relaxing homeopathic formula called Calmes Forte can be another soothing standby, day or night. It is a big seller at health food stores.

If the above supplements help but do not completely restore your strength and stamina and allow you to face stressful situations without feeling strained, drained, or overwhelmed, then it's time to move on to the ultimate supplement protocol. Our deeply stressed and exhausted clients take the basic supplements, the special blood sugar stabilizers and stress busters, plus the ultimate repair supplements, and are *very* glad they do.

The Ultimate Antistress Supplements

These supplements are potent. Please consult an expert while using them.

If your adrenals are in Stage I and your cortisol levels are too high:

One nutrient formula that is capable of quickly bringing cortisol levels down to normal is a supplement called Seriphos (phosphorylated serine).* This special compound works by reducing the ACTH (pituitary)

---

*Phosphatydal serine is a similar supplement available at health food stores, but is not nearly as effective as Seriphos.

messages that order the adrenals to release emergency amounts of cortisol and DHEA. We have seen it help with on problems like intractable insomnia that does not respond to melatonin or 5-HTP.

Unfortunately, Seriphos has many contraindications, including for pregnant and lactating women, in impaired kidney function, and with chocolate, caffeine, and other adrenergic agonist and alkaloid stimulant use. Another nutrient that can regulate cortisol levels is vitamin B_1, one of the most universally beneficial of all nutrients. B_1 has the remarkable ability to prevent cortisol excess or lower it in Stage I, as well as raise levels that are too low in Stages II and III. Be sure to take the B complex, which is one of your basic supplements, while you take this extra B_1.

For Stage I, II, or III of adrenal exhaustion, if DHEA is too low according to your saliva test:

DHEA. The hormone DHEA serves as a backup to cortisol in responding to stress and immune system needs and tests usually show that it needs to be supplemented in most stress-exhausted people. Your test results will clearly show whether or not you'll need supplements of DHEA. We have seen chronically fatigued clients respond strongly to DHEA within a week.

DHEA caution: Do not take DHEA if you have hormonally linked illness, such as breast or uterine cancer, endometriosis, or prostrate cancer. Monitor your testosterone and estrogen levels if you are taking DHEA because it can build up the levels of these hormones.

Since DHEA is a root hormone that can convert to testosterone and to estrogen, women should watch for acne or the growth of facial hair as signs that it's time to cut down or stop (but retesting should let you know before that happens). Both men and women should watch for headaches, stomach discomfort, light-headedness, and excess throat mucus.[7]

If your adrenals are in Stage II or III, your levels of cortisol are dropping abnormally low. Here are some remarkably helpful supplements to try.

Licorice. If you have *normal* to *low* blood pressure, not *high* blood pressure, you can raise your cortisol levels in a hurry by using the surprisingly potent herb licorice, in the form of licorice root capsules or liquid extract (*glycyrrhiza* is the name of the chemical in licorice that has this pro-adrenal effect). Excessive amounts of licorice can be toxic, but your dose won't go near the toxic level (more than 100 milligrams of glycyrrhiza per day). Reduce or stop your dose as you no longer need it; for example, if your appetite decreases, or if you feel too speeded up, or, especially, if you

> *Please do not take* whole *adrenal glandular supplements (which include the adrenal medulla from animal glands). The adrenaline (made in the medulla part of the gland) typically makes your problem worse by overstimulating you, adding to your stress level and exhausting your adrenals further.*

have heart palpitations or your blood pressure rises. (*Always* stop your supplements if you get adverse symptoms.)

Try whole licorice root extract, no more than one to two capsules per day or 5 to 10 drops under your tongue, one to two times a day taken only under professional supervision. If you take licorice after three P.M., your sleep may be affected. Do not get the licorice without glycyrrihiza, the only ingredient in the licorice that builds up cortisol.

Caution: If you have high blood pressure, you'll need to try homeopathic adrenal cortex, or low-dose prescription cortisone *instead of* licorice.

Cortisone. Homeopathic remedies for glandular problems are called sarcodes. Oddly, their lowest doses are indicated by higher numbers. For example, Dolisos Labs makes a 6C-strength homeopathic adrenal cortex, which is mildly elevating and sustaining (for Stage II), and a 4C, which is strongly elevating (for Stage III). (See chapter 19 for information on shopping for your master plan.) There is also prescription cortisone. William Jeffries, M.D., in *Safe Uses of Cortisone*, recommends low doses of 2.5 to 5 milligrams, two to four times per day. This dosage adds up to the same 10 to 20 milligrams a day of cortisone that your adrenal glands should normally produce themselves each day.[8] The amount of prescription cortisone that causes the "moon face" (swelling of the face) and other side effects is 100 milligrams or more per day—far in excess of any natural amounts ever produced by the adrenals themselves or recommended by Dr. Jeffries. We have had several clients use low doses of prescription cortisone for a few months with no adverse side effects at all, and considerable benefit. Cortisone can temporarily fill in for your own depleted hormone and rest your adrenals so that they can regenerate.

The Complete Adrenal Repair Protocol

Adrenal Support Supplements for All Stages of Adrenal Exhaustion

SUPPLEMENT	AM	B	MM	L	MA	D	BT
❑ Pantothenic acid 100–500 mg	—	1	—	1	—	—	—
❑ GABA 100–500 mg as needed for relaxation	—	—	—	—	1	—	1
❑ Calmes Forte as needed, for mild relaxation							

Ultimate Support Supplements
For Stages I, II, and III

❑ Vitamin B₁, 200 mg (three times per day in Stage I only, twice a day in Stages II and III)	—	(1)	—	1	—	1	—

For Stage I, II, or III of adrenal exhaustion, if DHEA levels are too low:

❑ Females: 5–10 mg   __1 dose __   __   __1 dose __
DHEA capsules or
sublingual drops

❑ Males: 10–15 mg DHEA.   __1 dose __   __   __1 dose __
Use capsules or
sublingual drops*

Take DHEA at the end of meals. Start with ¹/₂ the dosage for 1 week
to check your responses.

For Stage II or III of adrenal exhaustion, if cortisol levels are too low:

❑ Licorice root capsules or
liquid licorice root extract
(10 to 40 milligrams), 2 hours
before your test results show
you have a cortisol drop

❑ 5–20 mg pregnenolone per day
Take as recommended at the end of your meals.

❑ Homeopathic adrenal cortex 6c–4c

❑ Cortisone (by prescription)
Take as recommended 2 to 3 times per day.

---

*Rinse mouth and hold drops under tongue at least 30 seconds, allowing them to absorb in
your mouth. (Drops are twice as absorbable as capsules.) Don't drink or eat afterward for 30
minutes.

Pregnenolene. This root hormone of your adrenals (like DHEA) produces several hormones, notably cortisol and progesterone. Supplementing with it takes another burden off your adrenals. *Do not* use pregnenolene if you are taking progesterone in any form, particularly as a cream, without first testing your progesterone levels.

Pregnenolone caution: Do not use pregnenolone if you are hyperthyroid or if you have high levels of progesterone.

Retesting and Adjusting Your Supplements

While it can be very helpful to supplement as needed with DHEA and pregnenolone in capsules or as tinctures (tinctures contain either glycerin or alcohol), it should be done under a health practitioner's care and *only* after thorough testing. These are powerful hormonal supplements (and licorice is powerful, too). If your levels of cortisone, DHEA, estrogen, progesterone, or testosterone get too high because of supplementing with cortisone, licorice, DHEA, or pregnenolone, you could develop serious new problems. If you already, unknowingly, have too much estrogen, or progesterone, or testosterone, you could make a potentially hazardous hormonal imbalance worse.

My advice is to saliva test all of your sex hormone levels before using DHEA or pregnenolone. Then retest your morning cortisol and DHEA levels thirty days after treatment starts, and retest any excessively elevated or deficient sex hormones that have shown up on your first tests in 60 to 90 days and again in six months. (See chapters 6 and 14 for how to balance sex hormones.) Be sure to monitor your levels through *retesting.* Women, remember that too much DHEA can grow hair on your face! If you use DHEA, pregnenolone, licorice, or cortisone, it is particularly important to test the levels of your sex hormones, if you have been taking hormone replacement therapy of any kind, but especially if you've been using hormone creams, which we've found tend to store hormones excessively in the body. Increases or decreases beyond normal hormonal levels can pose problems for men as well as women.

Decrease your pantothentic acid, your licorice, adrenal cortex, or cortisone as you build yourself back up. Your retests will guide you there in as well as eliminating your DHEA and pregnenolone.

Addressing Stress Long-term

Anything that will rest and calm you can help restore your adrenals. Cutting out refined carbohydrates, which tax your adrenals, is crucial. So is eliminating any hidden stressors, like food allergies, yeasts, and parasites.

Now look at your lifestyle and de-stress it. Get counseling for emotional stress, if you need to. Don't overexercise. Learn to relax at least twice a day. Breathe quietly. Get massages. Learn yoga or other stretching-to-relax exercises. Get at least eight hours of sleep every night and, ideally, get to bed three hours after sunset. Have a light bedtime snack, if you tend to get hungry at bedtime or in the night. Take time off. Get away as much as possible. Do not overwork or push yourself, if at all possible. See the section on relaxation in chapter 21 for lots more de-stressing suggestions.

All of these helpful efforts aside, there will more than likely be many times when your stress levels will rise too high again. Life stress, perhaps even more than the stressful American diet, is a constant threat to maintaining our physical and emotional balance. But you can learn to keep ahead of it by using your stress-coping supplements for quick repair before the stress can do too much damage again. Keep your B complex, your panto, and your licorice around the house for the hard times. Don't forget!

ACTION STEPS

1. If you suspect diabetes, get your blood sugar and insulin levels tested and consult with a knowledgeable M.D. or D.O. You probably don't need to test your blood sugar if you suspect hypoglycemia.

2. Take your basic nutritional supplements as laid out in chapter 17, along with the extra supplements spelled out in this chapter.

3. Eat right to keep your blood sugar level even.
   + Don't skip meals.
   + Avoid sweets and white flour products forever.
   + Eat at least three solid meals per day.
   + Don't let more than four hours go by without food. Whole-food (low-carb) snacks may be needed in midmorning, midafternoon, and at bedtime.
   + Eat a substantial (at least 25 percent of the day's food intake), protein-rich breakfast.

✦ Stay away from refined sweets, starches, alcohol, caffeine, and NutraSweet. (It should be *easy* because of your supplements.)

4. If you have symptoms of adrenal exhaustion, consult a health care professional and test your adrenal function. Use saliva testing for cortisol and DHEA levels. If you are having hormonal problems or taking any hormones, you should also test for the hormones estrogen, progesterone, and testosterone.

5. Reduce, then eliminate your special blood sugar and adrenal repair supplements as you no longer need them.

6. Use them again during stressful times.

Readings

Bernstein, Richard K., M.D. *Dr. Bernstein's Diabetes Solution* (Boston: Little, Brown & Co., 1997).

Des Maisons, Kathleen, Ph.D. *Potatoes Not Prozac* (New York: Simon & Schuster, 1998).

Eades, Michael R., M.D., and Mary Dan Eades, M.D. *Protein Power: The Metabolic Breakthrough* (New York: Bantam, 1996).

Mitchell, Susan, Ph.D., and Catherine Christie. *I Could Kill for a Cookie* (New York: Penguin, 1998). This is a good guide to the causes and cures of stress eating.

Murray, Michael T., N.D. *Hypoglycemia and Diabetes* (Rocklin, CA: Prima Publishing, 1994).

Timmons, William, N.D. *Practitioner's Manual 1999* (San Diego: BioHealth Diagnostics). Available by calling (800) 570-2000. (Part of the education and training resources at Dr. Timmons's institute, where many of the adrenal repair protocols presented in this chapter were developed.)

Selye, Hans. *The Stress of Life* (New York: McGraw-Hill, 1978).

Resources

SUPPLEMENTS

To locate or order Source Natural's Coenzymate B complex, call (800) 777-5677 ext. 6497. For Country Life's Coenzymate B complex, call (800) 645-5768. Or send for both through NEEDS mail order, (800) 634-1380.

To order Seriphos, or liquid (alcohol tinctured) licorice, DHEA, or pregnenolone, you can call BioHealth Diagnostics, which developed the Complete Adrenal Repair Protocol, at (800) 570-2000. Licorice, DHEA, and pregnenolone capsules and nonalcohol licorice tinctures can also be found in most health stores. (Seriphos cannot.)

Call Dolisos for its homeopathic adrenal cortex of various strengths at (800) 365-4767.

All supplements included in this chapter are available through our clinic's order line (800-733-9293).

SALIVA TESTING

See Resources at the end of chapter 21, Essential Support.

TWELVE

Thyroid Solutions

By now, having read chapter 4, you have identified your low thyroid symptoms. You know that there are two basic types of thyroid dysfunction—hypothyroidism and thyroiditis—and that both types respond well to good food and to nutritional supplements. In this chapter you'll learn a lot about what nutritional supplements you can use to help correct your thyroid problem. You still need to know which of these two thyroid problems you have in order to be sure about which nutrients you should try and whether you'll need prescription medication. The difference between hypothyroid and thyroiditis symptoms is quite subtle: both can result in weight gain and low energy, but sometimes with thyroiditis you won't have weight gain or a low underarm temperature, even if you have cold hands and feet. To learn for certain whether you suffer from hypothyroid or from thyroiditis, you will need to find a physician who can test you properly as soon as possible. Also, you should test your adrenals at the same time, as they are often at the root of thyroid problems.

FINDING A PHYSICIAN

I recommend using the national physicians' directory that is available through the Broda O. Barnes, M.D. Research Foundation in Turnbull, Connecticut. Broda Barnes was an M.D. who spent his entire career studying and treating the thyroid. The foundation strongly promotes a thorough evaluation of both thyroid and adrenal function, and the use of Armour (animal) thyroid, though they do acknowledge that some people do better on synthetic thyroid. We have referred many people from all over the country to the Barnes Foundation list and have been more than satisfied with the results. Chapter 21 will give you several other good suggestions for finding wholistic physicians to work with.

You can call the Barnes Foundation (see Resources) and for a small fee, you can receive from them a list of the medical doctors, osteopaths, naturopaths, and others in your area who are associated with them. Keep in mind that whomever you see, you will have to use the information in this book aggressively to be sure you get all the care you need. Recovery Systems is the only clinic in the country that I know of that specializes in the wholistic treatment of eating, weight, mood, and addiction problems. You can't expect a health care provider seeing a wide range of problems to have the specialized information that you will get from reading this book. It will be important to find one who keeps an open mind on the animal versus synthetic medication question.

Any good physician will have valuable experience and ideas to add to *The Diet Cure*. My advice is to ask your doctors to follow the suggestions here before, or at the same time as, exploring other avenues. (See chapter 21 for a discussion of different types of physicians who can work with you.)

THE ADRENAL LINK

Many of my clients seem to have exhausted adrenals as well as malfunctioning thyroids. If you tend to be tired in the afternoon, or jittery, even though you are taking thyroid medication, or if you tend to be overly alert at night, have dark circles under your eyes, are easily stressed, among other symptoms, your adrenals may need help. (See the symptom list in chapter 3, page 47.)

The adrenals are energizing partners of the thyroid. If the thyroid fails, the adrenals get overworked and run down. The result is the stressed "tired but wired" sensation that we often associate with having too much "fight or flight" adrenaline in our system. If excessive stress has caused the adrenals to go into permanent overdrive, the thyroid will automatically turn down in an effort to calm the system. Furthermore, at this point the adrenals cannot regulate the immune system properly, and immune system problems like thyroiditis can result. See chapters 3 and 11 on diagnosing and treating adrenal exhaustion, and get your adrenals tested at the same time that you get your thyroid tests.

What to Request of Your Physician

1. A review of the symptoms and history that you have identified, including at least three underarm temperatures (take them according to the directions in chapter 4).
2. A manual examination of your thyroid gland.
3. An ankle reflex test.
4. Blood tests for thyroid functioning (described in detail in chapter 4): TSH, T_4 by RIA, T_3 by RIA, T_3 Uptake, FTI, Reverse T_3, two thyroid antibody tests by FAMA, plus basic bloodwork (a CBC, SMAC panel, and ferritin [iron] level). You'll need the CBC, SMAC, and ferretin tests to determine if you, like so many people with thyroid problems, have some form of anemia (low iron, low B_{12}, and/or low folic acid). This testing will also show cholesterol levels, which are often elevated in people with thyroid trouble.
5. For adrenal function, a saliva test and orthostatic blood pressure readings.

Your next step will be into a nearby lab to get your blood drawn if your doctor's assistant doesn't draw it in the office. Now you'll go home and focus on getting the foods and supplements you'll need for the next two weeks to start treating your symptoms, until all the lab test results are back and you can return to your doctor for test results and treatments that might be needed.

NUTRITIONAL STRATEGIES

Whichever thyroid problem you have, you should make sure that your first step in treating it is to eat high-quality food and use targeted nutritional supplements. If you have a mild thyroid problem, this nutritional boost alone may very well correct it.

Eat Plenty of Nutritious Food

To treat both low thyroid and thyroiditis, be sure you eat the following every day.

✦ **Vegetables:** At least 4 cups. Do not rely on lettuce alone, because of its bulk, but eat a variety of colored veggies. (Cabbage, spinach, rutabaga,

---

Urgent Warning Regarding Pregnancy

If you boost your thyroid function, you are likely to become more fertile because the thyroid can stimulate reproductive hormonal function quite dramatically. A 52-year-old nurse who had never conceived had a surprise pregnancy when her thyroid was treated. She was elated, but you should be very careful if you want to avoid pregnancy.

---

and turnip can inhibit the thyroid, so *don't* emphasize them if you have hypothyroidism.)

✦ **Protein:** At least 20 grams (3 to 4 ounces of lean meat, fowl, fish, or tofu) or more *per meal* (see protein content table on page 307, in chapter 20).

✦ **Healthy fats:** 2 tablespoons per day of good oils in foods like avocado, nuts and seeds, and in salad oils like canola, extra virgin olive, and flax.

✦ **Carbohydrates:** Be moderate in the amounts of fruit, potatoes, squashes, and whole grains that you take in each day. Two servings of fruits per day plus $1/2$ to 1 cup, one or two times per day, of other carbohydrates is usually adequate (see chapter 5 to make sure you don't have an allergy to some grains—many of us do).

To sum up, be sure to get enough protein and vegetables, then add good carbohydrates, like fruit, rice, and beans. (Have less pasta, bread, and other baked goods: *But don't avoid calories.*)

Weight and Thyroid Recovery

Many of you are undereating because your thyroid is so slow that you'll gain weight quickly on normal amounts of food. You'll find that on the kinds of foods I'm recommending that you'll be able to eat more. Sometimes it takes awhile to get your thyroid and metabolism going. But then you'll gradually increase your calories and lose weight. Getting enough protein, the builder of muscle and mind, is particularly important because low thyroid keeps you from benefiting fully from the protein food you eat, and many of you skimp on protein, anyway. You'll notice the difference right away: you'll feel lighter and better overall.

Drink Purified Water

Water is an invaluable nutrient, and you need at least eight 8-ounce glasses of it a day. But you may run into problems when you drink tap water, because chlorine, fluoride, and hydrocarbons, which are found in most water supplies, can suppress thyroid function—a big complication if you have low thyroid.[1] Ask your local purified-water expert about filtration devices that can eliminate all of the above contaminants. Filtration systems can be installed for your whole house or just under the kitchen sink.

The purity of bottled water is hard to judge. Plastic bottles easily overheat and emit biochemicals into the water (fake estrogens are of particular concern, as they can create hormonal imbalances that are linked to breast cancer). Use insulated water bottle covers with straps to keep your bottle cool and easy to carry.

Avoid Drugs and Druglike Foods

You may have been using drugs or sweet foods for energy, especially caffeine. Work with the amino acid chart in chapter 9 if you need to kill your cravings for these substances. If you are too tired without caffeine even after using the amino acid L-tyrosine, you'll probably have to wait until you get on some thyroid medication before you can quit.

WHEN THE TEST RESULTS COME BACK

Once you've been eating well and taking your basic nutritional supplements for two weeks, you should get your test results back and talk to your doctor about what to do next if you are unsatisfied with the results you've been getting from the dietary changes and basic supplements. Although over 90 percent of our clients stop any overeating or food craving and begin to feel better by this point, at least half need to add special supplements or medication to their programs, at least temporarily, once their test results are in.

Simple Low Thyroid (Hypothyroidism)

Your symptoms, basal temperatures, ankle reflex, and a thorough panel of blood and saliva tests should tell you if you have simple low thyroid (hypothyroidism). Three quarters of my clients who suffer from low thyroid function have classic hypothyroidism—their temperatures are low, their energy is low, their moods are often low, but their weight is usually high.

Elizabeth suffered from mild hypothyroid. She was an athletic 32-year-old strawberry blonde in recovery from a past eating disorder that had taken its toll on her body, as had many years of overwork and a stressful marriage and divorce. Elizabeth came to Recovery Systems after her energy had dropped and she had begun to gain unneeded weight. She was blood tested by our M.D., who found that her thyroid scores were below normal. He offered her a prescription for thyroid medication, but advised her to talk to one of our clinic's nutritionists first. At the nutritionist's suggestion, Elizabeth increased the amount of protein and vegetables she was eating and began taking the amino acid L-tyrosine and a thyroid-boosting supplement containing kelp, animal thyroid gland, and herbs; she also took the six basic supplements we recommend. She immediately regained her energy and vitality. In fact, she had to cut down on her dose of L-tyrosine and the thyroid booster in just a few weeks, because they soon made her *overly* energized.

Thyroiditis: When Your Immune System Is on the Attack

If you suffer from the second, more complex thyroid affliction, Hashimoto's autoimmune thyroiditis (HAIT, or Hashimoto's), in which your thyroid is attacked by your immune system, your thyroid antibody test results will usually show it. A needle biopsy can be done for a definitive answer, if you and your doctor are unsure.

If you have HAIT, first you'll need to do everything you can to calm down your hyperactive immune system. It will help to eliminate from your diet any foods that you are allergic to (see chapters 5 and 13), because continual allergic reactions provoke your immune system into hyperattack mode. You may also need special supplements and will probably also need medicine and/or acupuncture.

A Thyroiditis Story

The story of Dina's thyroiditis is a typical one. When I first met Dina, she was 34 years old, thin, and pale, with huge black circles under her eyes. She was very knowledgeable about nutrition and had been able to recover, on her own, from both anorexia and bulimia, which were an integral part of her life as a ballet dancer. She was working part-time and going to graduate school, but her energy was poor, she slept very badly, and was stressed and hypersensitive. "I'm just one raw nerve," she told me.

Dina's problems had started at age 14, about the time her periods had begun. (It is typical for thyroid problems to start during times of hormonal change.) Dina had recently been given a TSH test and scored in the low normal range, but she was declared to have no thyroid problem and told that no further investigation was needed. Twelve months later, Dina began having seizures and waking up in the night feeling suffocated, which terrified her. That was when she called us and we sent her to an M.D. with a comprehensive list of thyroid tests to request. The results were astonishing. Her thyroid antibodies, which should have been under 10, were over 20,000! Her blood test scores for anemia were off the scale as well. She was diagnosed with severe autoimmune thyroiditis. In fact, she had had it for twenty years, ever since she had stopped being alert and calm, and became "tired and wired" at age 14. Touching her neck, her doctor could feel a lump of scar tissue on her thyroid (no prior doctor had ever examined her).

Dina began her thyroiditis treatment with a strong dose of Synthroid, which made her symptoms worse. Next she was put on animal thyroid and, though she lost her appetite, she began to gain three pounds a week. Because of these adverse symptoms she was switched to very small amounts of Synthroid and Cytomel. She immediately dropped back to her original weight. Her dosages were gradually increased in tiny increments. In addition to these two medications, Dina took vitamin B_{12} shots and iron for her anemia, a rich multimineral and multivitamin for other thyroid support needs, omega-3 fish oil as an antiinflammatory, vitamin C with bioflavonoids, and vitamin E. She was assisted by a gifted Chinese acupuncturist, who gave her regular treatments with needles and herbs for her weak adrenals, and insisted that she cut back on her heavy exercise workouts for a while. All this brought her thyroid antibody score from 20,000 to 1,700 in six months. In one year it was down to 298! More important, she began glowing with health and vitality and was able to return to regular exercise. She gained five pounds in muscle, but her dress size stayed the same.

Curing her thyroiditis had another unexpected effect. Dina had been an A student until her thyroiditis hit at age 14. On her thyroid repair plan, she regained her concentration and proudly revealed to me that one of her graduate school professors had told her that her recent paper was the best he had ever read.

Thyroiditis is a very serious condition that can eventually destroy the thyroid gland and adversely affect every cell in the body. Dina had to continue working closely with her M.D. on her medication dose, but her office visits became much less frequent after the first year. Unfortunately, by the time her thyroiditis was diagnosed, her own confused immune system had destroyed the thyroid gland entirely, so she will need to stay on medication for life.

SUPPLEMENTS FOR THYROID PROBLEM

Because you've had an impaired thyroid you haven't been able to absorb nutrients from your food very efficiently. Whether you suffer from hypothroidism or thyroiditis, the extra nutrients found in the basic supplement plan (laid out in chapter 17) will help you now, and will help you even more later as your improved thyroid function increases your absorption over the next few months.

For low thyroid only: If you have low energy and are also agitated, wait until your test results are back before trying the following booster nutrients because you may have thyroiditis, which calls for calming the thyroid, not boosting it. If taking these boosters make you agitated, stop them until you get your test results.

To boost a low thyroid function, take the following. (Note that some special thyroid-boosting supplements contain all three of these basic boosters and may even include herbs as well, or you can buy the boosters separately.)

✦ **L-tyrosine.** This amino is the primary food that the thyroid uses to make all of its hormones. L-tyrosine is probably the body's most energizing food, being the source of not only thyroid but adrenaline, testosterone, and the body's natural caffeine—norepinephrine as well as dopamine. Low thyroid can drive many people to a dependence on stimulating drugs like caffeine and cocaine as their own natural energizers run down. Many of you have come to need coffee all day long to keep going, or sweets to give you a lift, or in some cases drugs like Dexatrim or ephedra, or even cocaine, to really get you moving. Tyrosine is the nutrient that relieves you of your need for these fake energizers. It can often jump-start the thyroid.

If your problem is just a mildly underactive thyroid, you'll feel the effects of tyrosine right away. Taking 500 to 2,000 milligrams before breakfast will usually eliminate your coffee cravings right away, too. Usually two to four 500-milligram capsules in early morning and midmorning (away from meals) is enough to get you reenergized. You can take the same amount of tyrosine in midafternoon, if it doesn't keep you awake.

	AM	B	MM	L	MA	D	BT*
❏ l-tyrosine, 500–1500 mg,* 1–3 times/day	1–3	—	1–3	—	1–3	—	—
❏ GF Thyroid or other thyroid glandular 50–100 mg	1	—	—	—	1	—	—

*AM=on arising; B=breakfast; MM=midmorning; L=lunch; MA=midafternoon; D=dinner; BT=bedtime.

✦ **Iodine.** You'll probably get enough in your basic multimineral/vitamin and you are already getting iodine in salted foods.

✦ **Thyroid glandulars:** Small amounts (under 100 milligrams) of the thyroid glands of animals, known as thyroid glandulars, can be helpful in stimulating and supporting your thyroid gland. Take them in the morning before breakfast and midafternoon along with your L-tyrosine. We have been very impressed by the effects of a supplement that we have used for years, which combines a small amount of glandular material with thyroid-nourishing herbs and homeopathics. It is called Gf Thyroid and is made by Systemic Formulas.†

THYROID MEDICINE

At Recovery Systems, we have seen close to a thousand people on many different kinds and doses of medication for both kinds of thyroid problems. For hypothyroidism or thyroiditis, most physicians exclusively prescribe Synthroid, (synthetic T_4—see below). In fact, in 1997 Synthroid was the second most frequently prescribed drug in America: 36 million Synthroid prescriptions were filled that year. Sometimes Synthroid often seems to work very well, but we have seen many cases in which Synthroid was not the most beneficial drug. Other forms or combinations of thyroid medication can be better for certain individuals.

Some doctors much prefer the original medication for thyroid that is made from animal thyroid glands. Pigs are the animals with the most humanlike thyroid glands. One difference: the ratio of key thyroid hormones in pigs (4:1) is not the same as it is in humans (10:1). That may be one reason that animal thyroid does not work well for everyone. When you start on thyroid medication, be patient. Finding the right medicine and

†GF Thyroid is available from our clinic's order line (800-733-9293).

> **Do you have trouble swallowing pills, especially tablets or large capsules?**
>
> This is not unusual for people with a thyroid problem because the throat can become congested and the thyroid gland can actually swell and hamper your swallowing capacity. Look for liquid, powder, or sublingual forms of the supplements you'll need. If necessary, you can blend them in a smoothie and you won't notice them. Or you can stir them into a little applesauce and/or mashed banana for between-meal doses. They'll be easier to swallow as soon as your throat congestion clears.

the right dose can take time and care. It can be difficult to determine how long each experimental course of medication should go on before the next higher dose or different medication should be tried. Some people feel benefits within days of their first dose. Others take weeks or even months to find the right dose or combination. This process is well worth the time. Be patient, but persistent. Perhaps your doctor will be willing to give you a schedule to follow on your own for increasing your doses at certain intervals, if your initial lower doses aren't strong enough.

Choosing and Experimenting with Medication for Low Thyroid

Here are the thyroid medications:

✦ Animal source (porcine—from pigs) of the four thyroid hormones: T_3 and T_4, plus T_1 and T_2; brands include Naturthroid Armour and Westhroid. (Of these, note that only Naturthroid is organic, meaning the pigs are fed organic food.)

✦ Synthetic T_4: for example, Synthroid, Lavoxal, and Levothroid. There can be some surprising differences in the way you react to different types of T_4. Try them all, if necessary.

✦ Synthetic T_3 (such as Cytomel), the most active, potent form of thyroid.

✦ Synthetic combinations of T_3 and T_4 (which provide the same 4:1 ratio of T_4:T_3 as the animal sources); examples include Euthroid and Thyrolar.

The animal-derived thyroid medications contain not only T_3 and T_4, they also contain T_1 and T_2. The Barnes Foundation points out that T_2 may be needed to prevent dry skin and problems with fibrous breast and uterine cysts. My female clients seem to divide evenly into those who do well with synthetic and those who do well on animal sources of thyroid. I have observed that male clients seem to do better on the animal-source medication.

Working with your physician, choose a type of medication and a starting dosage. Then monitor your reactions closely. If there is no response, your doctor can raise the dose gradually. If there is still no improvement at the highest safe dosage, your doctor will need to try another kind of medication and see how you fare on that.

Usually they will start with synthetic T_4 (Synthroid, but they may also try the equally potent Levothroid or Lavoxal). If T_4 medications alone don't help much, they may add the more potent T_3 medications, such as Cytomel. You may not have to be on thyroid medication for life. Consult with your physician after the first year to see if you can try going off it.

TREATMENTS FOR THYROIDITIS

If your test results show that you have thyroiditis you still have many treatment choices.

Acupuncture and Herbs for Thyroiditis

Many of our clients who suffer from thyroiditis have included acupuncture treatment along with their nutritional program and medication. The Chinese system of acupuncture does not have a thyroid-specific treatment. It restores thyroid indirectly through the adrenals and other glands like the liver. The more modern Japanese acupuncture system does directly treat the thyroid. Try to find an experienced acupuncturist who is recommended for his or her demonstrated skill. Usually acupuncturists trained in China or Japan are best at both herbal and needle work, especially those that have been practicing for fifteen years or more. They may put together herbal mixtures for you to brew as tea. See chapter 21 for suggestions on finding an acupuncturist.

Thyroiditis Medicine

Everyone I have worked with who has had elevated thyroid antibodies on their test results has needed medication, in addition to improved nutrition and often acupuncture. The most successful pharmacological protocol for

---

Low Thyroid Function and Anemia

Low body temperature can mean low hemoglobin. If your test results show you have anemia, you'll need B_{12}, B_1, iron, and/or folic acid. Weekly B_{12} shots taken over the course of several months can quickly help improve your energy and mood if you also have pernicious B_{12} (B_1 anemia responds to extra B_1) anemia, which occurs when you don't have adequate B_{12} and is common among people with thyroiditis (apparently thyroiditis blocks our digestion of B_{12}). Minerals are also crucial for thyroid function generally and especially crucial for thyroiditis, so be sure you're taking a good multivitamin/mineral. Finding extra-absorbable iron can be difficult. Try Slow Fe (available over the counter in drug stores) or Niferol (available only by prescription). Eat liver!

---

thyroiditis that we have seen includes a combination of synthetic T_4 (Levothroid or Synthroid) with very small amounts of synthetic T_3 (usually Cytomel). Doses start very low and go up and down as results indicate. You may need to work closely with your doctor on adjusting your doses over an extended period of time, probably several years.

A well-known San Francisco endocrinologist, Nathan Becker, M.D., after many years of treating thyroiditis with carefully monitored doses of Synthroid alone, found that then adding small doses of Cytomel, if needed, improved his results. We have worked with several of his patients and can verify the success of this approach. He also says that 30 percent of his patients can eventually go off of their medications because the treatment causes the immune systems to stop attacking their thyroid gland, allowing it to function normally.

We know of a number of women diagnosed with thyroiditis who were put on animal thyroid medication and began gaining weight very quickly. This stopped when they were switched to Synthroid (synthetic T_4) with or without Cytomel (synthetic T_3). But one of our consultants, Richard Shames, M.D., says that he has occasionally seen women with thyroiditis who do *better* on animal thyroid. It's an individual matter. Keep trying until you find the right solution for you.

ADVERSE SYMPTOMS OF THYROID MEDICINE AND SPECIAL CONCERNS

You may have been told in advance by your physician to reduce or stop your thyroid medication if any adverse symptoms showed up, and to come in for an appointment right away.

Be particularly careful if you are on medication that contains T_3, the most activating thyroid hormone. If you do get adverse symptoms from it, be sure to get very specific instructions from your doctor and pharmacist about cutting down or going off of thyroid medication. A gradual tapering off may be the safest and most comfortable way to stop using your medication if you need to.

Common Adverse Symptoms of Thyroid Medication

+ A wired, agitated, speedy feeling
+ Heart palpitations (If you have this symptom, check your adrenals, too.)
+ Sleep disturbances
+ Feeling overheated

Long-term Effects of Thyroid Medication

Are you afraid that thyroid medication will cause your gland to atrophy and never function on its own again? I have been reassured by many thyroid specialists that this does not happen, and I have personally watched many people go off of thyroid medication after a year or longer on it. Some of them return to the level of function that they had prior to going on the medication. Some have had better function on their own after a period on thyroid medication. None of them had worse function, but they *have* been very tired for a week or two after getting off their medications.

If your gland has been destroyed by thyroiditis or by radiation, or for other reasons just cannot function on its own, you will need to take medication for life. Dr. Broda Barnes discovered this from patients who had been forced, by cancer or overactive thyroids, to have their thyroid glands removed surgically. They all died young of heart disease unless they were put on thyroid medication. Although too much medication can cause heart palpitations, Dr. Barnes learned that the right amount of thyroid medication turns out to be extraordinarily heart protective.[2]

Without adequate minerals as supplements, too much thyroid medication, over a long period of time, *can* demineralize your bones. Discuss monitoring your bone density with your doctor.

What If You Have Already Been Treated for a Thyroid Problem, but You Didn't Get Better?

Many women come to our clinic saying, "Oh, yes, I thought it was my thyroid, but I'm on medication [usually Synthroid], and I'm still tired. I guess my weight problem must be caused by something else."

Usually the real problem is the medication. Of course, it helps a lot to eat plenty of high-quality, thyroid-activating foods like vegetables and protein, avoid allergy foods, and take supplements like L-tyrosine. But what can change the picture is a better dosage, type, or combination of medication. An evaluation of adrenal function often reveals a crucial deficiency that, when treated, corrects the problem (it wasn't the thyroid after all).

Many doctors who don't look carefully at symptoms use a standard dose of Synthroid, check to see that a single test indicator (usually TSH, again) is back in the normal range, and quit attending to the complaints of their patients. Then they resort to the same old diet advice. More attentive physicians are convinced by their patients' symptoms that, test scores aside, the thyroid isn't functioning properly, and they find a better treatment.

Thyroid Medicines and Allergies

Are you allergic to corn or milk? Armour (animal) thyroid contains corn, and Synthroid contains milk sugar and acacia (from a tree that many people are allergic to). Check with your doctor because thyroid medicines for food-sensitive people can be specially prepared through compounding pharmacies, which prepare medicines to the specific order of an M.D. or D.O. Compounders can also eliminate chemical coloring, binders, and additives. All major areas have compounding pharmacies. (For more on compounding pharmacies, see the resources at the end of chapter 21.)

Be sure to address any other imbalances right away, especially candida and food allergy. Both of these imbalances can block your recovery from low thyroid and thyroiditis. Now you are ready for action!

ACTION STEPS

1. Thoroughly review your symptoms, and your own history and that of your family members. Check your morning underarm temperature at least three times to see if it is under 97.8 degrees.

2. Choose a health care professional to work with. An endocrinologist (a specialist in thyroid and other endocrine glands) who is very competent (particularly if wholistic) would be ideal, especially if you have a serious problem with your thyroid, such as thyroiditis. See chapter 21 for more suggestions on finding a physician.

3. Visit the wholistic physician you decide to consult, and request a review of your symptoms and history and complete testing as described in this chapter and in chapter 4.

4. Basic Nutritional Support
  + Water: Daily, drink eight or more 8-ounce glasses of filtered water.
  + Food: Follow the guidelines in this chapter and in chapter 20 for increasing your intake of vegetables, protein, whole carbos, and healthy fats.
  + Supplements: Take the basic supplements outlined in chapter 17 and the extra supplements as per the charts in this chapter.

5. When your test results come back and you know whether you have hypothyroidism or thyroiditis, follow the directions in this chapter for using nutrients, medicine, and perhaps acupuncture.

6. If you are going to take medication, work with your physician until you have the right medication at the right dose. Continue paying attention to your symptoms and taking your basal temperature. Retest your thyroid and adrenal levels regularly, at least every three months, until you have stabilized.

7. Try tapering off your medication in a year or two in consultation with your physician.

8. Keep a food/medication/mood log to monitor your progress (see chapter 22).

Readings

Langer, Stephen E., M.D., and James F. Scheer. *Solved: The Riddle of Illness*, 2nd edition. (New Canaan, CT: Keats Publishing, 1995.)

Wood, Lawrence, David Cooper, and E. Chester Ridgeway. *Your Thyroid*. 3rd edition. (New York: Ballantine, 1995.)

Shames, Richard, M.D., and Karilee, R.N. *The Thyroid Connection* (New York: Morrow, forthcoming).

Resources

Broda O. Barnes M.D. Research Foundation
(203) 261-3017
The Broda Barnes Foundation has available articles, books, tapes, and conference information, besides their national directory of practitioners.
See chapter 21 for information on physician and acupuncture referrals.

THIRTEEN

Overcoming Addictions to Allergy Foods

By now you realize that while you love your favorite foods, they may be creating annoying symptoms, like gastrointestinal problems, headaches, low energy, and postnasal drip—not to mention the unneeded weight gain that comes from eating breads and sugary foods. In this chapter you'll learn how you can test for these allergies at home. I'll also tell you about other tests you can get that can help determine which allergies you might have.

When you learn what allergies you have, don't despair about never being able to eat "normally" again. Along with lists of foods to avoid, I'll provide lists of foods you can eat that you probably never thought of, foods you might end up enjoying more than the foods you're giving up. Once you've educated yourself about how to avoid your allergy foods, you can start with your basic supplements (as outlined in chapter 17) as well as anticraving supplements to make the transition to your new eating habits much easier.

TESTING FOR ALLERGIES

Home Testing

The easiest, fastest, and cheapest way to test for allergies to wheat, rye, oats, barley, and/or cow's milk products is to do a home test. In 1990, Dr. John E.

Postley, a Columbia University professor, made it clear in *The Allergy Discovery Diet* that the home test is also the most accurate way of all to identify food allergies. Here are important cautions for home testing:

✦ Keep a detailed food/mood log to monitor the testing process (see chapter 22).

✦ Reintroduce only one food or food group at a time.

✦ Wait two full days between tests of different foods. For example, if it turns out you are allergic to wheat, wait two days before you try rye. The reason for this is that sometimes you can get delayed allergic symptoms hours or days after your test. If that delayed reaction hits on the day that you try the next food, you won't know which food is the problem food. Some people have problems only with wheat, not with all gluten-containing grains. If wheat was not a problem, the other three gluten-containing grains—rye, oats, and barley—are not likely to be troublemakers either, and you probably don't need to test them. If you are intolerant to a food or food group, your body will react negatively to them.

✦ Women should test after their period and before PMS.

Here's how to do the test:

Days 1 to 7: Making the Break. Do not consume any of the foods that you have decided to test (either cow's milk products or the gluten-containing grains). Review the material in chapter 5 to remind yourself of hidden sources of these allergens so that you don't accidentally consume them. The supplements recommended at the end of this chapter will make sure your detox is short and mild, so don't dread this testing period. It won't be like any of the diets that you've endured. You won't miss the foods you eliminate and by Day 5 (if not before) you should be feeling better than you have in a long time. You may notice quick weight loss in this first week.

Day 8: The Challenge. On the eighth day, notice whether any of your bothersome symptoms have gone away. Then eat a regular serving of one test food for breakfast and again at lunch. For example, if you're testing for a milk allergy, have some milk at breakfast and a glass of milk with lunch. Make a note of how you feel. Also note your oral temperature, any food cravings, your mood, energy, digestion, respiratory symptoms, bowel function, appetite, skin changes, headaches, sleep patterns, and any and all information that your body imparts. You may have a very strong reaction, such as a migraine if you're prone to them. If you only get a little tired, bloated, or headachy after your challenge meals, don't ignore it. If you gain weight or start craving foods again, don't be surprised. It's not a coincidence.

When testing the gluten-containing grains, test first with wheat (bread, pasta, or another very plain form of wheat) because it is the grain highest in gluten and will therefore give you the clearest results. Do not eat any more of the food or food group for the next two days (after waiting two days, you can test another gluten-containing grain). Allergic reactions to milk products and gluten-containing foods can be very similar, so you'll get a clearer response to your testing if you eliminate both, then reintroduce them one at a time to see which one is the problem, or whether they are both problems. If it feels too overwhelming to let go of milk products and the gluten-containing grains all at once, start with testing, and removing, the grains first.

Do not eat any more of your convicted allergy foods as you go on to test others. It can help to test your foods while you are actually with someone who can help you notice your reactions. I've noticed many wives turn out to be the best observers of their husbands' changing symptoms.

If you have no leftover adverse symptoms from your first challenge, you can test another food. If you determine, after reintroducing grain and milk, that you need to avoid one or both of them permanently, you can expect to feel better for as long as you stay away from them. If you suddenly feel bloated or tired or achey again, you'll know that you've inadvertently consumed your allergen. Or perhaps you'll eat a little of them because of convenience or pressure when there's nothing else available on the menu or everyone's indulging in a traditional holiday treat—and you'll experience some of your old symptoms for a while. But they'll fade, and you can use two tablets of Alka-Seltzer Gold to get rid of them quickly.

Trust your body's messages. It will tell you what works and what doesn't.

Other Ways of Testing for Food Intolerances

At Recovery Systems, we rarely do other types of testing because the home test is so effective and convincing. But there are a few testing methods that we occasionally use when allergy symptoms continue even after the big-three allergens have been tested or eliminated.

Saliva Testing. This can identify allergies to all gluten-containing grains and/or cow's milk protein (but it cannot test for lactose—milk sugar—intolerance).

ALCAT. This new blood test measures many more reactions than other allergy blood tests.

Simple Pulse Test. Monitor your pulse to see if it increases or decreases by 12 to 20 beats right after eating a particular food.

Applied Kineseology. A muscle test developed by chiropractors, this test can determine if your muscle strength declines when you are exposed to certain foods (a treatment based on this test helps eliminate allergic reactions).

Skin prick testing. This wholistic procedure involves having the suspect foods injected under the skin or given as drops under the tongue. Reactions are then observed.

Further Testing for Severe Gluten Intolerance (Celiac Disease)

Blood Antibody. This test has been confirmed in European and British medical studies to be 98 percent accurate in measuring high blood antibodies to gliadin (gluten). Specialty Laboratories in Santa Monica, California, is one lab performing this test. It seems to detect only the worst cases of gluten intolerance. Any lab can send your blood sample to a lab like Specialty Labs that performs the test.

Biopsy. This is the most accurate way to diagnose celiac disease (the most extreme version of gluten intolerance). If you would like to know for sure if you have CD, see a gastroenterologist and ask for a small intestine biopsy. You are sedated, and it doesn't take long. You'll swallow a tiny tube. When it goes down past your stomach into your small intestine, it will snip out a sample of your intestinal wall for viewing under a microscope to see if typical damage has been done. For obvious reasons, only four of our clients have ever been willing to do this. (They were all men who had been unable to gain weight.)

AVOIDING ALLERGY ADDICTORS

If You Need to Avoid Gluten or Wheat

Becoming wheat- or gluten-free can alleviate your low energy, depression, agitation, digestive disturbances, cravings, and more, very quickly. You will not continue to feel deprived, even though you need to avoid many (mostly nutritionally negligible) foods, because there are so many delicious foods you *can* eat. Also, there are easy substitute foods that you'll love. I enjoy eating very much and always have, yet I haven't had gluten-containing food for more than ten years.

Common Gluten-Containing Foods to Avoid

Additives	MSG (monosodium glutamate); HVP (hydrolized vegetable protein); TVP (textured vegetable protein)
Breads	yeast, quick breads, muffins, scones, corn bread, buns, white or wheat bread, pancakes, bagels, biscuits, pizza, croissants, crackers, pretzels
Grains	wheat, rye, barley, oats, spelt, kamut, teff
Meats, poultry, fish	breading or batter on fried fish, fried chicken, corn dogs; anything floured before frying (to brown); dishes prepared "en croute" or "stuffed"
Pasta and others	macaroni, noodles, spaghetti, orzo, couscous, bulgur wheat, seitan (used as a protein source, it is 100 percent gluten)
Pastries	cookies, biscotti, cake, pie, crumb toppings, cobbler, doughnuts, brownies
Possible problem foods	quinoa and amaranth (There is some debate on whether or not these are gluten-containing grains.

	Our clients have not had prob-
	lems with them.)
Sauces	Mornay, cheese sauce, béchamel,
	white sauce, gravy, some soy sauce
Soups	barley and wheat varieties of miso
	soup, cream soups, bouillon,
	soups with bread in them (such as
	French onion), soups with pasta
	(minestrone, chicken noodle, and
	others)

Hidden Sources of Gluten

You probably wouldn't think to avoid these foods, but all contain gluten.

+ French fries (often dusted with flour before freezing)
+ Croutons on salad
+ Chinese crisp noodles (except rice noodles)
+ Processed cheese (like Velveeta)
+ Dumplings
+ Most soy sauce
+ Mayonnaise
+ Catsup
+ Some salad dressings
+ Distilled vinegar (If they just say *vinegar,* it is probably grain vinegar. Stick to the ones that state *wine vinegar, apple cider vinegar,* or *balsamic vinegar.*)
+ Caramel color
+ Modified food starch
+ Malt or malt flavoring
+ Sulfites
+ Seitan foods made in the same fryer as breaded foods
+ White and whole-wheat-flour tortillas

Read labels! The label for bakery products or mixes must say *Gluten Free,* not just *Wheat Free,* unless that is the only grain that causes problems for you. Don't get overwhelmed, just eat simply. Make sure that you do not consume allergens hidden in a recipe or disguised as something else. Ask whether there is wheat, or white, flour in any restaurant food. "Wheat" is often used to designate "whole wheat" as opposed to "white" flour, but white flour is made from wheat that has had its brown parts removed, and, therefore, it contains gluten.

What to Eat Instead of the Gluten-Containing Foods. If you're gluten intolerant, you must avoid gluten permanently. (Exception: if you go through a yeast kill-off (chapter 15) you'll be able to eat more carbohydrates afterward. Sometimes gluten intolerance can be confused with yeast overgrowth.) It takes months for your intestinal lining to heal. Any exposure can restart the damage. Stick to the safe grains: corn and rice.

Many ethnic cooking styles in this country are gluten-based, but corn- and rice-based cuisines do not usually contain gluten. Suppose that you lived in South America, where corn and beans are staples in wonderfully tasty dishes. Or that you lived in Asia, with the rice, vegetables, fish, coconut milk, and other foods used in all those richly varied cooking styles. It's easy to avoid gluten in those parts of the world. It can be easier here than you might think. There is a cornucopia of hearty, luscious eating possibilities. For carbohydrates, instead of the gluten-containing grains formerly in your diet, use rice and corn in all their forms, potatoes, yams, squash, taro, and other root vegetables, of all kinds. There are even creative recipes and ready-made mixes for pancakes, muffins, and yeast bread that are delicious.

A bread machine can be used to make delicious gluten-free breads that most people can't distinguish from wheat bread. In her book *More from the Gluten-Free Gourmet,* Bette Hagman includes some yeast bread recipes especially formulated to be made in a bread machine. She has also included a section with good suggestions for choosing a bread machine, if you don't already have one. Red Star Yeast has a pamphlet on making gluten-free bread in your bread machine.

Safe Gluten-Free Foods

Additions	nuts, seeds, beans, or dried vegetables sprinkled on salads, soups, and other dishes
Breads	made from rice, bean, and potato flours; corn tortillas; all-rice crackers

---

Special Note for Gluten Intolerants Who Also Have Yeast Overgrowth

You should follow the yeast dietary guidelines in chapters 7 and 15 for the first four weeks, before reintroducing foods. Do not home test for gluten or sugar intolerances while on the anti-yeast program.

Grains	corn, cornmeal mush, grits, brown rice, basmati rice, wild rice, creamy rice hot cereal
Grains tolerated by many gluten intolerants	millet, quinoa, amaranth, buckwheat
Meats, poultry, fish	sautéed, roasted, stewed, or braised (if not floured first); broiled, steamed
Pasta and others	made from rice, corn, and quinoa flours; polenta
Sauces	béarnaise, hollandaise, and others, *if* they are thickened with cornstarch, arrowroot, or gluten-free flour, like rice, potato, or garbanzo
Soups	split pea and potato, if no other thickeners are added; clear-broth soups: chicken rice, vegetable beef, and others
Sweets	fruit
Vinegar	apple cider, balsamic, and wine vinegars

See chapters 18, 19, and 20 for even more suggestions of fresh, delicious, nutritious foods you can enjoy.

Avoiding Sugar

Sugar can be extracted from many foods—corn, barley, sugar beets, sugarcane—and is called by many names. Here's a list of words from the Diabetes Friends Action Network (DFAN) that will let you know that a food contains sugar:

Common Sugar Forms

Words ending in -ose:
+ Dextrose
+ Fructose
+ Galactose
+ Glucose
+ Lactose
+ Levulose
+ Maltose
+ Sucrose

Words ending in -ol:
+ Mannitol
+ Sorbitol
+ Xylitol

Other Sugars
+ Beet sugar
+ Brown sugar
+ Cane sugar
+ Confectioner's sugar
+ Corn sugar
+ Corn sweetener
+ Granulated sugar
+ High fructose corn syrup
+ Honey
+ Invert sugar
+ Isomalt
+ Malto dextrins
+ Maple sugar
+ Maple syrup
+ Molasses
+ Raw sugar
+ Sorghum
+ Turbinado sugar

Avoiding Cow's Milk Products

What to avoid here depends on whether you react badly to lactose or to other contents of these foods, like the protein casein.

Foods to Avoid If You Have a Milk Allergy

✦ Butter and artificial butter flavor
✦ Buttermilk
✦ Casein and caseinates (sodium, potassium, magnesium, calcium, or ammonium)
✦ Cheese
✦ Cottage cheese
✦ Curds
✦ Galactose (a lactose by-product); this one's a problem for relatively few people, but be aware of the potential)
✦ Hydrolysates (casein, milk protein, whey, whey protein)
✦ Lactose (often sodium lactylate), lactalbumin, lactoglobulin, and other ingredients that begin with *lact*
✦ Milk
✦ Milk solids ("curds")
✦ "Natural ingredients" (Sometimes this refers to dairy products or by-products. Call the manufacturer—an 800 number is usually listed on the packaging—for further information.)
✦ Sour cream, sour cream solids, sour milk solids
✦ Whey
✦ Yogurt

Common Foods That May Contain Milk Products
✦ Bread
✦ Canned tuna (Watch for "hydrolized caseinate." You'll have better luck with tuna packed in water.)
✦ HVP (hydrolyzed vegetable protein; may use casein in processing.)
✦ Kosher parve desserts (May contain casein from nonanimal sources.)
✦ Margarine
✦ Medicines and vitamins (It's common to put lactose in coatings and binders; this is especially true of homeopathic medicines. Be sure to alert your physician and pharmacist about your allergy.)
✦ "Nondairy" products of all kinds ("Nondairy" is not the same as "milk free." It can contain as much casein as whole milk and still meet the dairy industry's definition.)

What to Eat Instead of Cow's Milk Products. Try goat's and sheep's milk products. They are delicious and much more easily digestible and less fatty than cow's milk products. Goat's or sheep's milk feta, a pungent, crumbly white cheese, is available almost everywhere. (It is sometimes made from cow's milk. Read the label carefully.) Goat's milk is available in super-markets as well as health stores, and comes fresh, canned and powdered. Goat's and sheep's milk yogurt (both fresh and powdered) is available at most health stores, as are many kinds of cheese—from Parmesan to ri-cotta, Cheddar, and Monterey jack. Cheese made from goat's or sheep's milk is made and prized all over the world.

Butter, which is low in lactose, can be tolerated by some people. Ghee (clarified butter) is the only kind containing no lactose at all. (Look for or-ganic versions to avoid antibiotics and pesticides.) You can also try the new cheeselike foods that are are being made from soy, almonds, and hemp oils, but be careful about ingredients if you are gluten intolerant.

For a milk substitute, you can try soy milk, though it doesn't agree with everyone. Be sure to get the unsweetened variety; most use rice syrup as a sweetener (Westbrae makes an unsweetened version). Or better yet, make your own delicious milks out of nuts or seeds that have soaked in water overnight. The next day, rinse them and blend them with a little wa-ter, until you make a cream. Dilute it to taste with more water—yummy, and very nutritious. (See the recipe for Seed or Nut Milk on page 318.)

Soy milk makes a very good substitute for milk in cooking and baking. You can substitute any liquid, including water, in recipes that call for milk. These substitutions can be delicious. For example, in sauce recipes, meat or poultry broth, or vegetable juice can substitute for milk, giving the dish distinctive flavors.

Instead of	Use
1 cup milk	1 cup water
1 cup milk (for baking)	1 cup water + 2 tablespoons canola oil
Light cream	Thick seed or nut milk (see page 318)
Heavy cream	Meringue (egg whites beaten until stiff)
Sour cream	Dairy-free mayonnaise or goat yo-gurt (if you can tolerate it)
Cream cheese	Dairy-free mayonnaise
Condensed milk	Powdered soy or goat milk + water. Add a little water at a time until the mixture is the same thickness as condensed milk.

	AM	B	MM	L	MA	D	BT*
❏ L-glutamine 500 mg	1–2	_	1–2	_	1–2	_	1–2†
❏ Aloe vera juice, 8 oz	_	1	_	1	_	1	_

(George's or other good-quality brand)
(drink before meals)

*AM=on arising; B=with breakfast; MM=midmorning; L=with lunch;
MA=midafternoon; D=with dinner; BT=at bedtime.
†If you get sweets cravings at bedtime

SUPPLEMENTS THAT CAN HELP YOU RECOVER FROM FOOD ALLERGIES

The Allergy Detox Supplements

Even after you go off the special allergy-detox supplements after a few days or weeks, you'll still be taking the supplements on the basic supplement plan. This is the core of all eight of the rebalancing protocols in this book, and the permanent nutrient support that will help you to remain rebalanced for good. (See chapter 17 for your master supplement plan.)

For Sweet and Carbo Cravings

If you crave sweets and doughy foods, chromium (the blood sugar–normalizing mineral included in your master supplement plan) and the amino acid L-glutamine (which also helps heal any digestive problems) are your answer. They will usually eliminate any cravings for sweets and starches in twenty-four hours. Check the Amino Acid Therapy chart in chapter 9. If your cravings persist, you may need a few other aminos.

For Milk Allergy

Lactase (Lactaid) is an enzyme product available from your drug store that helps the body digest milk sugar. (If your problem is the casein, or protein, in milk, this will not help.) It comes in three strengths of caplets to be taken with the first bite of dairy food. See the package for detailed directions. Of course, Lactaid containing milk is available everywhere now.

For Allergic Reactions That Cause Digestive Distress

The aloe vera plant heals the damage to the "skin" of your digestive tract in the same way it can heal your external skin. Aloe juice can get sluggish bowels moving normally, too. Look for George's brand juice.

For Quick Elimination of Allergic-Reaction Symptoms from Food or Inhalants

Use Alka-Seltzer Gold (2), as needed during detox week for headaches or digestive discomfort. Use it any time you have an adverse reaction to allergy food.

ALLERGIES ARE STRESSFUL: REPAIRING DEEPER DAMAGE

If you are allergic to common foods like the allergy three, your body might have been engaged in a struggle every day for most of your life. This chronic stress has strained you in ways beyond the obvious postnasal drip, stomach bloating, or food cravings. You have been dealing with constant assault, and the troops are probably very tired. Thankfully, taking the supplements and changing your diet will relieve the pressure that your immune system and stress emergency system have been under. But if you continue to feel a lack of vitality and to have a tendency to feel too easily overwhelmed, please consider a simple test for adrenal-stress function. If your adrenals (your stress and immunity guardians) are worn too low, you won't be able to revive them without a special supplement protocol that can be determined only after you get your saliva test results. (See chapters 3 and 11.)

ACTION STEPS

1. Review your symptoms, as discussed in chapter 5 and decide which foods you are probably allergy-addicted to.
2. Do your home elimination and reintroduction tests for the big-three foods. Keep a food/mood log to record the process.

3. Consider getting the backup saliva, skin prick, or blood tests, especially if you think you might have severe gluten intolerance (that is, celiac disease), or allergies to foods other than the big-three.
4. Learn how to avoid any of the big-three foods you have adverse reactions to on your home tests. Review the guidelines in this chapter.
5. Learn how to enjoy all the other foods that you can eat without injury. See chapters 18, 19, and 20 for suggestions on what to eat.
6. Start on your anticraving supplements as well as your basic supplement plan.
7. Check your adrenal-stress symptoms if you benefit by removing any of the big-three allergy foods but continue to feel wound up and overwhelmed (see chapters 3 and 11).

You may not believe it now, but you will soon find that avoiding these foods, though inconvenient, will become second nature. And feeling better, and probably looking better, will keep you motivated. What's more, you'll still enjoy eating.

Reading

Appleton, Nancy. *Lick the Sugar Habit.* (Garden City, NY: Avery, 1997).

Cutler, Ellen. *Winning the War Against Allergies.* (Albany, NY: DelMar, 1997). Cutler advocates new allergy testing and elimination technique.

Gittleman, Anne Louise. *Get the Sugar Out.* (New York: Crown Publishing, 1996).

Hagman, Bette. *More from the Gluten-Free Gourmet.* (New York: Henry Holt, 1993).

———. *The Gluten-Free Gourmet Cooks Fast and Healthy.* (New York: Henry Holt, 1997). Hagman is the author of three gluten-free cookbooks. In her latest, she has put priority on cutting the amounts of fats and sugars, which are often pretty high in the recipes in her other cookbooks.

Lowell, Jax Peters. *Against the Grain: The Slightly Eccentric Guide to Living Well.* (New York: Henry Holt, 1995).

Philpot, William H. *Brain Allergies: The Psychonutrient Connection, Including Brain Allergies Today: An Update.* (New Canaan, CT: Keats, 1987).

Postley, John, M.D. *The Allergy Discovery Diet.* (New York: Doubleday, 1990).

Rapp, Doris, M.D. *Is This Your Child?: Discovering and Treating Unrecognized Allergies in Children and Adults.* (New York: William Morrow, 1992). By a wholistic allergist.

Rivera, Rudy, M.D., and F. Deutsch. *Your Hidden Food Allergies Are Making You Fat.* (Rocklin, CA: Prima, 1998).

Taylor, John, Ph.D. *Helping Your Hyperactive ADD Child.* (Rocklin, CA: Prima,

2d ed., 1997). For information about Dr. Taylor's national workshops and materials on nutrition and ADD call (800) 847-1233.

Resources

GOAT'S MILK PRODUCTS
Myenberg's (800) 343-1185
This company sells fresh and powdered goat milk to health food stores and some supermarkets. Call to find a store near you that carries their products.

ORGANIZATIONS
Something to Moo About (Nondairy)
10425 S.W. 114 Court
Miami, Florida 33176
(305) 598-0374 or
Canada and the United States (416) 733-2117
Its Web site ("The No Milk Page"): *http://www.panix.com/~nomilk/*
Provides info and resources on milk intolerances. Browse though its Web site's links to personal, scientific, educational, and commercial sites.
The International Society for Orthomolecular Medicine
For referrals to wholistic allergy specialists.

For ALCAT blood testing for food allergies (800) 881-AMTL
To order a test kit from:

AMTL
1 Oakwood Blvd.
Hollywood, FL 33020

Specialty Laboratories
2211 Michigan Avenue
Santa Monica, CA 90404-3900
(800) 421-7110
Specialty Laboratories is one lab that performs the celiac blood test.

The American Academy of Environmental Medicine
For wholistic allergy testing and treatment
(215) 862-4544

The Celiac Sprue Association (CSA/USA)
P.O. Box 31700
Omaha, NE 68131-0700
(402) 558-0600

Contact CSA/USA for more complete food lists, books, and other information on how and why to avoid gluten

LABS
Saliva testing for gluten and milk protein:
Bio Health Diagnostics
(800) 570-2000

Diagnos-Techs, Inc.
U.S. (800) 878-3787; fax: (425) 251-9520
U.K. 011-44-179-246-4911; fax: 011-44-179-247-2466

FOURTEEN

Hormone Help

As debilitating as your PMS or menopausal reactions might be, if you follow the advice in this chapter you may be completely free from adverse symptoms in a few months. By your *very next* period, if you have a few weeks running start with the right nutrients and foods, your PMS problems—from food cravings to cramps, bloating, and mood swings—will be gone. Menopausal mood swings, food cravings, and weight gain usually desist quickly, too. But other menopausal symptoms (like low energy and hot flashes) can take somewhat longer to eliminate.

If you are suffering from PMS, you'll learn how supplements and food can even out your hormone levels and eliminate your symptoms. If you are perimenopausal or menopausal, you will learn how to test your hormones and find natural hormone replacements to alleviate your symptoms. I'll also explain how nutritional support, acupuncture, exercise, and stress management can help rebalance your hormones.

FOOD CRAVINGS

Do you experience powerful cravings for sugars and fats before your period or as you approach menopause? Most of these hormonally inspired food cravings will disappear when you stop eating "drug" foods. Chocolate, sugar, refined flour products, caffeine, and NutraSweet all contribute to hormonal mismanagement. They have got to go if you are going to escape from PMS or menopausal cravings and weight problems. I know that it is not enough to tell you to just quit eating these foods. If you start taking the supplements I recommend, you will lose interest even in chocolate.

Once your cravings are gone (and it won't take long), you will feel satisfied, not deprived, by highly nutritious food. Green, purple, yellow, and red vegetables will delight you. Fish, tofu, chicken, eggs, and meat will satisfy and please you. You will enjoy, but not overeat, wholesome carbos like beans, potatoes, rice, and polenta.

The trouble is that addictive druglike foods are everywhere; we call them "convenience" foods. It can be inconvenient to eat well, but it is more inconvenient to have PMS and hot flashes! It takes time to prepare fresh food or to find healthy places to eat. You will need to make it a priority, because the time you have now is being spoiled by the hormonal imbalances that are probably being magnified by your current diet in a real vicious circle: unbalanced hormones make you overeat and overeating further unbalances them.

Amino Acids

These nutrients are just what you need to break the cycle. Whether you are pre- or postmenopausal, amino acids will reduce your sugar cravings and mood swings. These nutrient heroes are described in more detail in chapters 1 and 9, but I'll summarize here. Hormonal changes, particularly drops in estrogen and progesterone and rises in stress chemicals, can radically reduce the supply of all of your four mood-enhancing brain chemicals: serotonin, endorphin, norepinephrine, and GABA. You won't need aminos for long, because your new eating style and other changes will stop the hormonal imbalances within a few months.

✦ **L-glutamine** stops cravings for sweets, starches, and alcohol and is mildly calming. Use it if you have cravings that go on all day.
✦ **5-HTP** is particularly needed for late afternoon and evening cravings, and when PMS includes moodiness. Many studies have made it clear that low serotonin, common during the week (or two!) before your period, is a primary cause of irritability, negativity, depression, and insomnia. Chocolate and other drug-carbos can indirectly trigger a serotonin surge (at a high price, as we mentioned earlier). Using 5-HTP or prescription L-tryptophan, the body's natural precursor to serotonin, is a much healthier way of raising levels premenstrually.
✦ **St. John's Wort** helps 5-HTP raise serotonin levels faster.
✦ **GABA supplements** can relax your muscles like a natural Valium. Levels of both the relaxing brain chemical **GABA** and the pain-relieving

---

For cravings and mood swings of PMS; use as needed

	AM	B	MM	L	MA	D	BT*
❑ L-glutamine, 500 mg	1–2	—	1–2	—	1–2	—	—
❑ 5-HTP, 50 mg	—	—	1–2	—	1–2	—	2
(or prescription tryptophan, 500 mg)							
❑ St. John's Wort, 300 mg	—	—	1	—	1	—	1
(with 900 mcg (0.3%) hypericin)	—	—	1	—	1	—	1
❑ GABA 100–500 mg	—	—	1	—	1	—	1
❑ DLPA 300–500 mg	1–2	—	1–2	—	1–2	—	—
❑ or DPA 200–500 mg	1–3	—	1–3	—	1–3	—	—
❑ L-tyrosine, 500 mg	2–4	—	2–4	—	2–4	—	—

*AM=upon rising; B=with breakfast; MM=midmorning; L=with lunch; MA=midafternoon; D=with dinner; BT=at bedtime.

---

endorphins have also been shown to drop during PMS, which helps explain why some of us experience so much painful cramping and emotional misery in the week before menstruating. Too much can make you drowsy.

✦ **D-phenylalanine** (DPA) will increase your endorphins, which help you to tolerate pain and stress. It is most easily found as DL-phenylalanine (DLPA) in combination with energizing L-phenylalanine, which should help you stop craving chocolate and NutraSweet. If the DLPA is too stimulating, get DPA by itself.

✦ **L-tyrosine,** another amino acid energizer, can help you with caffeine cravings.

Too much will make you jittery. See Amino Acid Therapy, page 120, and decide which aminos you will need, based on your particular PMS mood symptoms.[1]

TAKE YOUR SUPPLEMENTS

Many research studies have confirmed that even the moderate doses of nutrients in multivitamins/minerals can provide dramatic improvements in PMS and help in menopause too. Along with an improved diet, the Diet Cure's basic supplement plan in chapter 17 will provide all the extra nutrients you'll need to decrease or eliminate most PMS symptoms: the B vitamins (especially vitamin B_6) and the minerals calcium, magnesium, and zinc all play a role. Most of us are deficient in these nutrients, because we have not been eating enough fresh, whole foods, and our produce comes from mineral-depleted soils. Another of your basic supplements, fish oil, can also stop PMS symptoms cold and heat us up in menopause. PMS, among other things, is a nutrient-deficiency problem, but such deficiencies can be easily rectified.

Herbal Help for PMS. The six basic supplements and the aminos usually stop junk-food cravings so that you can start eating well, even before your period. If you continue suffering from PMS, add an herbal formula that includes the herbs angelica (dong quai, an herb that has helped to regulate estrogen levels in women in China for thousands of years) along with other herbs with long histories of hormonal helpfulness for women like sassparilla and blue cohosh. Our clinic uses the Systemic Formulas Bio Function brand Female Plus, which combines all of these herbs; take it once a day, every day, with or without food. You can try to find similar combination herbal formulas at your health food store, or you can order it from us.

Herbs in Menopause. We have tried many herbal formulas that feature dong quai and black cohosh. They are easy to find in health stores and they make women feel so much better, typically eliminating hot flashes and insomnia. Research confirms this. But these herbs do not seem to fully normalize hormone levels in many, perhaps most, women. We find osteoporosis, for example, in women who, because they'd lost their hot flashes, assumed that all was well. When their saliva test results come in, they show that estrogen, progesterone, and DHEA levels are low. Please get your own hormone levels tested now for a base line and then every six months until you are consistently in the optimal hormonal ranges, and annually after that.

EAT WELL AND STOP DIETING

You will need to eat at least three times a day from now on. By eating more vegetables, protein (such as meats, fish, and eggs), and good fats; eliminating sweets and white flour starches like white bread, cereal, and noodles; and taking your supplements, you'll find yourself free of carbo cravings and weight gain, even premenstrually, within two months. (See

The Soy Story

Does the soy story have a happy ending?

Once upon a time researchers found that women of the Far East had low breast cancer rates. Why? Was it that they ate soy products? Was it that they ate 20 percent more calories than we do? Was it because they ate few refined, processed foods and more vegetables? Less fat? Less animal protein?[2]

Somehow soy became the focus of the excitement. Soy is a *very* complex bean that contains many nutrients. Some of these nutrients, the phytoestrogens, act like estrogen, fooling our cells. One cup of tofu provides the estrogen equivalent of one dose of Premarin,[3] the potent estrogen brew made from horse urine. Initial research suggested that soy might be protective against breast cancer, osteoporosis, and Alzheimer's in menopause.

But what about premenopause? When should someone start taking soy as a medicine? The Japanese use it all their lives. Many U.S. children are now becoming vegetarian and using soy all their lives, too. Yet low estrogen is not a problem in youth. We don't need more estrogen then. What does soy do to people who are not close to menopause?

These are some of the increasing questions about soy. Some disturbing answers are starting to come in.

1. Despite their high soy intake, Japanese women have *much* higher rates of osteoporosis than we do (one in three versus one in eleven). Moreover, bone mass deterioration begins in Japanese women at age 20, not, as in the United States, at age 35.[4]

chapters 17, 18, 19, and 20 for specific suggestions.) *Just keep in mind that too many high-carb foods and any dieting will keep you hormonally unbalanced.* One example: The insulin that is triggered by too many carbohydrates lowers testosterone in men, who gain fat and lose muscle, and sex drive, as a result. Insulin does the reverse in women, raising testosterone levels, thus contributing to male-pattern (apple shape) weight gain and polycystic ovarian disease, among other things (see adverse effects of high and low testosterone on page 88).[9]

The combination of supplements and improved eating does the trick

2. Soy increases the growth rate of cancerous breast cells in women (in vivo) and in test tubes (in vitro)![5]

3. Soy increases progesterone activity and more breast cell growth in menstruating women.[6]

4. Soy decreases thyroid (T_3) and DHEA levels in menstruating women and others (both of which are central to energy, health, and weight maintenance) as well as estrone, LS, and FSH (female reproductive hormones).[7]

5. Breast cancer specialist Dr. Susan Love cites studies indicating that soy has anti-estrogenic effects on premenopausal women, and pro-estrogenic effects in menopausal women.

6. One study found soy to be a factor in disturbances in menstruation in a group of premenopausal women.[8]

The upshot is that good health in the Far East is likely to be due to factors other than soy. Remember that all people on simpler diets (and with simpler lives) have much better health than we do in the United States, and most of them do not use soy. And hundreds of fresh fruits, vegetables, and grains contain phytoestrogens similar to soy's.

If you are eating soy, be aware that the soy protein is very difficult to digest. This is why tofu and tempeh are so popular in the East. They are fermented, which makes them easier for the stomach to break down. You may tolerate tofu and tempeh better than soy beans, soy milk, or soy protein powders, which are not fermented and often cause stomachaches. We don't recommend that people force down soy products that they can't digest or that they don't really need. On the other hand, soy is very high in protein—for those who can digest it.

for 80 to 90 percent of Recovery Systems' clients who suffer from PMS. If you still have premenstrual cravings or mood swings after two months, the following information will take care of any remaining, stubborn problems.

Be sure to watch for your body's reaction to the proteins you feed it. Some of us seem to be genetically programmed to do best with animal protein, despite our vegetarian or health ideals. Remember that red meat is a source of easily absorbed iron and zinc, two minerals that are very important if you are menstruating (they are flushed out of your body in menstrual blood). This would explain why many of our vegetarian clients dream of hamburgers before their periods each month—their bodies are sending them a message to get more iron and zinc. Be sure to supplement with these two minerals if you are vegetarian *and* premenopausal and your multivitamin/mineral doesn't contain both minerals.

TEST YOUR HORMONES WHEN PMS OR MENOPAUSAL SYMPTOMS JUST WON'T GO AWAY

While the supplements and new eating plan can do wonders for relieving PMS and menopausal food cravings for most women, others need more help. If you've experienced little or no relief in your PMS or other symptoms after two months on this program, I suggest you have your hormone levels tested. You should also have them tested if you are experiencing any perimenopausal symptoms. Since serious hormonal imbalances can begin ten years before menopause (and sometimes earlier), I encourage hormone testing at any sign of adverse hormonal change, which is what perimenopause is. For example, if you've never had PMS before and you suddenly start experiencing it in your mid- to late thirties, or your periods start getting heavier or crampier, you should test your hormones. I think some women are shocked at how early their periods can become irregular, sporadic, or absent. Most of you will not have to test your hormone levels because these nutritional strategies will alleviate symptoms of PMS and perimenopause; only about one in ten of our PMS sufferers at Recovery Systems need hormone tests. But if you do need to check your hormone levels, please read about testing later in this chapter.

The symptoms of low and high testosterone levels in men have been thoroughly studied, but there have not been equally definitive studies done on women to determine just exactly what symptoms would let you know for certain whether it was your estrogen or your progesterone levels that were out of balance. For example, there is considerable debate about whether estrogen causes or prevents hot flashes. There are whole camps of wholistic clinicians who are either anti-estrogen and pro-progesterone, or the reverse (though this camp is thinning as the need for progesterone in HRT—hormone replacement therapy—to protect against cancer caused by estrogen replacement alone has become evident).

You'll need to be very careful to subscribe to any rigid ideas about your hormones. The real issue is, do you have enough of all your hormones, and are they in balance? You could experiment, trying first an estrogen supplement, then, if that didn't work, a progesterone supplement. Both are avail-

PMS, Menopause, and Stress

Stress can disrupt your hormonal life in newly understood ways. It is very important to get saliva testing for your adrenal function, especially if you are in perimenopause or menopause. During these periods your ovaries are making less estrogen and progesterone, and your adrenals are having to take over the job, on top of making twenty-four other hormones. The adrenals are mighty, but if they have to attend to too much stress, they can't do their new jobs very well. Coping with stress (emergencies) always takes priority. Several of my infertile clients found that their adrenal function was very low. Two of them were having frequent panic attacks as a result. The stress of junk-food eating, low-calorie dieting, and other health and life problems can exhaust your adrenals, reducing their ability to help you and our body cope with menopause and PMS. Adrenal exhaustion is often the cause of hormonal deficiencies. Don't overlook it! See chapters 3 and 11 for more on stress and the adrenals.

able in natural, nonsynthetic, easily absorbed, plant-based products. But I don't recommend this. I would much prefer that you test your hormone levels before you do anything else. The most reliable tests, in my experience, are done using saliva. You know from chapter 6 what symptoms to watch for so that you have an idea of what your hormone tests should reveal. If you end up taking natural or synthetic hormones, you can be sure they are addressing the problems they were supposed to address. Your hormone tests will clarify what your actual levels are and you can compare them to your symptoms. Be sure to keep a food/mood log for this purpose (see chapter 22).

When you have a rough idea, from symptoms, of whether your hormone imbalance involves estrogen, progesterone, testosterone, DHEA, or a combination of the four, get some accurate testing to confirm the imbalances before you act to correct them. If you are menopausal, even if you have no discomfort but particularly if you do, I believe that saliva testing is well worth your while. You should also have your hormone levels tested if you have, or suspect you have, fibroid tumors or any other hormone-related problems, such as endometriosis, or if you want to know more about your fertility. Always retest six months later if you start taking any hormones, or anytime that you have new symptoms of hormonal imbalance. Continue to retest at least annually for the rest of your life. Saliva testing for hormone levels is considered to be the gold standard by the World Health Organization.

Blood Testing versus Saliva Testing. You could ask an M.D. or D.O. for blood tests for estradiol, progesterone, testosterone, and DHEA. This would only give you another rough idea of your hormone levels, though, because blood testing measures inactive as well as active hormones. Unfortunately, the inactive ones are ten times more prolific, but have no effect on you. There are blood tests for active hormones, but they are wildly expensive. Saliva testing only measures active hormones.

If you are premenopausal, perimenopausal, or have been menopausal for less than seven years (because menopausal women can continue having hormonal fluctuations each month for seven years after they quit having periods) your blood levels will be compared to the levels that are considered normal for the time of the month that you tested in. If you have PMS, I suggest you test premenstrually, while you are having symptoms. Your results will be measured against "normal" premenstrual (or luteal) levels. Your early morning body temperatures can give you menopausal cycle-mapping clues. If you keep a record of them for two to three months, you should spot estrogen peaks that raise your temperatures for a day or so. You can determine, by the number of days in between, how long your menopausal cycle is and test appropriately. Check with your testing lab for other suggestions. I don't want you to start hormone replacement therapy (HRT) based on a single day's hormone picture if you are still varying a lot in your levels of estrogen and progesterone.

If you have been menopausal for at least seven years, you'll be measured against "normal" menopausal levels. Be sure to retest after thirty days and then every six months after you start your hormone supplements, until your levels are normal and you feel great!

A better solution is to test saliva, which, surprisingly, yields a treasure trove of biochemical information. You can order these tests directly yourself, or you can ask your practitioner to arrange it for you (see the resources for chapter 21 for a list of labs that do saliva testing). Some labs will discuss your results with you by phone or refer you to practitioners in your area who will help you interpret and treat your imbalances. They will often consult extensively with health professionals by phone, on your behalf. (Estrogen and testosterone in the natural form are available only by prescription, so you'll need an M.D. or D.O. at some point if your levels of those hormones are low.)

You may need to be quite assertive about getting tested and using natural HRT, if your physician is not wholistic. If you're in this situation, read chapter 10 in *The HRT Solution*, which was written by Marla Ahlgrimm, a pharmacist who specializes in wholistic hormone replacement and works with M.D.'s constantly.

You can collect a single sample of your saliva anytime, during PMS or advanced menopause. If you are still getting menstrual periods, you can chart your whole monthly cycle by collecting saliva samples every day over the entire course of your cycle.

The Results of Your Tests. The lab will send you back a map showing you exactly what your hormones are doing, which can be a fascinating revelation. Some women have two or three ovulations per month, for example. Some have none. Some have plenty of estrogen or progesterone, except during PMS. This is information you should have. Your map will change as you get closer to menopause and experience new symptoms that your saliva tests will help you understand.

You can test one sample of your saliva for any or all of the following hormones: estradiol, estriol, estrone, progesterone, testosterone, DHEA, and cortisol (the last two hormones will tell you if adrenal exhaustion is at the core of your hormone imbalance). I recommend that you test for all of the above hormones before considering HRT and at intervals after embarking on HRT. Results come with interpretations and suggestions from most labs.

Why Testing Is Important. Most of the hormone-troubled women who come to our clinic have never had their hormone levels tested, even the ones who are seeing gynecologists and on potent hormonal drugs! Since Premarin (horse estrogen) has typically been prescribed for menopausal women at a whopping 625-milligram dosage regardless of symptoms or body size, it can easily raise estrogen levels too high if not closely monitored, especially if low estrogen was not the problem to begin with.

Because your own body's hormones can become unbalanced in hazardous ways, you really must test them before you consider adding any additional hormones, however natural, whether you are experiencing PMS or are menopausal. As several studies have shown, unnaturally high estrone, estradiol, and testosterone can cause breast cancer. Other studies show that low estriol is associated with breast cancer. Testing can give you early warnings. If you do take hormone replacement of any kind, testing can monitor your levels, helping you keep them in safe ranges. Clients with PMS usually show a steep drop in progesterone at the end of their cycle. Menopausal

---

PMS, Menopause, and Low Thyroid Function

You'll certainly need an M.D. or D.O. if you need blood testing to measure your thyroid function. Low thyroid is often implicated in PMS, in menstruation that is heavy or irregular, and when sex drive and energy are generally low. Other clues to thyroid trouble are that you tend to be chilly, or you started menstruating early or late in life. (See chapters 4 and 12 for a complete list of low thyroid symptoms and testing information.) Low thyroid is a factor in the problems of many of my menopausal and PMS clients. A sluggish thyroid can result in all of the sex hormones being at low levels. Estrogen can inhibit thyroid function, while progesterone enhances it. In both menopause and PMS, progesterone levels tend to drop faster than estrogen levels.

We know that progesterone increases metabolic rate. That's why premenstrual chocolate bingeing often results in little or no weight gain: Progesterone levels are supposed to be at their height before your period, both triggering cravings and burning calories more quickly (in preparation for a possible pregnancy). But it can drop very low instead, causing PMS symptoms. I have seen many clients who could not lose weight after a pregnancy or after menopause. Progesterone levels tend to drop then, and thyroid is often low as well. Measure both and get treated accordingly.

---

clients usually test low in both estrogen and progesterone, but a significant number test much lower in progesterone.

Testing Your Bones. As Marla Ahlgrimm, author of *The HRT Solution,* points out, your bones hold secrets to navigating perimenopause and menopause osteoporosis-free. Your bones will start shrinking slowly at age 35, then quickly for the first ten years of perimenopause, then slowly again. A new nonradiation method is available using ultrasound technology to measure your current bone density, and a simple urine test, the Dpd test, will tell you if, and at what rate, your bones are now breaking down. This test can be repeated to make sure that your hormone-rebalancing program is working, or whether you'll need to increase your hormone supplements. High cortisol and low estrogen, progesterone, testosterone, and DHEA can all contribute to bone loss—another reason to be sure your hormones are in balance.

Special Hormonal Repair Supplements

SUPPLEMENT	AM	B	MM	L	MA	D	BT*
Herbs for PMS							
❑ Female Plus†	1	—	—	—	—	—	—
Herbs for Menopause							
Take as recommended on bottles:							
❑ Dong Quai and/or	—	—	—	—	—	—	—
❑ Black Cohosh	—	—	—	—	—	—	—
Ultimate Hormonal Protocols							
Take as recommended by your health professional:							
❑ Progesterone	—	—	—	—	—	—	—
❑ Estrogen	—	—	—	—	—	—	—
❑ Testosterone	—	—	—	—	—	—	—
❑ DHEA	—	—	—	—	—	—	—
❑ Pregnenolone	—	—	—	—	—	—	—

*AM=on arising; B=with breakfast; MM=midmorning; L=with lunch; MA=mid-afternoon; D=with dinner; BT=at bedtime.
†This Systemic Formulas supplement is not availabe in stores. You can order it through the clinic order line (800-733-9293).

HERBAL AND OTHER SUPPORT FOR MENOPAUSE

The basic supplement plan plus amino acids and healthy foods will usually stop your cravings, allowing you to avoid the excessive carbos that further deplete your already sinking hormone levels. But you will probably need more help. Herbs can go a step beyond this basic plan to help normalize your hormonal life. Their most notable effect is on PMS and hot flashes. Though their means of restoring more normal hormone function is somewhat mysterious, they have been studied extensively for safety and effectiveness. Dong quai is China's chief female tonic. A Native American herb, sold under the name Remifemen, is now the strongest selling alternative to menopausal hormone replacement in Germany, Australia, and the United States. Its real name is black cohosh. It has been known to relieve emotional symptoms as well as physical ones. An herbal combination that includes black cohosh as the main ingredient is Change-O-Life from Natures Way. It is often effective in relieving hot flashes and is widely available from health food and drug stores, and in some cases from supermarkets.

Although these herbal tonics can be helpful, I prefer that you test your hormone levels *before* you start taking them, or any other hormone regulator. You need to be sure that you should be raising estrogen levels instead of progesterone levels, for example, before you begin. If you just can't stand waiting and want to experiment, go ahead while you wait for your test results. Stop taking herbs if they have no obvious positive effect within a few weeks. Herbs have not been thoroughly tested for reversing osteoporosis or heart disease, though they are well known to ease or eliminate other menopausal problems, such as hot flashes, mood symptoms, and carb cravings.

USE NATURAL HORMONES: THE ULTIMATE HORMONAL PROTOCOLS

Once you know from your symptoms and test results where the hormonal trouble lies, you can move very carefully into balancing your hormones. Natural hormones used to be impossible to absorb by mouth, but the micronized (microscopic in size) forms, routinely used in Europe and available in the United States, are fully absorbable. Better yet, they have none of the side effects of horse urine estrogen (Premarin) or the synthetic progesterones (called progestins) found in birth control pills and drugs like Provera.

Are you a refugee from Premarin or Provera, or the birth control pill? You could hardly do worse on natural hormones than has probably been done to you with various kinds of prescription pharmaceutical hormones. Horse's urine is as far away from human estrogen as Provera is from human progesterone (to say nothing of what the mares suffer in the extracting of this hormone). Usually, these products have been handed out in high doses without benefit of hormone testing to help identify which, and in what amounts, they might be needed (though a trend toward lower dosing does seem to be under way now).

Natural estrogen replacement made from soy and wild yam in the micronized formulations are available and have been eagerly used in countries like Germany for many years. Natural progesterone is available in conventional U.S. pharmacies, but your M.D. or D.O. will have to order natural estrogen or testosterone from special compounding pharmacies. Many of them are wholistic mail-order pharmacies specifically catering to women's health needs. (Names and phone numbers are listed in the resources for chapter 21.) There are three types of naturally occurring es-

Bearded Ladies: The Power of Hormone Therapy (Even the Most Natural)

You know personally how intense hormonal effects can be: Just think of sexual arousal, menstruation, pregnancy, and PMS. Before you consider natural hormone replenishment, I want to be sure that you understand how powerful hormones are. The synthetic hormones clearly have more hazardous effects than the plant-based hormones. But the natural soy- and wild yam–based hormones are very potent, too, and can be overused, creating imbalances that can be dangerous.

There is one other thing that worries me. The pathways between hormones are not entirely predictable. For example, the very popular hormone supplement DHEA can just as easily convert to unneeded estrogen or testosterone as to new DHEA. That is why ladies using DHEA (as well as testosterone and progesterone) can grow beards. (This also can happen naturally in menopause as estrogen levels drop.) Yet if truly deficient and carefully monitored (by symptoms and testing), DHEA supplementation can be a boon.

If you use progesterone augmenting creams, be especially careful. Do not overuse them, and be sure to retest your hormone levels every three to twelve months. Retest immediately and stop using any hormone if you begin to get adverse effects, including facial hair. It is easy to absorb too much hormone through the skin. One of our clients used progesterone cream as body lotion, instead of the one eighth to one quarter teaspoon recommended, and grew soft, downy sideburns. It took her several months, off of progesterone, to get rid of them.

trogens: estradiol, estriol, and estrone. Compounders can make a blend of the three to your doctor's specifications. There is some controversy over what the best proportions should be. The hormone 17-beta estradiol alone has quite a good track record, but combining it, as the body does, with estriol and estrone is the ideal.

Natural Hormone Supplements for Perimenopause and Menopause. You'll really need your saliva-testing map to figure out how to deal with this hormonal mystery zone. You'll also need your bone density test results, because you may have raised your hormone levels enough to relieve your obvious menopausal symptoms but not enough to protect your bones from eroding. If you already know you have osteroporosis, help is available through supplementation with estrogen, progesterone, testosterone, and DHEA, as well as vitamin K and medicines like Fosamax.

If your saliva test shows that you are too low in estrogen, progesterone, or testosterone, you'll need to work with an M.D. or D.O. to bring your levels up with natural hormones. But creams build up quickly. Please test regularly if you use creams. Watch for quick improvement in any adverse symptoms you're experiencing with oral hormones or patches. Retest in one month and again every six months until you seem to be symptom-free and testing well. Retest at any sign of discomfort, or if your Dpd bone status test shows you're bones are still shrinking or starting to again.

If your cortisol and DHEA levels are low, this could be the real key to your hormonal problems, because it's a sure sign that your adrenals are too exhausted by stress to make adequate amounts of estrogen, progesterone, or testosterone. (Remember, in perimenopause and menopause, your adrenals take over as your ovaries quit producing as much estrogen and progesterone.) Use the suggestions in chapter 11 to restore your adrenals to working order as soon as possible. Retest everything over the next few months to see if raising your cortisol and DHEA has brought your other hormones up to a point where you might need to cut back on your HRT (estrogen, progesterone, etcetera).

If your testosterone levels are low, a low-dose prescription can make a wonderful difference. But keep retesting regularly. Excess testosterone can be dangerous.

Where to Find Natural Hormones. You can buy natural progesterone in creams, drops, and pills or pellets over the counter (or by prescription from compounding pharmacies); the same is true for DHEA and pregnenelone. Natural estrogen and testosterone are only available through compounding pharmacists.

The strengths and combinations in compounding pharmacists' repertoires are extensive. And they can pay attention to individual cases. Many of them are wholistically oriented. You'll need to find a physician (M.D. or D.O.), who will prescribe from a compounder for you. Compounding pharmacists will consult with you and your physician by phone about what and how much of any hormone to use, depending on your symptoms and test results. Be ready to call the compounding pharmacist yourself first, since many physicians don't seem to be aware that these com-

Herbs for PMS
❑ Female Plus   — — — — — — — —
Herbs for Menopause
❑ Dong Quai and/or   — — — — — — — —
   Black Cohosh   — — — — — — — —
   as recommended on
   product label   — — — — — — — —
Ultimate Hormonal Protocols
❑ Progesterone   — — — — — — — —
❑ Estrogen   — — — — — — — —
❑ Testosterone   — — — — — — — —
❑ DHEA   — — — — — — — —
❑ Pregnenolone   — — — — — — — —

pounders and their valuable hormonal products and advice exist. I have seen many women successfully switch from synthetic hormonal medications, like Premarin and Provera, to natural prescription hormones with the help of compounding pharmacists.

Compounders usually can send out prescriptions through overnight mail. Madison Pharmacy also arranges for saliva and other testing and can help your physician prescribe based on the results. Beware of compounders who do not advise hormone testing before prescribing. (See the resources for chapter 21 for a list of compounding pharmacies.)

If Your Levels of Any Hormones Are Too High. There are a few things that will help you to reduce excess hormones in your body:

✦ Stop taking any foods, herbs, or supplemental hormones that might be encouraging excess (hormonal creams are especially suspect).
✦ Increase the amount of vitamin C you are taking to 5 grams per day.
✦ Use a gentle fiber, like pectin, (Jarrow's fiber product is very good) daily. Mix it in plenty of water. Be sure to eat plenty of fiber-containing foods—fruit, beans, and crunchy vegetables.

✦ Try Seriphos, a nutrient supplement that can bring down excessive cortisol levels (see chapter 11, page 163) if your own levels are elevated.*

If you have tested your hormones and found imbalances, but you decide that you do not want to use even the natural hormones, you might consider homeopathic remedies. They are well laid out in *Menopause and Homeopathy*, by Ifeoma Ikenze, M.D., a Harvard-trained, wholistic women's health expert. At Recovery Systems, we have not used homeopathic remedies yet for reproductive hormonal rebalancing, but we have seen homeopathy help with many other imbalances.

If you have hormonal problems that don't respond quickly to nutritional supplementation, improved diet, and natural hormone balancing, you might want to try acupuncture. Acupuncturists can also prescribe herbs and order saliva hormone tests. (By the way, the needles don't usually hurt.)

Julie learned firsthand the curative effects of acupuncture. Julie had been in menopause for two years. She ate well and had been using hormone creams for two years. Most of her hot flashes and insomnia had disappeared as a result, but a large and uncomfortable fibroid tumor had not subsided. Because we had seen acupuncture help with hormonally related problems, including infertility and the side effects of chemotherapy after breast cancer surgery, we suggested she try it for her fibroid. She went to an acupuncturist who specialized in women's health problems. After two sessions in which the acupuncturist used fifteen painless needles in her pubic area, the fibroid and its symptoms subsided and did not return. The acupuncturist told Julie that similar treatments for fibroids are successful about 50 percent of the time.

GET ENOUGH EXERCISE AND RELAXATION—AND SUNLIGHT!

Descending estrogen levels during menopause bring three feel-good brain chemicals down with them. Exercise can bounce them all up again,

---

*These last three methods were suggested to us by Dr. William Timmons of Bio Health Diagnostics in San Diego, California, where we have done a lot of our saliva testing and have been well educated about interpreting results and implementing and monitoring treatment.

especially serotonin. You have to almost kill yourself to get an endorphin high from exercise, but serotonin levels will rise nicely, though only temporarily, after moderate exercise. If you feel much better after exercise, you've probably had a serotonin boost. The supplement 5-HTP will keep your levels up much longer than exercise will, so you won't have to suffer from depression if you can't exercise. Sunlight (or very strong lamps, 2000 lux or brighter) will raise serotonin levels, too. So exercise outdoors without sunglasses whenever you can. Raising serotonin often helps with food cravings, mood swings, as well as insomnia in PMS and menopause.

Menopausal exercisers can lose some of their newly created fat cells by building muscle. Muscle burns fat for a living; it uses fat as fuel for its activity. But we put on menopausal fat for an excellent reason: we need it so that we can feed our adrenals the special fat-storage estrogen, called estrone, that helps them replace the estrogen that used to come from our ovaries. So don't get too buff. We were meant to soften with age. Before menopause, women's higher estrogen levels minimize abdominal fat, but not when estrogen levels start dropping in menopause unless they are balanced with supplemental estrogen.

Stress will block muscle building, causing muscle to be lost (and bone, too). If you are tired after a workout, stress has probably worn out your adrenal glands and you'll need to slow down your exercise program, at least for a while. Moderate exercise is actually a proven stress fighter. Don't forget that stress can destroy the hormones that should be coming from the adrenals (when your ovaries aren't making them) to stop your menopausal symptoms. They can easily get rerouted into stress-coping functions instead. Anything that de-stresses you keeps your estrogen, progesterone, testosterone, and DHEA levels up. See chapter 21 for more on exercise, relaxation, and stress-busting.

ACTION STEPS

1. Use the symptoms lists in chapter 6 to get a sense of which hormones may be out of balance.
2. Use supplements and herbs for PMS and menopausal cravings, mood swings, and other adverse symptoms.
3. Follow the food recommendations—pay attention to what to avoid as well as what to consume.
4. If you suffer from PMS, and the supplements and food recommendations don't eliminate your symptoms, work with a health care

professional and get hormone testing as per the testing suggestions in this chapter.

5. If you are in perimenopause (premenopause) or menopause, nutritional supplements and the Diet Cure's food recommendations will alleviate many of your menopausal symptoms (such as cravings), but you should also get your hormones tested.

6. Find a health care practitioner to work with you.

7. Order hormone testing, thyroid testing, adrenal testing, or bone-density testing, as needed.

8. When results are in, decide which hormone supplements or prescriptions to try.

9. Consider acupuncture or homeopathy.

10. Be sure to get exercise and plenty of relaxation.

11. Keep track of your symptoms and retest to monitor your levels and adjust hormone replacement therapy as needed.

Now that you have access to amino acids, herbs, acupuncture, saliva testing, and natural hormones, you don't need to go on blindly suffering hormonal havoc. You can be freed from discomfort, ill health, and premature aging as a result.

Readings

Ahlgrimm, Marla, R.Ph., *HRT Solution: Optimizing Your Hormone Potential.* (Garden City, NY: Avery, 1998).

Ford, Gillian. *Listening to Your Hormones: From PMS to Menopause, Every Woman's Complete Guide.* (Rocklin, CA: Prima, 1997).

Ikenze, Ifeoma, M.D. *Menopause and Homeopathy.* (Berkeley, CA: North Atlantic Books, 1998).

Laux, Marcus, N.D. *Natural Woman, Natural Menopause.* (New York: Harper Perennial, 1997).

Love, Susan, M.D. *Dr. Susan Love's Hormone Book: Making Informed Choices About Menopause.* (New York: Random House, 1997).

Murray, Michael, N.D. *Premenstrual Syndrome.* (Rocklin, CA: Prima, 1997).

Northrup, Christiane. *Women's Bodies, Women's Wisdom.* (New York: Bantam Books, 1998).

Vliet, Elizabeth, L., M.D. *Screaming to Be Heard: Hormonal Connections Women Suspect and Doctors Ignore.* (New York: M. Evans and Co., 1995).

Waterhouse, Debra, MPH, R.D. *Outsmarting the Midlife Fat Cell.* (New York: Hyperion, 1998).

Resources

See chapter 21 for information on saliva testing and compounding pharmacies and chapter 17 for supplement ordering information.

FIFTEEN

Repairing the
Damage Caused
from Yeasts

All of the other imbalances covered so far in this book have had relatively quick and straightforward solutions that can be implemented
easily, often without professional advice or help. But yeast overgrowth de-
tection and elimination are quite a bit more difficult. Have you been trying for a long time to get rid of this cruel pest? At Recovery Systems we've
spent years developing techniques that would do the job. At first there were
really no effective natural remedies available in health food stores (we tried
them all), so we had to go further afield in ordering supplements. In fact,
our head nutritionist, Timothy Kuss, ended up creating two of his own
products, because he could not find what he needed anywhere.

But now there are some really effective natural remedies available.
What I have done in this chapter, with Tim's help, is to point to the best
supplements available in stores as well as give a description of the methods for killing yeasts that we use at Recovery Systems that may not be available in stores, but that can be ordered from us.

I recommend that you work with a knowledgeable health professional
on this problem. All health professionals have their own ideas about what
works best against this pest. The information here will let them know
what our nutritional staff has found most effective. We haven't varied our
anti-yeast protocol in years, because it kills the yeasts so gently that you
won't feel uncomfortable in the process—and you won't have to restrict
your diet as much as earlier protocols required. (We used to think that
starving the yeasts out by withholding all carbs was the way to go, but it
rarely worked.)

To control yeast overgrowth, you must do five things:

1. Eliminate parasites first, if there is both a yeast and a parasite infection (take a saliva and/or stool test to find out).
2. Gradually but significantly reduce the yeast population of the body with supplements and/or pharmaceuticals.
3. Starve the yeasts by eating fewer carbohydrates (and raising protein and fat).
4. Strengthen the immune system.
5. Rebuild the health of the intestinal tract, which may have been damaged by an extensive yeast (or parasite) infection.

THE ANTI-YEAST EATING PLAN

Your diet holds the key to your becoming yeast-free quickly. It is difficult, if not impossible, to overcome yeasts without avoiding certain foods that promote yeast overgrowth and emphasizing foods with potent anti-yeast qualities. The good news is (1) that anti-yeast supplements are quite effective and allow you to eat a diet with plenty of variety, and (2) this diet does not go on forever. As you kill off the yeast you can gradually start eating all kinds of healthy foods again.

Immune System Boosters

To control and conquer yeasts, the best bet is to make the immune system as strong as possible. Try the following immune system boosters.

✦ Get plenty of dry heat and sunlight. Yeast thrives in wet, cold, and damp conditions; it is less of a problem in hot, dry climates. Homes with little natural sunlight or that have mold or mildew promote yeast overgrowth. Get out and enjoy the sun for a short while every day to boost your natural immunity. Avoid damp, cold, poorly ventilated places.
✦ Avoid exposure to toxins. Toxins that can lower immunity include chemical sprays and solvents as well as highly processed foods (you know, the ones that have ingredients on the label that you can't pronounce). Be sure to read chapter 18 to bone up on the best foods for keeping your immune system strong.
✦ Exercise. Lymph, the fluid that removes bacteria from the body (our "immunity" fluid) doesn't move much unless we move our leg muscles and arm muscles.

✦ Relax. Any form of relaxing activity, whether it's meditation, yoga, or massage, or doing something you love, such as gardening or walking in nature, actually boosts immunity. Test your adrenal function to see if stress has lowered it so much that it cannot support your immune system. See chapters 3 and 11 for testing and adrenal repair information.

✦ Get acupuncture. This ancient Chinese art of healing helps restore the immune, digestive, and eliminative systems as well as the adrenal glands. Acupuncture also eases the discomfort of detoxifying considerably, which makes it very helpful when you are eliminating yeasts and the toxins they have created in your body.

✦ Consume more garlic. Garlic, in food or as a supplement, boosts immunity overall as well as fights yeasts and parasites.

✦ Drink plenty of fluids. Purified water and teas such as ginger, pau d'arco, hyssop, spearmint, or raspberry all boost immunity. A ginger and pau d'arco blend is particularly therapeutic, and the ginger flavor makes the pau d'arco more appealing. If you don't like ginger, substitute spearmint instead.

Restore Your Digestive Fire

According to Oriental and Ayurvedic medicine, the digestive process is supposed to be a "hot" one. To break down food, the stomach requires ample hydrochloric acid, and other digestive enzymes. When you have too much yeast, this digestive fire is squelched or reduced. An effective way to rekindle that flame is to use warming foods, such as ginger, oregano, cinnamon, cloves, and black pepper, all of which increase gastric secretions and assimilation of nutrients.

(Caution: Do not use the these warming foods if you have an ulcer or tend to have stomach sensitivity, or find them too stimulating.)[1]

Foods to Avoid

Alcohol and yeast-containing foods	alcohol, alcohol-containing foods, baker's yeast.
Dairy	milk and cheese from cows, cottage cheese, sweetened yogurt (Remember: the lactose in these foods is a form of sugar, which the yeasts feed on, and cheese is a fungal product, which encourages

	yeast growth.) However, butter and unsweetened yogurt are usually okay.
Fermented food products	apple cider vinegar, other vinegars (except rice vinegar), hops, malts, soy sauce, pickles, pickled vegetables.
Fruits	Just in the beginning, you won't be able to eat any fresh fruit at all, let alone dried fruit or fruit juices (which I hope you will mostly avoid, even off the anti-yeast program).
Mushrooms	ALL types.
Processed meats	marbled meats, all processed and smoked meats, bacon, sausage, corned beef, ham, MSG (because it causes meat cravings), and others.
Starches	grains in general (with the exception of whole rice, corn, and millet), bread, cookies, gravies, muffins, pancakes, pasta, sauces, tapioca, waffles, French fries.
Sweets	(Things you won't eat anyway for your Diet Cure) candy of all kinds, soda pop, desserts, sugar (white, brown, raw), honey, molasses, turbinado sugar, maple syrup, rice syrup, sweeteners (malt, corn sweetener, date sugar, sucrose, fructose, high fructose corn syrup, mannitol, NutraSweet or aspartame, saccharine), catsup, mayonnaise, barbecue sauce.

This list is not comprehensive because while there are many theories about foods that can introduce yeasts into the system, a lot is still unknown. If you're unsure about a particular food, check with a nutritionist or other experienced health professional.

The First Four Weeks

For the first four weeks, you will need to emphasize the nutrient-rich foods listed below. And it will help a lot to incorporate the foods known to have anti-yeast and anti-fungal properties.

Safe Foods

Eggs	cooked at a low temperature
Freshly prepared soups	without cream or milk
Fresh nuts and seeds	preferably soaked in water overnight
Goat cheese, unsweetened yogurt made from cow's milk, and buttermilk	For those not dairy intolerant, they supply good bacteria and are not sweet
Legumes	beans, lentils, peas (one serving per day)
Protein	fish, antibiotic-free poultry, beef, lamb
Tofu	Soft or hard
Vegetables	particularly steamed or lightly sautéed
Whole grains	basmati rice, millet, amaranth, quinoa, or corn (one moderate serving per day)

Anti-Yeast, Anti-Fungal Foods

+ Broccoli
+ Brussels sprouts
+ Cabbage
+ Cinnamon, cloves, oregano, rosemary, sage, thyme, tumeric
+ Collards
+ Fresh lemon as a flavoring (to help the body detoxify)
+ Garlic
+ Kale
+ Olive oil, flax oils
+ Onions

What Is the Recovery Process Like?

If you slip on the eating plan, don't despair: *just stay with the program*. You haven't blown it. The supplements will still be working.

As the anti-yeast supplements and your special diet kill off and neutralize the organisms, you should quickly lose your cravings, bloating, and other symptoms. However, occasionally the process of eliminating yeasts can cause adverse reactions such as diarrhea and flulike symptoms caused when so many yeast organisms are killed quickly that your eliminative organs have trouble removing them. If necessary, cut back or stop the supplements for several days. The good news is that these uncomfortable reactions usually don't last long. And on the supplement plan that we use now, these "die-off" reactions are very rare. But one of the reasons that I recommend you work with an experienced yeast die-off expert is so that you'll have someone to talk to about the process. How long you need to stay on the anti-yeast program depends on how long yeast overgrowth has been present; the state and competency of your immune, digestive, and endocrine systems; and how closely you stick to the anti-yeast diet. It can take up to six months to overcome yeast overgrowth, but normally it takes from two to three months. How do you know it's gone? Retake the questionnaire and retake at least the saliva test after three months of your yeast-killing program. If you stop too soon, your yeast will just grow back and quickly make you feel bloated and miserable again. This has happened to many of our clients before they came to us.

Other Steps
+ Use flavorings such as onion, curry, and pepper (in moderation).
+ For oils, use flax, olive, canola, Better Butter (half butter, half oil), grape seed, sesame, and sunflower oils.
+ Be sure to drink eight 8-ounce glasses of water a day. Squeeze a little lemon juice into water and drink it before meals to support the liver in its yeast-expulsion effort. Other liquids to enjoy are vegetable juices and teas (pau d'arco, ginger, and/or spearmint).
+ Chlorophyll products, such as Chlorella, Spirulina, alfalfa, or barley, can be used as supplements or added into smoothies.

After the First Four Weeks

Now add a piece of fruit and observe the response. If you bloat up and crave more sweet things after the experimental apple (or other fruit), wait another week or two before adding fruit back in. The same goes for starchy grains or beans. Experiment and see for yourself. You'll usually be ready by week four to expand the amount of carbohydrate you can eat.

Alcohol, sugar, and some other substances cannot be reintroduced. The only reason fruit can be added back in so quickly is the effectiveness of the anti-yeast supplements used in our program. Without them, fruit would have to be withheld for an additional four to six weeks or longer.

SUPPLEMENTS FOR TREATING YEASTS

Please note: This program is only for yeast and fungal infections that have gotten out of hand, not for the rare vaginal infection or a bout of athlete's foot.

One of our yeast recovery success stories was Risa, a blue-eyed brunette who played the violin professionally and who had suffered with chronic yeast infections. For three years they flared up every month before her periods. She sometimes bloated so much that people thought she might be pregnant. She ate almost nothing but carbs and was spacey and miserable. Her score on the yeast questionnaire—the same one that you have on page 93—was 300! (It's supposed to be under 100.) On our anti-yeast program, she lost her cravings and most of her bloat in the first week. She used a special douche in addition to the oral supplements so that by her next period she was free of her vaginal symptoms, too. When she retook her questionnaire, her score was 59!

Risa, like other Recovery Systems clients, took combination herbal remedies to fight her infection. A number of outstanding herbs exhibit potent and proven anti-yeast properties, but most herbalists agree that combination herbal remedies are much more effective than taking any one herb alone. The following herbs are generally available through both health professionals and health food stores.*

---

* You can send for the exact supplements used in the Recovery Systems program. It contains most of the "generic" supplements plus others not available in stores. See the resources section for this chapter.

Ingredients for Your Anti-Yeast Supplement Program

✦ Multiflora. This is one lactobacillus-bifidus product. It restores and maintains normal intestinal flora.

✦ Pau d'arco. This South American herb contains three anti-yeast compounds that are active against *Candida albicans* and fungi. Pau d'arco is effective in tea, liquid extract, and capsule form.

✦ Grapefruit seed extract (GSE). GSE kills yeasts but is nontoxic to humans. GSE, which comes in liquid concentrate form or in capsules, may also be used as a skin cleanser, gargle, douche, and as a traveler's aid to minimize gastrointestinal problems (it discourages parasites, too).

✦ Garlic inhibits microbes of all kinds, including yeasts and parasites. Garlic is most active in raw form, fresh, on food, or it may be taken in capsule form: one to three times daily, with meals. Most people use a combination of the two (3 capsules is equal to a medium clove of fresh garlic). To help counter the powerful smell, chew one or more of the following herbal breath fresheners: parsley, fenugreek, or fennel.

✦ Oregano oil packs a wallop against a wide range of fungi and yeasts and has antiparasitic properties as well. Caution: The vast majority of oregano oil is mislabeled, because it is actually derived from thyme and marjoram, and is not nearly as effective. If you use the oil form instead of the capsules, you can place 2 drops, the equivalent of 1 capsule, into soup, or put it into an empty capsule if you dislike the taste.

✦ Ginger inhibits both fungus and yeast while promoting the growth of friendly bacteria like lactobacillus acidophilus.

✦ Biotin is a B vitamin that helps stop sugar cravings and has a surprisingly inhibitory effect on yeasts.

An Anti-Yeast Protocol

✦ *Upon arising:* Take 2 capsules of a combination of the good bacteria— lactobacillus acidophilus and bifidus, on an empty stomach. (The best, like DDS, are found in the refrigerator in health stores.)

✦ *With meals:* 1 to 2 capsules of grapefruit seed extract, 1 capsule of biotin (1,000 micrograms), 2 capsules or a small clove of garlic, and oregano oil.

✦ *Anytime:* Drink pau d'arco and ginger tea.

✦ *Optional:* Include one or more of the other herbs just mentioned.

Yeasts That Won't Go Away

If you have been treated for a yeast overgrowth for three months or longer, and you are not well on the road to recovery, one or more of the following conditions may be a factor that you'll need to discuss with a health professional:

✦ Epstein-Barr virus (EBV), cytomegalovirus (CMV) or chronic fatigue syndrome
✦ Parasites or microbial organisms (Giardia, amoebas, and others)
✦ Hepatitis C
✦ Overly alkaline body pH
✦ Chronic gallbladder problems
✦ Allergies to foods listed above, and to supplemental therapy

---

You will need to work closely with a health practitioner on a program that should include combining these yeast fighters with the foods described earlier. At Recovery Systems we use these nutrients and a few others that are not available in stores in a three-month protocol that you can send for from us. (See Resources at the end of the chapter.)

DRUG TREATMENT FOR YEASTS

In a small minority of cases, certain people do not respond as expected to the herbal-based anti-yeast program. If these individuals have also been tested for parasites and none have been found, we usually refer them to a physician for a course of the anti-fungal medication Diflucan (Fluconazole). Diflucan is the most effective drug treatment for yeast and fungal overgrowth. It is also less toxic to the liver than Nizarol (Ketoconazole) and Nystatin, the other two common anti-yeast, anti-fungal drugs.

Unfortunately, Diflucan is quite expensive. At the time of publication in early 1999, a single 200-milligram tablet costs $17.85. For yeast/fungal overgrowth it is usually taken once a day for one to three months; you can do the math. If you take Diflucan, you are likely to experience a die-off reaction in the third week of taking the drug. Be prepared for this; otherwise, you may conclude you're getting worse. To minimize the die-off reaction, drink extra fluids, get plenty of vitamin C, and/or take epsom salt soak baths (3 cups of epsom salts to a bathtub of water).

*   *   *

It will take a few months and some hard work to get rid of your yeasts once and for all, but I promise that you will start feeling better right away, which should encourage you to finish the kill-off meticulously. There is life after yeasts!

ACTION STEPS

1. Get a saliva and/or stool test.
2. Find and organize your special supplements as you get started with the basics in chapter 17.
3. Start the anti-yeast diet for four weeks.
4. After four weeks, gradually liberalize the diet.
5. Retest at four months.
6. Use an alternative medical approach, if needed.

Readings

Crook, William G., M.D. *The Yeast Connection Handbook* (Jackson, TN: Professional Books, 1999).

De Schepper, Luc, M.D., Ph.D., C.A. *Candida* (Santa Monica, CA: DeSchepper Publishing, 1986).

Galland, Leo, M.D. *The Four Pillars of Healing* (New York: Random House, 1997).

Murray, Michael, N.D. *Chronic Candidiasis: The Yeast Syndrome* (Rockin, CA: Prima, 1997).

Tips, Jack., N.D., Ph.D. *Conquer Candida: Restore Your Immune System* (Austin, TX: Apple-a-Day Press, 1989).

Resources

For help finding a health professional and testing for yeasts and parasites, see the resources for chapter 21.

For saliva and blood antibody testing for yeast and parasites:

Immuno Sciences

(800) 950-4686

For stool testing for yeasts and parasites:

Institute of Parasitic Diseases

(602) 955-4211

Great Smokies Lab

for practitioners: (800) 522-4762

for individuals: (888) 891-3061

For anti-yeast and anti-parasite protocols, or Recovery Systems' yeast- or parasite-control supplements, call (800) 733-9293.

SIXTEEN

The Fatty Acid Fix

Y ou're probably more than ready to turn off your fat cravings. Start out
by getting familiar with the symptoms in chapter 8, so that you'll have a
sense of whether you are essential fatty acid (EFA) deficient, have a lack of fat-
digesting enzymes, a liver–gallbladder problem, or parasites. Because you've
probably been eating too many junk fats and carbohydrates, you should get
your cholesterol tested right away, along with other tests I'll detail here.

In this chapter you will learn how to get more of the essential fatty
acids into your diet and less of the junk fats and carbs that you don't need.
You'll also learn about supplements that end those powerful cravings for
rich or greasy foods. I'll also fill you in on a few ways to boost your liver
function if it is not up to speed, so that you can be sure your body is handling fats properly and you are not risking damage to these vital organs.

If you think you're incapable of giving up doughnuts, chips, or ice
cream, please don't despair. I know you'll be pleasantly surprised by how
little they tempt you once you start getting your fatty acid fix.

TESTING

If too many fats (especially junk fats) and carbos have been on your
menu, it's time to find out if they have elevated your cholesterol. Get blood
testing done to check for:

✦ Elevated cholesterol levels, and, more important, a determination of the
 ratio between the two kinds of cholesterol (the ratio of LDL to HDL,
 which should be less than 2 to 5).

✦ Elevated homocysteine levels. (These are the very best indicators of too much fatty buildup in your arteries.)

✦ Deficient levels of the two essential fats, omega-3 and omega-6, in your blood.

Your wholistic physician can arrange this test for you and work with a lab like Great Smokies (see the resources at the end of chapter 21).

You'll see elevated blood levels come down as you start to use the nutritional techniques recommended in this and other chapters. Retest in three to six months and dazzle your doctor.

If you suspect a liver or gallbladder problem, it's a good idea to get a physical examination, to see if your liver is oversized or hard, as well as a blood test. Check the levels of your liver enzymes, and check for hepatitis A, B, and C. (Liver enzymes are not usually elevated in the blood except in conditions like alcoholism.) If you suspect a parasite, see the end of chapter 7 for specific suggestions for testing and treating parasites.

FOODS THAT DISCOURAGE FAT CRAVINGS AND RESTORE OMEGA FAT BALANCE

Essential Fish

To be sure you are getting enough healthy fat and to get rid of fat cravings, you'll need to monitor your intake of essential fats. First, to restore omega-3, at least twice a week you should eat the fish listed in chapter 8. (If you have "fishy" genes, that is, if you come from ancestors who were fish eaters, you should eat this type of fish more often.) These fish include salmon (especially the meat near the skin),* sardines (especially those packed in their own oil), fresh tuna (most canned tuna has had the fat extracted), mackerel, and herring. (See chapter 8 for a complete list.)[1]

Getting enough omega-6 is easy. Have a small handful of raw seeds or nuts every day or put them in a breakfast smoothie with fruit and protein powder. Any vegetable oil contains plenty of omega-6, too.

Oils

Almost all oils contain some of all of the four basic kinds of fats—the two essential fats and two nonessential fats—in some ratio, but oils with a good balance of omega-3 to omega-6 are rare.

---

*While this is the part most likely to be contaminated by pollutants, it's also, unfortunately, the best source of omega-3 in the fish.

Get the Fat!

Eight to 10 percent of our food intake should be composed of omega-3 and omega-6 fats in a ratio of 1 to 2 or less.[2]

For your salads, use oils with the best ratio of omega-3 to omega-6: flax, hemp (it's legal, and no, it doesn't contain the intoxicant THC), canola, walnut, and olive. Vary them as much as possible. Although olive is the lowest in omega-3 content, it's even lower in omega-6 oils (which is good). It lowers cholesterol and does not block omega-3 function, as other vegetable oils do. For cooking, use canola or olive oil. Also, note that olive oil burns at a lower temperature than canola. (Grapeseed oil burns at an even higher temperature than canola does, and it reduces triglycerides, though it is low in omega-3.)

Dark Green Leafy Vegetables

Dark green leafy vegetables are another source of omega-3. To eat more of these, try chard, kale, spinach, arugula, collard, mustard greens, dandelion, and mesclun salad mix.

Walnuts

Walnuts are the only nut besides the Brazil nut with enough omega-3 to balance omega-6 effectively. Most nuts and seeds are much higher in omega-6 than omega-3 oils. Eat walnuts only when they are fresh, in the fall and winter, unless they are left in the shell and cracked just before eating. You can try freezing them as well. The packaged, shelled variety get rancid faster than any other nuts.

FATTY FOODS TO
MODERATE BUT NOT SHUN

Butterfat, Animal Fat, Vegetable Oils
(Soybean, Peanut, Sesame, and Others)

Butter is a neutral fat that has a few health benefits used in moderation. Fats that we used to think were safer than butter are the fragile vegetable oils, like corn and safflower. They actually become rancid quickly when exposed to heat and light, because they are overrefined. Though they contain good amounts of the omega-6 fatty acids, we can easily get too much of them, causing the omega-3 deficiency symptoms that are so common now. Unrefined, early press versions, which are available at health food stores, contain unprocessed elements, like vitamin E, that keep these oils more stable.

The junk fats are the chemically fried fats: margarine and other "partially hydrogenated" vegetable oils (that is, shortening), found in most packaged foods like cookies and crackers. Read labels, because hydrogenated, even partially hydrogenated, means that the oils have been fried with hydrogen and metal for six to eight hours. This converts them from their natural liquid state into solid, indigestible trans-fats that are unquestionably linked to heart disease. (Why are these fats still served in our hospitals?) A trans-fat is a mystery fat. Your body doesn't know what to do with it, so it gets in the way of your blood flow—*seriously* in the way—clogging your arteries.

Oils that are used repeatedly for deep-fat frying become health hazards, even if they are basically stable, like coconut or palm oils. (Most other oils are damaged by even one deep frying. All of these fried fats block or destroy the essential omega fats and the fat-soluble vitamins D, E, A, and K).[3]

So run from margarine and any other fully or "partially hydrogenated" trans-fats.[4] Read your labels! Avoid fried foods. Moderate your use of butter and omega-6 vegetable, seed, and bean oils—soy, corn, safflower, peanut, sunflower, and cottonseed. Favor canola, flax, and olive oils.

Alcoholism, Depression, and Oil

As I explained in chapter 8, if you are from a family that is Scandinavian, Irish, Scottish, Welsh, or coastal Native American, you are more likely to suffer from alcoholism and depression, because of a lack of fish oils in your diet. Depression and cravings for alcohol, as well as fat, can usually be relieved by the use of supplements containing DHA from fish oil. No matter what your genetic background, if you crave fats, try some omega-3 fish oil.[5] If you belong to one of these groups but do not want to use fish oil, use flax and algae oils together as described below to get the same effect.

Supplements That Stop Your Fat Cravings

The following supplements should be added to the basic supplements in chapter 17:

✦ **Fish oil** capsules contain the essence of the omega-3 oils: EPA and DHA. Remember, 95 percent of us are deficient in these precious oils. And some of us cannot break down omega-3 vegetable oils (like flax) into these two precious breakdown products and must get them directly from fish. (Red and brown seaweed are the only other direct sources.) Take 2,000 milligrams per day.

If you are a vegetarian or can't digest the fish oil caps, flax seed oil is the next closest thing to fish oil (only without the EPA and DHA that some genetic types need). But you can supplement your flax oil by ordering supplements made from DHA-rich algae oil. A dose of 100 milligrams twice per day (at breakfast and dinner) gives the same DHA as that in two fish oil capsules.

✦ **Lipase** is the specific digestive enzyme that helps you break down the fats you eat. You can find it as part of a complete digestive enzyme supplement that also includes enzymes that help digest proteins and carbohydrates. But you can get it by itself, too. Look for a product containing lipase with 8,000 USP units.

The nutrients that are most crucial for helping you to utilize all of your essential and other fats are included in the basic supplement plan. Vitamins A and E (both fat-soluble vitamins) work together with vitamin C and the mineral selenium to protect all the fats in your body from oxidation (that is, rancidity). Vitamin A is especially instrumental in keeping your skin moist and oiled. Most of the oils that you use have had their protective vitamin E removed so that they'll look pretty in their clear bottles. You'll have to put vitamin E back in. Vitamin E will repay your effort generously by protecting you from stroke and cataracts. It will also prevent the vitamin E–deficiency brown spots on

Supplements

	AM	B	MM	L	MA	D	BT*
❏ Omega-3 (fish oil caps with DHA and EPA), 1,000 mg	—	1	—	—	—	1	—
OR:							
❏ Flax oil caps, 1,000 mg	—	1	—	1	—	1	—
or liquid with	—	2 tbs	—	—	—	2 tbs†	—
EPA-rich algae oil, 100 mg	—	1	—	1	—	1	—

For Liver and Gallbladder Problems

❏ Milk thistle 300 mg	—	2	—	—	—	2	—

As a Fat Digestion Aid:

❏ Lipase, at least 8,000 USP units	—	1	—	1	—	1	—

* AM=on arising; B=breakfast; MM=midmorning; L=with lunch; MA=midafternoon; D=with dinner; BT=at bedtime.
† Down to 1 T (4 caps) two times a day in three months. If you need to, start at this low dose, too.

the backs of your hands from collecting in your brain as well. Selenium may have earned its reputation as a cancer fighter from its ability to guard the layer of fat around every one of our bodies' cells. All the B vitamins tremendously enhance the effectiveness of the omega oils that you take in.

Liver and Gallbladder Problems

Consult a wholistic professional about any liver and gallbladder problems. Acupuncturists, in particular, can often be effective in diagnosing and treating liver and gallbladder problems. They are actually the only health professionals I know of who can successfully treat the liver for hepatitis C (which is stumping Western medicine entirely) and help with liver cirrhosis, too (though milk thistle has a good track record there). When we see symptoms of liver problems, the first thing we do is to suggest an herb that has convinced even the medical community that natural methods can be remarkable: milk thistle. This herb is tremendously helpful to the liver in its vital job of filtering toxic or useless substances out of our bodies. If it is clogged with toxins, the liver can't process fats properly. Take 300 milligrams of milk thistle twice a day.

I hope by now I've gotten you over your fat fear. As you will discover in chapters 18, 19, and 20, there are plenty of delicious foods you can eat without triggering fat cravings or causing weight gain—foods that will give you a fatty acid fix without jeopardizing your health.

ACTION STEPS

1. Review your symptoms to decide whether you need to explore essential oil supplements, liver/gallbladder repair, fat-digesting enzymes, or possible parasites.
2. Test for your essential fatty acid levels now, and retest after you've been on your program for three months.
3. Test for your cholesterol and homocysteine levels.
4. Test for any liver or parasite problems.
5. Take fish or flax oil, and oils with a good omega-3 and omega-6 ratio.
6. Avoid unhealthy fats.
7. Select and begin your supplement program.
8. Get acupuncture, if you need to, for liver and gallbladder problems.
9. Be sure to read chapter 2 on the dangers of low-calorie dieting and chapter 18 on selecting the best foods for your special biochemistry.

Readings

Gittleman, Ann Louise, M.S. *Beyond Pritikin* (New York: Bantam Books, 1996).

Kuss, Timothy, Ph.D. *A Guidebook to Clinical Nutrition for the Health Professional* (Pleasant Hill, CA: Institute of Bioenergetic Research, 1992).

Pizzorno, Joseph, N. D., and Michael Murray, N.D. *The Encyclopedia of Natural Medicine* (Rocklin, CA: Prima, 1998).

Rudin, D., M.D., and Clara Felix. *Omega-3 Oils: A Practical Guide* (Garden City, NY: Avery, 1996).

Simopoulos, Artemis, M.D. *The Omega Plan* (New York: HarperCollins, 1998).

Udo, Erasmus. *Fats That Heal, Fats That Kill.* (Burnaby, BC, Canada: Alive Books, 1993).

Resources

For directions on how to contact wholistic health practitioners, see Resources in Chapter 21.

SUPPLEMENTS

Fish oil capsules are widely available, as are flax. Vegetarians can supplement their flax oil by ordering supplements made from DHA-rich algae oil. Call (800) 522-5512. Martek Biosciences Corporation sells both retail and to practitioners.

Part III

Your Master Plan for the Diet Cure

SEVENTEEN

Your Master Nutritional Supplement Plan

U p to now, you've been identifying your body's imbalances and learning how to use supplements to correct each of them nutritionally.
Now it's time to put it all together in a master supplement plan. Your master supplement plan will be laid out in two parts: (1) the basic supplements
that you'll be taking regardless of which imbalances you have and that
you'll need to take long-term, and (2) the special repair supplements targeted at specific imbalances, which you'll be taking short-term.

Every one of the supplements recommended in this book will be listed
here in this chapter. The basic supplements list will include suggested
amounts. The special repair supplements list will be left blank so that you
can fill it with the amounts you decide to take, based on the recommendations in part II, chapters 9–16.

I have tried to list supplements that you'll be able to find in health food
stores, through mail order sources, and in some drugstores. Starred (*)
supplements need to be special ordered (by you or through your health
consultant) because they cannot usually be found in stores or catalogs. I
have listed these less accessible supplements only when I knew of no other
supplement that worked well for the particular purpose. This doesn't
mean that good options don't exist, but that at our clinic we have not discovered or used them. These less accessible supplements or any of the exact supplements we use for our clients can be ordered from our clinic's
supplement order line: (800) 733-9293.

YOUR MASTER SUPPLEMENT PLAN

You'll need to take quite a few supplements at first. Then over the next three to twelve months, as you establish consistently more nutritious eating habits, you'll cut down to the six most basic supplements. These you should probably continue to take permanently. You should always reintroduce your special repair supplements again, if you need them temporarily in the future to get you over any rough times.

The Basic Supplement Plan

I have been alluding to the basic supplement plan throughout the book because it really is the basis for your Diet Cure, along with your new foods. The broad collection of supplements included in this basic plan are intended to restore any nutrient depletions you have (we all have them) and to keep your nutrient levels strong permanently.

One of our nutritional consultants has been doing very detailed diet analyses for years. She has never found any diet, including the rich and healthy diets of superathletes, that contains 100 percent of the essential nutrients at even the most minimal (R.D.A.) levels. There are just too many obstacles— among them heat, light, age, processing, and inadequate soil—between you and the amount of nutrients it takes to keep you happy and healthy.

This basic collection of vital nutrients is intended to be safe enough to take permanently yet potent enough (in combination with your new foods) that they can actually correct a few of your imbalances without any additional special repair supplements.

Multivitamin/mineral: A good multivitamin/mineral really is crucial and is the crown jewel of your basic program. Look at the results of just two of many studies on the use of multis like the one you'll be taking (for the rest of your life, I hope).

1. A study of four hundred women found that taking a multi gave a 50 percent lower risk of having babies with any congenital abnormality![1]
2. A ten-year study of nine hundred people found that taking a multi lowered the risk of colon cancer by half![2]

Our clinic used and discarded dozens of multis as better formulations appeared, until five years ago when we finally found a multi that satisfied us. This supplement, Glucobalance, is wonderful for most people who need

Nutrient Contents for Suggested Dose per Day

	GLUCOBALANCE	MY FAVORITE MULTIPLE	ALLERGY MULTI
Number suggested to take per day	In 6 capsules:	In 6 capsules or 4 tablets:	In 6 capsules:
❏ Vitamin A	5,000 IU	5,000 IU	10,000 IU
❏ Beta carotene		5,000 IU	15,000 IU
❏ B₁ (thiamin)	50 mg	50 mg	25 mg
❏ B₂ (riboflavin)	25 mg	50 mg	25 mg
❏ B₆ (pyridoxine)	30 mg	50 mg	50 mg
❏ B₁₂	50 mcg	50 mcg	100 mcg
❏ Niacin	30 mg	50 mg	
❏ Niacinamide	120 mg		100 mg
❏ Pantothenic acid	100 mg	50 mg	50 mg
❏ Biotin	3000 mcg	300 mcg	150 mcg
❏ Folic acid	800 mcg	400 mcg	400 mcg
❏ PABA		50 mg	25 mg
❏ Choline		50 mg	25 mg
❏ Inositol		50 mg	25 mg
❏ Vitamin C	500 mg	250 mg	1000 mg
❏ Vitamin D	100 IU	400 IU	400 IU
❏ Vitamin E	600 IU	400 IU	400 IU
❏ *(Vitamin E needed in addition to multi)*	*(200 IU)*	*(400 IU)*	*(400 IU)*
❏ Chromium	1000 mcg	200 mcg	200 mcg
❏ *(Chromium needed to add to multi)*	*(none)*	*(600 mcg)*	*(600 mcg)*
❏ Calcium	200 mg	1000 mg	1000 mg
❏ *(Calcium needed in addition to multi)*	*(500– 700 mg)*	*(250– 350 mg)*	*(250– 350 mg)*
❏ Magnesium	400 mg	400 mg	500 mg
❏ *(Magnesium needed in addition to multi)*	*(400 mg)*	*(400 mg)*	*(400 mg)*
❏ Potassium	99 mg	99 mg	99 mg
❏ Zinc	30 mg	25 mg	30 mg
❏ Manganese	20 mg	2 mg	10 mg
❏ Copper	2 mg	2 mg	2 mg
❏ Vanadium	20 mcg		
❏ Selenium	150 mcg	50 mcg	200 mcg
❏ Iodine		150 mcg	

	GLUCOBALANCE	MY FAVORITE MULTIPLE	ALLERGY MULTI
Number suggested to take per day	In 6 capsules:	In 6 capsules or 4 tablets:	In 6 capsules:
❏ Boron		200 mcg	
❏ Molybdenum		50 mcg	500 mcg
❏ Iron	None	Optional 18 mg	10 mg
❏ L-carnitine	30 mg		
❏ Bioflavonoids		150 mg	
Available from*			
NEEDS	Yes	Yes	Yes
The Vitamin Shoppe	Yes	Yes	Yes
Vitamin Express	Yes	Yes	Yes
L & H Vitamins	No	Yes	Yes
General Nutrition Center	No	Yes	Yes
Your local health store	Some, or by order	Many, or by order	Many, or by order
Your local drugstores	No	Some	Some

*See Resources in chapter 19 for supplement source information.
Note: Those of you who hate swallowing pills can find sublingual, chewable, powdered, and sprayed supplements through knowledgeable health practitioners and employees of good health stores. Your trouble swallowing may be due to an enlarged thyroid (the thyroid gland sits in your throat). That's been the case with a number of our clients.

a Diet Cure. Health food stores and supplement mail order houses can get it for you if they don't actually carry it in stock. In case you need an alternative to Glucobalance, I will also list two other multis our nutritionists have determined to be high in quality. So that you'll know exactly what a good multi is, I'm going to lay out the contents of all three multis, as well as give you information on how to locate them. Get your knowledgeable supplement specialist to help you make sure you get a multi that is equivalent in quality to these three. Unfortunately, it is impossible to get enough of the nutrients you need in good multis without taking four to six of them per day. If you just can't manage to take a lunchtime dose, you could divide your whole day's dose in two and take half at breakfast and half at dinner.

You'll see in the foregoing chart just how many valuable nutrients are packed into a multi. But even the best multis plus the best foods can't provide enough of certain nutrients. The chart also includes the amounts of four basic nutrients you'll need to take in addition to your multi. When selecting a multi, keep in mind that *men and menopausal women who regularly eat red meat should avoid more than 18 milligrams of added iron.* (Menstruating women can handle iron safely because they are always losing any excess in menstrual fluid.) For enormously readable and up-to-date details on why you need each of the vitamins and minerals in your multi, read *The Vitamin Nutrient Solution* by Robert Atkins, M.D.

Here are our recommendations:

NAME OF MANUFACTURER	NAME OF MULTIVITAMIN/ MINERAL PRODUCT
1) Biotics Research (Probiologic)	Glucobalance* (no iron)
2) Natrol	My Favorite Multiple capsules/ tablets; My Favorite Multiple capsules/tablets w/o iron
3) Twin Lab	Allergy Multi (little iron)

Basic Magnesium and Calcium. Even very good multis, such as the three I've presented here, rarely contain enough of the minerals calcium and magnesium. These two minerals are too bulky to fit into a multi capsule or tablet along with all the other nutrients, since you need quite a bit of both. Glucobalance lacks enough of both calcium and magnesium. Twin Lab's and Natrol's contain enough calcium but not enough magnesium.

Calcium's importance for building and protecting bone is now well established, but you may not know that calcium also helps with sleep and protects against colon cancer. Calcium has an inseparable mate, the mineral magnesium, that is deficient in 80 percent of us yet is even more vital than calcium. It protects us from heart attack, Alzheimer's, constipation, low blood sugar, diabetes, eating disorders, chronic fatigue, low thyroid, PMS, and osteoporosis (to name only a few of its 325 benefits.)[3]

Also, like all minerals, calcium and magnesium need to come from well-absorbed sources that need to be carefully chosen. (This is particularly important for magnesium, which can otherwise causes diarrhea.) The most reliably absorbed minerals are chelated; that is, they are bound to tiny amino acids that transport them into your bloodstream. Solgar and

Special Note for Vegans

If you eat *no* animal products including fish, chicken, milk products, or eggs, your basic supplement plan may not give you all the extra nutrients you'll need. Check your multi's contents against the following suggested amounts of key nutrients and get any extra supplements you'll need to get up to these levels.

Vitamin B_{12}	100–400 mcg daily (less, if you are under 40)
Vitamin D	400 IU daily
L-carnitine	500–1000 mg daily
Zinc	25 mg daily
Selenium	100–200 mcg daily

People with blood type A (the natural vegetarians) are often deficient in hydrochloric acid (HCl) and may have to take extra, up to 600 milligrams per meal total. Do not take *any* HCl if you have an ulcer.

Carlson brands provide superior (Albion) chelated calcium and magnesium. Their products can be found in stores or ordered easily.

Calcium and magnesium are listed right underneath your multi on your basic supplement plan below. Magnesium is to be taken with breakfast and lunch while calcium should be taken at bedtime.

Basic Vitamin B Complex. All eight imbalances require the B complex vitamins for repair and permanent balance maintenance. The B content of your multi won't be high enough to do the job without extra B complex taken between meals to keep levels constantly optimal.

The coenzymate form of the B complex is rapidly utilized by your body. It won't upset your stomach and will reliably do its priceless work. Because coenzymated vitamins are already bound to the necessary amino acid and mineral cofactors, you'll need to take only half as much as you would of a standard B vitamin. Source Naturals' Coenzymate B Complex, sublingual (dissolve under the tongue) peppermint- or orange-flavored, has been excellent with our clients.

Others with extreme blood sugar sensitivity may respond poorly to the sweetener in the Source Naturals' product. Country Life's version, Coenzyme B-Complex, is available in capsules without sweetener.

Master Supplement Plan

Basic Supplement Plan

Supplement	AM	B	MM	L	MA	D	BT*
❏ Multivitamin/mineral	—	2	—	(2)†	—	2	—
❏ Calcium 250–350 mg	—	—	—	—	—	—	1–2
❏ Magnesium 200 mg	—	2	—	2	—	—	—
❏ B complex 10–50 mg	—	—	1	—	1	—	—
❏ Vitamin C with bioflavonoids (1,000 mg C and 200–500 mg bioflav.)	—	1	—	—	—	1	—
❏ Vitamin E 400 IU	—	1	—	—	—	—	—
❏ Fish oil or flax oil 1,000 mg	—	1	—	—	—	1	—
❏ Chromium 200 mcg (not needed with Glucobalance)	—	1	—	1	—	1	—

Special Repair Supplements

Supplement	AM	B	MM	L	MA	D	BT*

Chapter 9: Refueling Your Brain Chemistry

	AM	B	MM	L	MA	D	BT*
❏ L-Glutamine, 500 mg	—	—	—	—	—	—	—
❏ GABA 100–500 mg‡	—	—	—	—	—	—	—
❏ L-tyrosine, 500 mg	—	—	—	—	—	—	—
❏ L-phenylalanine, 500 mg	—	—	—	—	—	—	—
❏ DLPA, 500 mg or DPA, 500 mg	—	—	—	—	—	—	—
❏ 5-hydroxytryptophan (5-HTP), 50 mg or L-tryptophan (by prescription) 500 mg	—	—	—	—	—	—	—
❏ St. John's Wort, 300 mg (with 900 mcg [0.3%] hypericin)	—	—	—	—	—	—	—
❏ Complete essential amino acids, 500 mg	—	—	—	—	—	—	—

*AM=on arising; B=with breakfast; MM=midmorning; L=with lunch; MA=midafternoon; D=with dinner; BT=at bedtime.

†If you are taking My Favorite Multiple tablets, it won't be necessary to take any at lunch as there are only four a day to take.

‡GABA Calm by Source Naturals and Amino Relaxer by Country Life combine GABA with calming aminos taurine and glycine.

Supplement	AM	B	MM	L	MA	D	BT*

Chapter 10: Nutritional Rehab for the Ex-Dieter

Anorectics and bulimics add the following supplements:

❏ Liquid Zinc (only Ethical
   Nutrients' Zinc Status or
   Metagenics' Zinc Tally) 40 mg __ __ __ __ __ __ __
❏ George's Aloe Juice (8 oz) __ __ __ __ __ __ __
❏ EmergenC Lite packets
   1,000 mg C with electrolytes
   (*instead* of the C in the basic
   supplement plan) __ __ __ __ __ __ __
❏ Vitamin B_1 100–200 mg** __ __ __ __ __ __ __

Chapter 11: Balancing Your Blood Sugar

❏ Biotin 1,000 mcg __ __ __ __ __ __ __
❏ L-glutamine 500 mg __ __ __ __ __ __ __
❏ Vitamin B1 100–200 mg __ __ __ __ __ __ __

Adrenal Support Supplements for All Stages of Adrenal Exhaustion

❏ Pantothenic acid 100–500 mg§ __ __ __ __ __ __ __
❏ GABA 100–500 mg __ __ __ __ __ __ __
❏ Calmes Forte __ __ __ __ __ __ __
❏ Vitamin B1 200 mg** __ __ __ __ __ __ __

Ultimate Adrenal Stress Protocol

Add as per your health professional's recommendations:

❏ Licorice __ __ __ __ __ __ __
❏ DHEA __ __ __ __ __ __ __
❏ Pregnenolone __ __ __ __ __ __ __
❏ Homeopathic Adrenal
   Cortex 6C–4C __ __ __ __ __ __ __
❏ Cortisone (by prescription)
   2.5–5 mg __ __ __ __ __ __ __

Chapter 12: Thyroid Solutions

Thyroid boosters, if you have hypothyroidism, but not *thyroiditis:*

❏ L-tyrosine 500 mg __ __ __ __ __ __ __

**If you have more than one imbalance that calls for extra vitamin B_1, do not take more than 600 milligrams per day as an additional single nutrient supplement, in doses of 100 to 200 milligrams.
§Source Natural or Country Life Brands.

Supplement	AM	B	MM	L	MA	D	BT*
❏ Thyroid Glandular 50–100 mg	—	—	—	—	—	—	—

Chapter 13: Overcoming Addictions to Allergy Foods

❏ George's Aloe Vera Juice
  8 oz, between meals   — — — — — — —
❏ Alka-Seltzer Gold (2)
  as needed   — — — — — — —

Chapter 14: Hormone Help

Herbs for PMS
❏ Female Plus   — — — — — — —

Herbs for Menopause
❏ Dong Quai and/or   — — — — — — —
❏ Black Cohosh   — — — — — — —

Ultimate Hormonal Protocols
Add as per professional recommendation.
❏ Progesterone   — — — — — — —
❏ Estrogen   — — — — — — —
❏ Testosterone   — — — — — — —
❏ DHEA   — — — — — — —
❏ Pregnenolone   — — — — — — —

Chapter 15: Repairing the Damage Caused from Yeasts

(See separate lengthy protocol for yeasts at the end of chapter 15.)

Chapter 16: The Fatty Acid Fix

❏ Lipase, at least 8,000 USP   — — — — — — —
❏ Milk thistle (Silymarin)
  300 mg   — — — — — — —

Other Supplements

❏ _____   — — — — — — —
❏ _____   — — — — — — —
❏ _____   — — — — — — —

After your first three months, switch to a standard, cheaper, B complex containing 11 to 12 of the Bs from B₁ to choline and inositol, with no added C or other nutrients. The ideal dose of the Bs in the first three months is 25 to 50 milligrams and 10 to 25 milligrams thereafter as needed.

Basic Vitamin C with Bioflavonoids. In nature, vitamin C and bioflavonoids are always combined; they work best together that way as antioxidants which help prevent cancer, heart disease, asthma, and stress burnout, among other things. Our nutritionists generally recommend 2,000 to 3,000 milligrams per day—no more than what you'd get if you added two 1,000-milligram doses to the vitamin C in your multi.

Basic Vitamin E. This extraordinary longevity anti-oxident has been heavily researched. Among other things we know it can cut your risk of stroke and cataracts by 40 percent! If you have a family history of stroke, heart, or liver problems, you'll really need this vitamin.

Basic Fish Oil (or flax oil, if you're vegetarian). These are the super omega-3 nutrients that enhance your health from brain to colon. Vegetarians can combine 1,000 milligrams of flax oil along with 100 milligrams of a seaweed extract to get a fish oil effect.* (See chapters 8 and 20.)

Chromium. Chromium is a mineral that eliminates sugar cravings by improving your blood sugar balance, relieving stress, and helping to build muscle. Take extra doses to bring yourself up to 1,000 micrograms a day total (there's some chromium in the multi) for at least three months until your cravings are gone for good. (If you use Glucobalance as your multi, you won't need this extra chromium.)

Please make several copies of the master supplement plan I've provided here and write in pencil, so that you can revise your plan over time, as you change doses and start dropping supplements that you no longer need or start trying new ones. Review chapters 9 through 16 and fill in each special supplement section below that pertains to you, based on the suggestions in the pertinent chapters.

Supplements are *foods,* and inherently safe. But like foods, not all nutritional supplements are needed by everyone, nor do they all agree with everyone. We are each unique, biochemically and genetically. Our reactions to supplements vary accordingly. In addition, supplements have gone

*To order seaweed extract (DHA), call Martek Biosciences at (800) 522-5512.

Are Your Supplements Safe?

The U.S. death rate due to prescription and over-the-counter medications: 106,000 per year (290 deaths per day), according to a study published in the *Journal of the American Medical Association* in April 1998.[4]

Death rate due to supplements: one death in 1995–96, according to the most recent report by the American Association of Poison Control Centers (and even that one death is still being hotly contested.)

---

through an elaborate pharmaceutical preparation process that leaves some tiny impurities that bother a few people. If you tend to be sensitive to medications or have many food sensitivities, you may already know whether you can or can't tolerate nutritional supplements. About 1 in 100 through an elaborate pharmaceutical preparation process that leaves some tiny impurities that bother a few people. If you tend to be sensitive to clients at our clinic has some adverse reaction to a supplement even though he or she obviously needs it. More have adverse reactions, such as mild headaches, to supplements they don't need.

So although supplements are rarely dangerous, they often let you know quickly if they are not appropriate for you. If, for example, at first you love magnesium for its relaxing and laxative effect but then begin to experience loose bowels, it's time to cut the dose.

Nutritional supplements are known for their safety, but there are some exceptions. If you have any concerns or questions, consult with a knowledgeable health professional before starting your supplement program. Your master supplement plan will not provide overdoses of any nutrients, but I'd like you to know which nutrients could conceivably cause adverse symptoms at excessive doses:

Iron. This is the only truly hazardous supplement: Just a few adult-dosage pills can kill a child. Men and menopausal women shouldn't take iron without careful supervision of their heart function. With more than 18 milligrams per day, constipation and stomach upset can occur. At more than 100 milligrams per day, fatigue and weight loss can occur too.

Vitamin A. Doses above 50,000 IU can cause dizziness, blurred vision, headache and nausea. If you're pregnant, too much or too little can cause birth defects.

Vitamin B₃ (niacin). Doses as low as 300 milligrams at one sitting can cause headache, nausea, and a brief hot flush. (Doses over 2 grams may cause liver damage.)

Vitamin D. Daily doses above 1,000 IU may cause nausea, headache, fatigue, diarrhea, dry mouth, loss of appetite, and possibly irreversible kidney and heart problems. Spending a few minutes in the sun is a much better way to get plenty of vitamin D.

Zinc. High doses (over 50 milligrams) cause nausea, anemia, dizziness, lower immunity and HDL (good cholesterol), and block copper absorption.

Vitamin B₆. Over 250 milligrams per day for prolonged periods can cause temporary nerve damage.

Selenium. Over 800 micrograms per day causes brittle hair, nails, dizziness, fatigue, nausea, diarrhea, liver disease.

Copper. More than 2 milligrams (the RDA*) can cause nausea, headache, and jaundice.

Magnesium. Over 1,000 milligrams per day can cause diarrhea, low blood pressure, and nausea.[5]

Amino Acids. You should consult a physician before taking *any* amino acids if:

+ You have lupus
+ You have serious physical illness
+ You have severe liver damage
+ You have an inborn error of amino acid metabolism
+ You have an overactive thyroid
+ You have an ulcer (aminos may be too acidic)
+ You are pregnant
+ You are on methadone
+ You are taking many medications
+ You have schizophrenia or other mental illness

*Recommended daily allowance.

If you:	*You should consult a physician before taking:*
have high blood pressure	tyrosine, DL-phenylalanine, or L-phenylalanine*
take MAO inhibitors	tyrosine, DL-phenylalanine, or L-phenylalanine†
take MAO inhibitors for depression	L-tryptophan or 5-hydroxytryptophan (5-HTP)‡
have an overactive thyroid (hyperthyroid)	tyrosine, DL-phenylalanine, or L-phenylalanine
have Hashimoto's thyroiditis	tyrosine, DL-phenylalanine, or L-phenylalanine
have PKU (phenylketonuria)	tyrosine, DL-phenylalanine, or L-phenylalanine
get migraine headaches	tyrosine, DL-phenylalanine, L-phenylalanine, or 5-hydroxytryptophan (5-HTP)
have melanoma	L-tryptophan or 5-hydroxytryptophan (5-HTP)
taking SSRIs (selective serotonin reuptake inhibitors)	L-tryptophan or 5-hydroxytryptophan (5-HTP)§
have manic depression (bipolar disorder)	L-glutamine lifts depression but can trigger mania
have low blood pressure	GABA, taurine, or niacin

If you are being treated for any serious illness or are on any medications, consult with your doctor about taking amino acids. Should you get permission from your doctor to try amino acids but experience discomfort of any kind taking them, discontinue taking them immediately.

TAKING YOUR SUPPLEMENTS

Once you are clear on which supplements to take and have used the suggestions here and in chapter 19 to purchase them, you'll be ready to start taking them.

---

*Consult your physician; these amino acids have also proven helpful in *lowering* blood pressure!

†You must ask you doctor when it would be appropriate to start taking any of these aminos after discontinuing MAO inhibitors.

‡You must ask your doctor when it would be appropriate to start taking any of these aminos after discontinuing MAO inhibitors.

§You must ask your doctor if you can take these aminos with your SSRIs. Many M.D.s are open to doing this. After the phen-fen scare, no one wants to risk any serotonin-related problems.

✦ Whether you have one or more than one imbalance, you can and should start taking all of your rebalancing supplements at once, unless you are very sensitive and reactive to supplements.

✦ Watch your reactions to the supplements carefully.

✦ If there is a range of doses given, please start with the *lowest* dose of all of your "supps" (supplements). Do this just to make sure you get no adverse reaction to too high an amount of any of them.

✦ If you've tried all your supps at the lowest dose and tolerated them well but got little benefit from them, go up to the next highest dose and watch your reactions again. But don't increase over the maximum doses recommended here without expert consultation.

✦ Record your body's responses in your food/mood log (see page 362) to help you tune in and track progress or problems. If you've had a positive reaction to an amino acid at the lowest dose, for example, you may find that a higher dose is too much. (Most of our clients do better on the higher doses.)

✦ If you have any adverse symptoms (e.g., headache that starts only after certain supplements), check the troubleshooting tips below and stop taking or lower the dosage of the supplement that is the most likely culprit. If the symptoms don't stop quickly (in twenty-four hours), stop all supplements and, when the symptoms have disappeared, reintroduce your supplements one by one until you find the culprit. (Our clients have to do this only very rarely.)

✦ To keep track of what you're taking, it can be very helpful to lay out your supplements in either small labeled plastic bags or in plastic boxes with dividers designed to hold all your supplements for several days (see Resources in chapter 19).

✦ For help in adjusting your doses of supplements for best effect, read chapter 22 carefully, where I walk you through your first few weeks on your supplements.

✦ If you mistakenly take your breakfast, lunch, or dinner supplements *without* food, your multi may nauseate you. If you forget your between-meal supplements, just take them with your next meal. Don't skip them. They'll still work, just not as well.

✦ It can be hard to remember to take the supplements between meals. Use an alarm watch, a pager, or a computer reminder.

Supplement Troubleshooting Table

Troubling Symptom	*Supplements That May Be Implicated*
Stomachache	hydrochloric acid (HCl), B complex
Headaches	L-tyrosine, DLPA, L-phenylalanine, L-tryptophan
Diarrhea	magnesium, vitamin C
Nausea	B complex
Burping	fish oil (you can take extra lipase to aid digestion)

ELIMINATING YOUR SUPPLEMENTS

Once you have corrected your imbalances and your symptoms are gone, you can begin to experiment with going off your special repair supplements, one at a time. If your symptoms come back, you'll know that you still need that particular supplement for a while longer. Eliminate it again in a month and see what happens. Continue to do this until you no longer need any of your special repair supplements, but be ready to take them again, short-term, during stressful times, should you need to in the future. Continue with your basic supplements. Experiment with varying your multi once or twice a year by trying a new one when your old multi runs out, to get a different ratio of nutrients. Notice any differences in how you feel after you buy your new multi.

In the next chapter you'll get some help in buying your Diet Cure supplies and getting ready to go into action.

Readings

Atkins, Robert, M.D. *Dr. Atkins' Vita-Nutrient Solution* (New York: Simon & Schuster, 1998). A readable, fascinating tour of basic supplements.

Braverman, Eric, M.D. *The Healing Nutrients Within* (New Canaan, CT: Keats Publishing, 1997). This is the most complete book on amino acid therapy I know.

Crayhon, Robert. *The Carnitine Miracle* (New York: M. Evans and Co., 1998). This is a great book for vegetarians in particular.

Hausman, Patricia. *The Right Dose* (New York: Ballantine, 1989).

Lieberman, Shari, Ph.D. *The Real Vitamin and Mineral Book: Using Supplements for Optimum Health* (Garden City, NY: Avery, 1997).

Murray, Michael T., N.D. *The Encyclopedia of Nutritional Supplements: The Essential Guide for Improving Your Health Naturally* (Rocklin, CA: Prima, 1996).

Resources

See chapter 19 for complete information on sources for supplements.

EIGHTEEN

The Best Foods for Your Special Biochemistry

Your Master Eating Plan

THE FOOD WE EAT

Before I go into detail about how you can identify which foods will nourish you best, I want to try to free you from the question "how *much* food should I eat?" I don't believe that anyone knows the answer to that question about any particular person. We are each unique, especially in the United States where genetic histories are so varied, to be calorically predictable.

What we do know is that *eating too little is hazardous.* The very least number of calories you should eat is 2,100 calories; after all, the World Health Organization has declared that below that you are experiencing starvation. And that number is literally all inclusive: it indicates our needs in the West as well as the needs of other peoples, like the generally smaller-boned Chinese (who actually eat 20 percent more calories than we do).[1] So be brave. Raise your calories like a flag. Wave it over 2,100 calories high and keep going.*

In chapter 20 you'll see what the proportions on your plate should look like. It will be crowded with delicious foods. The proportions are

---

*Anorectics need to take it slower and need to start lower. They also need to be weighed standing with their backs to the scale.

important, but there is some debate over them: Should you eat almost as much protein as carbohydrates or should carbos predominate, and by how much? I would like you to find out for yourself what feels best for you.

The proportion of protein to healthy carbohydrate most successful with our clinic clients over more than ten years is 1 gram protein to 2 grams carbohydrate. Any individual variations tend to lean toward less carbohydrate. This ratio of food has been found to maintain the critical balance between incluin and glucagon, keeping us stable in energy, mood, and weight.[2]

Examples of 1:2 protein to carbohydrate meals:

2/3 cups cottage cheese with 1 1/2 cups fresh fruit
1 turkey sandwich on whole grain bread with celery sticks
2 bean tostadas

Vegetarian eaters will probably eat a higher proportion of carbohydrates because their protein sources, such as beans and rice combined, are not carboless, like meat, fish, and chicken are. Nuts, seeds, eggs, and cheese are carboless, but not all vegetarians eat eggs and cheese. Beans and, especially, grains contain lots of carbohydrates along with less protein, so it will be harder for you, if you are vegan (and eat absolutely no animal products) to get enough protein to keep your protein-carbo balance. Fruits and vegetables contain very little protein at all. Please watch very carefully to see that you get enough protein to keep you free of cravings and health problems.

As for fat, about a third of your total calories will come from foods like avocados, salad oil, nuts, seeds, and fish. Eating this way won't make you feel heavy or gain weight. In fact, it will help you lose by making you satisfied and full, rather than continuing to eat indefinitely because you don't ever feel really satisfied. And good fat will help you burn fat more effectively, too, if you need to. Every cell in your body needs its coat of fat maintained so that it protects what's inside. Every cell needs a *good* coat, not a moth-eaten, leaky one, so enjoy your healthy fats. And don't worry about weight gain. Dr. Atkins and numerous studies proved long ago that fat is not the problem in weight—excess carbohydrates are the problem.

Food as Nourishment

Your body must have water and at least forty-five minerals, vitamins, fats, amino acids (protein), and some kind of carbohydrates to sustain your health. Are you getting them? Gladys Block, Ph.D., at the University of California at Berkeley, recently summarized data from three major nationwide nutrition surveys and discovered that one of every two American women consumed inadequate amounts of almost every vitamin and mineral studied. On any four consecutive days, only 14 percent of women ate *even one* dark green vegetable. Almost 50 percent of all women avoid fruit. No wonder our risk of contracting cancer, heart disease, and stroke continues to skyrocket. Only one in five children eat the recommended five servings of fruits and vegetables daily, and nearly 25 percent of all the "vegetables" they consume are French fries.[3] Four out of five Americans believe it is all right to eat whatever they want, whenever they want it.[4] I wish this were true.

Bad Food, Good Food

Many billions of advertising dollars are spent each year to entice you to buy one processed food after another. The sole motivation is sales, not concern for your health. Food marketing preys on your emotional needs with superstitions, misconceptions, and half truths. So we get Coca-Cola promoted as "the real thing," and products that are loaded with refined flour and sugar promoted as healthy because they are "low fat."

Yet at no other time in history have there been so many nutritious foods available, and we now know more about foods and their effects on the body than ever before. Research proving the value and benefits of particular foods and nutrients is being done at a tremendous rate and the news media reports on it almost daily. We're starting to realize that the most important element in the prevention and treatment of disease is diet and lifestyle. But we've also been getting conflicting information for years about what foods are good and what foods are bad. So we still don't know what to eat. Though most of us know that we need vegetables and fruits, we can't say no to the sweet, starchy junk foods that keep us unbalanced.

The first sixteen chapters of *The Diet Cure* teach you how to free yourself from the tyranny of empty but addictive foods. In this final section I help you learn what to eat instead—to keep yourself healthy and trim. The good news is that unlike other diet plans, with the Diet Cure you won't find yourself craving forbidden foods (thanks to those anticraving supplements). You will enjoy the foods you eat; many will be old favorites while others will be delicious new discoveries. In these next three chapters, I'll teach you about what types of food to eat and give you specifics about what you can cook, or assemble at a salad bar, or order at a restaurant, or snack on between meals. Let's start by looking at the foods that will minimize or maximize your health.

Our Four Biggest Dietary Problems

The four biggest dietary problems we face today:

1. We don't eat enough fresh vegetables and fruits. Less than 10 percent of the population eats five servings a day. Fresh vegetables and fruits supply many health-enhancing and disease-preventing substances, including enzymes, minerals, vitamins, antioxidants (which protect against cellular deterioration and prevent diseases, including cancer), and phytonutrients. Eating plenty of vegetables and fruits can also help overcome other dietary problems.

2. We eat too much sugar. Diabetes and blood sugar problems caused by eating too much sugar are almost at epidemic proportions and contribute to many other diseases as well.

3. We skip far too many meals. Without regular meals the body must constantly borrow nutrients from muscles, bones, and vital organs to maintain the proper nutrient balance in the blood. Skipping a meal and depending upon stimulants such as coffee, soda, sweets, or Power Bars to momentarily pump up your blood sugar create new and deeper problems.

4. The majority of Americans eat an unbalanced diet. One or more of the three basic foods (protein, carbohydrates, and fat) is out of balance in most Americans' diet. Some eat too little or too much protein. Some scrupulously avoid fat and are deficient, whereas others eat it to excess. But worst of all, as a nation, we eat far too many carbohydrates, especially processed and fast-food carbs. Excessive carbs can also cause blood sugar imbalances and slow down our metabolisms, leading to fatigue and weight gain. Consequently, a large majority of adults lack energy and/or are overweight.

THE SIX NUTRIENT GROUPS

There are six nutrient groups essential to life that, ideally, we should all have plenty of in the food we eat. In order of importance, they are water, proteins, fats, carbohydrates, minerals, and vitamins. On average, fat makes up about 28 to 40 percent of the total weight of a woman and 11 to 25 percent of a man. Proteins account for about 12 percent of the total body weight of both men and women. Excess dietary protein is converted into stored fat, or, if you exercise, into muscle. Carbohydrates only contribute about 0.5 percent of body weight. They are either burned for energy or converted into fat. Minerals make up about 3.5 percent of your body weight with water accounting for the remaining 62 to 69 percent.[5]

1. Water

Water is the most precious liquid on earth. Every living thing depends upon water for its life and sustenance. Every cell of our body requires water to carry nutrients and energy to them and to carry away toxins and metabolic wastes. The human body itself is about two thirds water.

Today, obtaining pure drinking water is ever more challenging. Whenever we drink water with additives, flavorings, sweeteners, and carbonation, our overworked liver must spend time and energy to filter and remove the additives. Only then can we use the water that is contained in the drink. In contrast, pure water requires no special processing by the body. It can be absorbed and used right away as soon as it touches our lips.

Choices in Drinking Water. Despite claims from regional water treatment officials, tap water isn't a very good source of drinking water anymore, because it contains large amounts of chlorine to kill the bacteria and protozoa in it. Chlorine is toxic, especially to the kidneys, liver, and heart, and it depletes the body of vitamin E and other vital nutrients. Carbonated water is much too high in phosphorus (which can leach calcium from the body) to drink more than occasionally. Bottled spring waters are good choices, when they are low in TDS (total dissolved solids; i.e., sludge). Higher quality bottled waters print their TDS in parts per million (ppm) on their labels. Look for brands like Canadian Glacier and Chippewa Springs Water from Wisconsin that have TDS ratings below 100 ppm.

It's okay to drink distilled water, but only occasionally. It's good for cleansing and detoxifying the body, but unlike spring water, or purified water treated with a reverse osmosis filtration process, it is lifeless, so don't drink it regularly. Reverse osmosis filtered water is very good quality as the water has been treated with a combination of two filtration systems, plus ultraviolet light. Carbon-block filtration units, which can attach to your faucet or are part of a water pitcher, are okay because they remove chlorine and some harmful chemicals. But make sure to change your filters regularly, as directed, as once they are full they will begin to recirculate wastes back into your drinking water. Buying your own faucet or under-the-sink water filter is an invaluable investment in your health: it's cheaper, more convenient, and safer than using plastic containers.

2. Fat

Believe it or not, fat *is* truly beneficial to your health. For most people, fat is the most abundant substance in the body next to water. Of the forty-five known essential nutrients, two are fatty acids: alpha-linolenic (omega-3) and linoleic (omega-6).

The biggest problem with fats is that most people eat too many poor-quality fats and not nearly enough of the essential fats. A hamburger and French fries or even a chicken or turkey sandwich contain fat, but are devoid of *essential* fats. Furthermore, one of the essential fats, omega-3, is so rare in what we eat that most of us are quite deficient in it. The best omega-3 sources are fish, fish oils, and flaxseed or hemp oil. Omega-3 oils have an amazing array of benefits: they protect us against many dangers, including cancer, arthritis, stroke, and cardiovascular disease. Canola oil is the only commonly used oil with significant amounts of omega-3.

The other essential fat, omega-6, is readily available in most bottled vegetable oils, such as grapeseed, canola, sesame, and sunflower. For optimal health, you should consume 1 part omega-3 oils to 1 to 2 parts omega-6 oils. Realistically this means you need to eat oceanic fish two to four times a week and use at least 2,000 milligrams of fish or flax oil daily as supplements.

A final group of healthy oils are oils rich in omega-9 fatty acids. Extra-virgin (first pressing) olive oil is the best known of these and makes a wonderful salad oil as well as a tasty cooking oil. It is quite stable kept at room temperature and plays a central role in one of the world's most healthy diets—the Mediterranean diet, with its low risks of cancer, arthritis, and stroke.

An Engineering Masterpiece. Fat and fat cells are engineering masterpieces. They offer the most ideal and efficient way to store energy for future use. Each gram of fat stores more than twice as much energy as a gram of protein or carbohydrate.

Fat is vitally important for the health and nourishment of every cell in the body. Essential fats are necessary for the cell wall, as well as cellular energy production. Your brain is 60 percent fat. See chapter 8 and 16 for more information on the function and importance of fat.

3. Protein

In Greek, the word *protein* means "of primary importance." Protein supplies the building blocks of your body, the amino acids, which are so critical to constructing and maintaining the healthy structure of the body, from its muscle to its hormones. Foods containing protein have different kinds and amounts of amino acids. Our bodies require twenty-two different amino acids for proper function. A complete protein contains nine essential amino acids—tryptophan, lysine, methionine, valine, leucine, isoleucine, phenylalanine, threonine, and histidine.* These nine amino acids are essential because they *must* be derived directly from our diets. Our bodies cannot manufacture them from other aminos.

Certain foods supply all the essential amino acids in sufficient amounts. These foods are called complete proteins—meat, fish, poultry, eggs, milk, and cheese. Soy is the only plant-based complete protein. All other plant-based proteins are missing one or more amino acids and are called incomplete proteins. But two or more plant-based proteins can be combined together to create a complete protein. For example, beans with whole grains, nuts, or seeds combine to create complete protein.

In reaction to previous generations' overconsumption of red meat, protein, like fat, has suffered a bad reputation over the past several decades. But the simple fact remains that without adequate protein, the body will be unable to provide sufficient muscle, hormones, and mood-regulating chemicals for the brain.

Adults normally require between 50 and 100 grams of protein on a daily basis. Bodybuilders, heavy exercisers, and those under great stress may at times need more.

4. Minerals

There are twenty-two minerals that we know of that are vital to health. Over time several additional trace minerals will likely be added to the list. Leading health authorities tell us that more than three out of four Americans are deficient in one or more minerals.[6] Without minerals, the foods we eat and the vitamins we take do little or no good because our body can't make use of them unless it has minerals. Although the body can manufacture a few vitamins, it cannot manufacture a single mineral. Minerals must be supplied through the foods that are taken in.

Despite the importance of minerals, calcium is the only mineral whose function is widely known and accepted. (Clearly, the remaining minerals need a better publicist!) Every cell of every living organism requires minerals for proper function and structure. Minerals act as catalysts for many

---

*In addition, arginine is considered essential in infancy.

biological reactions, including muscle response, nerve transmissions, digestion, energy production, growth, and healing.

Minerals are present in a wide variety of foods, but are most richly supplied in vegetables, fruits, and legumes. Of course this assumes these foods are grown in mineral-rich soils, which is often not the case. Therefore, a balanced multiple-mineral supplement can fill in certain inevitable mineral deficiencies.

5. Vitamins

Vitamins are absolutely essential to life. Their discovery in 1910 was one of the most important scientific achievements of the twentieth century. Vitamins promote growth, health, and life itself as well as regulate the metabolism and assist the biochemical processes that release energy from digested food. Vitamins are considered micronutrients because we need relatively small amounts of them as compared to the macronutrients: protein, carbohydrates, fat, and water.

With a few exceptions, vitamins must be supplied daily in our diets or as supplements because our bodies can not synthesize them. The vitamin content of food can vary greatly depending upon where it was grown, when it was harvested, and how it has been stored and processed. Vitamin content is highest when food is fresh and minimum heat is applied. For example, heating food in a microwave destroys significant vitamin content.

Vitamins work on the cellular level. A lack of one or more vitamins can cause a variety of deficiency symptoms and health problems. A deficiency interferes with many bodily processes and how the body utilizes other nutrients as well. Because vitamins are essential to the body's energy production, when we're low in them we feel fatigued or lethargic. But much worse effects show up if deficiencies continue. A terrible vitamin B deficiency syndrome called pellagra killed ten thousand Americans in the south after 1915 and sent thousands of others to mental institutions.

There are currently thirteen recognized vitamins: The fat-soluble ones include A, D, E, and K; the water-soluble vitamins are C and the B-complex (thiamin, riboflavin, niacin, pantothenic acid, B_6, B_{12}, biotin, and folic acid). Additionally, choline and inositol are two water-soluble members of the B-complex family. Fat-soluble vitamins can be stored in the liver and the body's fatty tissue. However, we need to take in water-soluble vitamins daily because our bodies cannot store them and they will be excreted in one to four days.

6. Carbohydrates

Carbohydrates are the best source of energy for all body functions. (Although protein and fat can also be burned for energy, it takes more work to do it.) They are stored in the body as glycogen in almost all body tissues, but especially in the liver and muscles. The glycogen is a ready source of reserve energy instantly available to be metabolized into glucose, which fuels all of the body's cells as well as the brain and red blood cells. In this way, carbohydrates supply the body's immediate needs for calories to burn as energy. When you consume more calories than your body requires, a portion of the excess carbohydrates are stored for future use as fat.

Carbohydrates are divided into simple and complex carbohydrates. Simple carbohydrates are often called simple sugars and include table sugar (sucrose), fruit sugar (fructose), and milk sugar (lactose). Most simple carbohydrates are refined sugars, which you should avoid, as you know. Your body reacts to the simple carbohydrates in candy, cookies, sugar-coated cereals, canned fruits in syrup, catsup, fruit drinks, and juices as if they were drugs. In contrast, fruits are beneficial simple carbohydrates, supplying levels of essential nutrients and fiber along with its fructose sweetener.

Complex carbohydrates also consist of sugars, but the sugar molecules are made up of longer, more complex chains. Foods rich in complex carbohydrates include vegetables, legumes (beans, lentils, and peas), and whole grains. Complex carbohydrates are the ideal carbohydrates to meet the body's short-term energy needs. They metabolize quickly, but contain many nutrients and, combined with the right ratio of protein provide sustained energy.

BETTER FOOD HABITS

Eat Organic and Fresh Food Whenever You Can

Sales of organic food have increased more than 20 percent in each of the past six years. Now one in six Americans buys organic.[7] Many supermarket chains now offer organic produce as their customers demand it. While more costly than nonorganic food, organic fruits and vegetables are not only more rich in minerals than other produce, they are devoid of pesticides and chemical residues. And they taste better!

Consider Eating for Your Blood Type

Each of us is biochemically unique. One man's meat is another man's poison. Food I thrive on may make you sick, or vice versa. Your blood type offers a key that may unlock the door to the mysteries of individual health, disease, and longevity. Understanding what impact your blood type has on your eating can make a difference in your overall vitality. What your ancestors ate in the past still has a direct bearing on your present health as you have genetically inherited their digestive strengths and weaknesses.

If your blood type is O—the oldest, the original blood type—you'll probably thrive on a "caveman" diet—meat, fish, vegetables, nuts, seeds, and fruit. It is very difficult for an O type to be a successful vegetarian. Dairy products and grains, especially wheat, seem to present significant digestive problems for type O's, so you may want to avoid or eat minimal amounts of them. Protein seems to be particularly essential to people with blood type O (you'll need 20 to 40 grams at each meal, depending on your body size, metabolism, and activity level).

If your blood type is A, you can usually handle certain grains much better than type O's, as your ancestors were the original agrarians—planting crops for food. Legumes are also good—beans, lentils, and tofu, among others. In fact, A types make the best vegetarians, although fish is often wonderful for them as well. A types usually do best to avoid most dairy, except for yogurt and the more recent grains in our evolution—wheat, rye, barley, and oats, especially if weight loss is an issue.

If your blood type is B, you are the only blood type that seems to thrive on dairy products, as your more recent ancestors regularly consumed and adapted to them. A widely varied diet is best for B types, including meat and fish, though they don't seem to be able to digest chicken and the gluten-containing grains very well.

If your blood type is AB, you may have inherited the strengths and weaknesses of both type A and B. Your immune system is probably strong and you can adapt to a variety of different foods, but don't need as much animal protein (meat) as type B and may have trouble digesting chicken. ABs have a better tolerance for dairy and for gluten than some other blood types (but it may prevent them from losing weight).

For further information on eating for your blood type, check out two books on this subject: *Your Body Knows Best*, by Ann Louise Gittleman, and *Eat Right for Your Type*, by Dr. Peter J. D'Adamo. Order a blood-type test through a physician (it costs about twenty dollars) or order it yourself (see the resources for chapter 21).

Get Plenty of Those Vital Vegetables

This is one area of diet that most of us can definitely improve on. And yes, our mothers and grandmothers both were right: For optimal health, we do need to eat more vegetables. They are the perfect carbohydrate source. Ideally the majority of dietary carbohydrates will come from vegetables. Four cups a day should do it.

Veggies not only supply carbohydrates for energy, they are the richest source of minerals and phytonutrients in our diet. They also provide enzymes, vitamins, and some protein. Moreover, they are alkalinizing, making them an ideal counterbalance to heavier acid-forming foods such as meats and grains. In our many years of nutritional counseling, one simple fact has consistently proven true: People who eat the most vegetables do the best on our program, and are the most healthy people of all. The largest study of women's health ever done found that one serving per day of certain vegetables cut women's stroke risk by 40 percent. Scientists are now intently studying the special nutrient content of vegetables to understand why they protect health so effectively. For example, tomatoes and peas protect against prostate cancer while phytonutrients in soy help prevent breast cancer. The most intensely colorful vegetables (such as red beets, purple cabbage, yellow squash, collard greens, and spinach) contain the highest levels of nutrients, which boost the immune system and protect from degenerative disease. One of our clients who started to eat a large multivegetable salad and two cooked vegetables per day during Christmas break startled her classmates when she returned to graduate school, because her cheeks were so pink and her eyes so bright—from all the color in her veggies.

Cooked or Raw: The Enzyme Question

The best convenience, or "fast," food is uncooked fresh ripe fruits and some vegetables. Foods containing high levels of nutrients and digestive enzymes are best consumed in the raw state. This group contains most ripe fruits and some vegetables including avocados. Unripe fruits, many vegetables, and most grains contain enzymes that can negatively impact digestion. With these foods, ripening, sprouting, or cooking enhances nutrient absorption and provides a higher nutritional value. An example of these foods include carrots, tomatoes, and potatoes, all having higher digestibility of proteins and starches after cooking.

Supplemental digestive enzymes can be very helpful for all of those in recovery from dieting and eating disorders. Starving, bingeing, and purging all ravage the body's ability to properly digest food. As soon as your body can tolerate raw vegetables, have lots of them. It's best to include *both* raw and cooked veggies in your meals, but find what works for you—and your lifestyle. It seems to work best to eat more raw foods in the warmer months and more cooked in the cooler months. Optimally, half of the vegetables you eat will be raw, assuming you digest them well. So don't overlook the raw veggies, as they supply many nutrients that cooked vegetables do not. But if you find you feel hungry or unsatisfied after a meal, especially after eating only raw foods with protein, it's a sign that the next time you should add more cooked vegetable to the meal. This small addition will usually leave you feeling more satisfied and fulfilled after the meal.

Also, make sure you eat a *minimum* of four cups of vegetables daily. This may sound like a lot, but it's actually easier than it appears. For instance, a large salad with two cups of lettuce, a cup of raw vegetables, a half cup of peas or beans, and three quarters a cup of turkey, cheese, or nuts at one meal and a cup of veggies at another will fulfill your daily vegetable requirement. Preparing raw, steamed, or lightly sautéed veggies with a meal, or even as a snack, is also excellent. Just be sure to leave a little crunch still in the vegetables to maintain sufficient nutrient value. Adding a tasty sauce to the vegetables makes them even more appealing: Try curries, pestos, salsas, avocado, or any salad dressing. You can make them yourself or buy them in health food stores—Annie's Naturals tasty dressings for cooked or raw veggies are excellent. Try a number of them until you settle on your favorites.

Homemade soup is another great way to enjoy your veggies. It's easy to make soup stock, or you can buy it; health food stores carry broths that are free from additives (like MSG and extra sodium), which you can turn into delicious soups in a matter of minutes. (See chapter 20 for recipes.)

Feast on Fruit

Fresh fruit is delicious as well as energizing and easy to digest. Fruit is an ideal source of quick energy, offering the extra bonus of valuable enzymes, minerals, vitamins, and fiber. Moreover, fruit makes a great snack food (especially when eaten with protein), requiring little or no preparation. Choose fruits you enjoy, such as apples, grapefruit, and oranges, but experiment with more exotic fruits such as pomegranates, mangoes, and kiwi.

Food Combining

Many nutritionists have set up elaborate rules concerning food combining; that is, what foods should be eaten together. For some people with sensitive digestive tracts, it can be helpful to follow the protocol of proper combining. For others it doesn't seem to matter much at all. If you have a sensitive digestive system, you'll usually feel better when you eat simply and don't combine many different foods into one meal. The basic food-combining principle is this: Eat fruit alone, vegetables and fat with anything, and avoid eating protein with starchy food.

If yeast and hypoglycemia are not a problem, eat two to four raw fruits or their equivalent per day (1 apple equals 1 cup of berries). Fruit provides more digestive enzymes than any other food because we tend to eat it raw. Fruit is important for its vitamins and minerals (which cooking also reduces). It is a better source of fiber than grain and as alkaline as vegetables. Try to eat it between meals or before a meal for better digestion.

Get Enough Fiber

Diets high in fiber help lower cholesterol levels and reduce the risk of heart disease. Fiber has also been shown to prevent colon and other cancers. In general, populations that consume high-fiber diets have small hospitals and less disease. Make fiber a part of all your meals. Fiber, or "roughage," is found almost exclusively in plant foods—vegetables, fruits, legumes, whole grains, nuts, and seeds. Beans, lentils, peas, corn, prunes, blackberries, and blueberries are exceptionally rich in fiber. Avoid wheat and oat bran fiber if you are gluten intolerant. Remember that processed foods lack fiber, and cooking vegetables and fruit to the point of being mushy destroys much of their fiber.

Fiber has a lot of other good qualities, too: it binds with toxins and wastes and helps neutralize them before they cause bodily damage. It also adds bulk to the stool, which assists in maintaining regular bowel function. Without enough fiber, you will experience constipation, which is a contributing factor in many diseases.

(Caution: If you have a digestive disorder, consult with your physician before embarking on a high-fiber diet.)

FOODS AND FOOD ADDITIVES TO AVOID

Aspartame (NutraSweet)

This sweetener is two hundred times sweeter than sugar. It increases the appetite in general and the desire for sweets in particular. Incredibly, aspartame accounts for 75 percent of all nondrug complaints to the FDA. Yes, you should avoid sugar, but aspartame isn't a good substitute. (See chapter 2 for more details on aspartame's side effects.)

Caffeinated Beverages

Coffee, black tea, and colas are powerful stimulants that overstress the body in many ways. They deplete nutrients such as vitamin B_1 (thiamin), biotin, inositol, vitamin C, calcium, potassium, and zinc. Caffeine also increases thirst; overstimulates and weakens the kidneys, pancreas, liver, stomach, intestines, heart, nervous system, and glands (especially the adrenals); and overacidifies the pH (causing potential premature aging). Coffee is laced with pesticides and free-radical-producing hydrocarbons that weaken cell membranes. Studies show individuals who drink the most coffee often suffer chronic depression.[8] What's more, it only takes a small amount of coffee before the negative effects start kicking in—as little as two small cups or one mugful a day. (Decaf coffee is a better choice but not the best, because it contains a small amount of caffeine as well as all the pesticides and hydrocarbons.)

Carbonated Beverages

In the carbonation process, phosphorous levels in beverages increase significantly. If you regularly drink carbonated beverages you will upset the mineral balance in your body. If the body doesn't have enough calcium to buffer higher phosphorus intake, it will "borrow," or leach, calcium wherever it can be found—from muscles and bones. The net result may be a gradual weakening of bone structure, contributing to osteoporosis. Furthermore, the sugar content in carbonated sodas is very high, and diet sodas with aspartame and artificial sweeteners aren't any better.

Fried Food

Avoid fried foods in all forms, including French fries and fried chips from the health food store. (Japanese tempura is probably the healthiest fried

---

Soda Pop Facts

Americans drank twice as many soft drinks in 1997 as they did in 1973. Soft drink companies produce 54 gallons a year for every American—that's 19 ounces a day. The average teenage boy gulps 42 ounces daily. Girls also get their share, consuming 75 percent as much as the boys. Male teenagers consume enough caffeine in sodas to equal 1¹/₂ cups of coffee daily.

A 12-ounce can of nondiet cola has about 10 teaspoons of sugar and 150 calories. Soda serving sizes have grown from a 6-ounce bottle in the 1950s to 20-ounce bottles today. At McDonald's, a "child"-size soft drink is now 12 ounces and a small is 16 ounces. At 7-Eleven stores, the Double Gulp is 64 ounces.[9]

---

food, but even so, it should be only an occasional treat.) Because fried foods are exposed to heat for long periods of time, the food enzymes and essential fats break down, and in the body they clog the blood vessels and weaken circulation, among other things. It's okay to stir-fry, however, because the heat is lower and the food is exposed to it for a much shorter time period.

Hydrogenated Oils

This oil is the grocer's dream because it has an almost infinite shelf life, but it's the liver's nightmare. Hydrogenated oils (like margarine) raise cholesterol, cause heart disease, and are being linked to the development of other degenerative diseases such as cancer and arthritis. Hydrogenated oils are what you find in most packaged crackers, cookies, baking and cooking mixes, and other packaged goods. Margarine contains hydrogenated oils, which contribute to heart disease and obesity and promote inflammation while suppressing immune function.[10] A biochemist I know called margarine "one molecule away from being a plastic." Although butter is high in saturated fat, it's better for you because it's more stable than margarine. Butter can be used in moderate amounts: a pat or two a day as a seasoning. New information about health-promoting buterates found in butter make it an even better option. If you can, choose organic butter.

The Facts on Red Meat

Red meat has been much maligned for several reasons. First, American meat is full of hormones, like diethyl stilbestrol (DES), which is used as a growth stimulator. This is why most other countries do not allow its importation. Second, men who eat red meat, especially ground meat, five or more times a week also have four times the risk of colon cancer and two times the risk of prostate cancer as do men who eat red meat less than once a month. But women need the easily accessible iron and zinc in red meat, especially when they are menstruating. Less fatty cuts are better because they contain fewer hormones and antibiotics and pesticides, although this isn't an issue with organic red meat.

Another concern with red meat is that eating meat cooked rare can harbor dangerous *E. coli* bacteria, but overcooking is not healthy either. Well-done steaks and burgers contain ten times the amount of the cancer-causing chemical heterocyclic amine than is found in meat cooked medium.[11] When preparing red meat, use a meat thermometer to be sure the inside reaches 180 degrees; this way, you'll avoid *E. coli* and overcooking.

Iceberg Lettuce

Iceberg lettuce, originally developed so that it would ship well, will keep for a month or two in the vegetable crisper in your refrigerator—far longer than any other lettuce. It degrades very slowly, and likewise has a correspondingly slow transit time in your bowels, contributing to constipation and other intestinal problems. Choose more colorful, tastier lettuces, such as red or green leaf, and romaine, which improve bowel transit time rather than slow it down.

Monosodium Glutamate (MSG)

This flavor enhancer is responsible for CRHS (Chinese Restaurant Headache Syndrome). No wonder so many people have negative reactions to it: glutamate is a neurotoxin that destroys brain cells in laboratory animals and potentially in humans. Check food labels; it shows up in a lot of unexpected places.

Microwave Cooking: Zap and Be Zapped

In our fast-paced society, the microwave oven is an incredible convenience factor in preparing food. Unfortunately, there are some health risks associated with its use. German studies show microwaving of food is associated with a drop in hemoglobin and lymphocyte levels in the blood and a significant rise in white blood cell counts. An increase in white blood cells is an immune response that usually means the body is fighting some type of infection or inflammation. Some researchers feel that heavy reliance on microwaved food may be linked to the significant increase in autoimmune disorders. Moreover, the microwave kills almost all enzymes present in the food. Because enzymes, which are biochemical catalysts that contain the "life force" of food— the key to all life processes—the loss of enzymes is a real problem. I have observed many people feel more tired and lethargic after eating too much microwaved food. So use your microwave to reheat or defrost, or even to cook, food only occasionally; don't rely on it. It is far better to dirty a pot and cook on the stove (a little water at the bottom will help keep the food from sticking when reheating).

Pesticides

Seventy of 300 pesticides used on U.S. crops are known to be probable or possible human carcinogens. The following produce has the highest levels of pesticide residues (in order of greatest contamination): strawberries, bell peppers, spinach, cherries (U.S.), peaches, cantaloupe (Mexican), celery, apples, apricots, green beans, grapes (Chilean), and cucumbers. Rinse produce thoroughly. If you can, soak them in vinegar and water for a few minutes.

Processed Meats

These include bologna, salami, hot dogs, most sausages, and smoked meats and fish. The problem with processed meats is that they are very high in saturated animal fat, cholesterol, and sodium. Smoked, cured, and pickled foods are also high in nitrates, which form potentially carcinogenic byproducts.[12]

Sugars, Sugars, and More Sugars

The sugar content in foods is alarmingly high and going higher. We get plenty of naturally occurring sugars in milk or fruit, but then the food industry adds sugar to an incredible array of foods, including salad dressings and almost all processed foods. Sugar is often hidden on the label, disguised with other names such as corn syrup, corn starch, sucrose, and fructose, among many others. Eating sugary foods causes exhaustion and depletes vital nutrient reserves, especially essential minerals and B vitamins. Most alarmingly, sugars found in junk foods such as soft drinks, cookies, and cakes squeeze out and replace healthier foods in our diet. Just as Mom always said, when we eat sugar, we spoil our appetite for dinner. (For more on sugar, see chapter 3.)

Be a label reader. It's a primary means of survival. Just because a substance is allowed in food does not mean it is safe or nutritious.

BENEFICIAL FOODS TO EMPHASIZE—AND TRY OUT

A diet rich in vegetables, fruit, and protein helps reduce the risk of all the major causes of illnesses and death. As you begin to change your eating habits and eliminate problem foods, you will discover that there are many other foods you've never heard of, or never thought to eat regularly, that will improve your health. Here's a list of foods that increase vitality and supply a superior source of nutrients. Some will be familiar, while some might sound a little strange. But why not give them a try and see if you don't enjoy their taste and their effect on your body? Just remember that each of us is unique and no one single food works for all people. Some of these foods may not agree with you. If so, listen to your own body.

Beans

Beans are high in protein, minerals, and fiber. Most beans possess 80 percent of the calcium content of milk, by weight. And the calcium in milk is not the most easily absorbable for humans. Soak beans overnight and discard the original water to prevent flatulence. Cook in fresh water below the boiling point to enhance digestibility. A crock pot is ideal for preparing all sorts of beans. Try these beans and legumes:

+ Adzuki beans
+ Black beans
+ Black-eyed peas
+ Cannelloni beans
+ Chick-peas (garbanzo beans)
+ Cranberry beans
+ Fava beans
+ Great Northern beans
+ Lentils*
+ Mung beans
+ Pinto beans
+ Soybeans
+ Flageolet beans
+ Kidney beans
+ Lima beans
+ Navy beans
+ Red beans
+ Split peas*

Eggs

Disparaged for two decades, eggs are now beginning to make a comeback. Eggs are one of the most nutrient-rich of all foods. They are an excellent source of protein, minerals, and B vitamins. New research suggests only those people with both high cholesterol and high triglycerides should limit their eggs to four per week (those who have coronary heart disease should avoid them completely). According to studies, those with high cholesterol only (not high triglycerides) are not adversely affected by eating two eggs per day. So about 80 percent of the population can enjoy eggs with no limitations. When they are poached or soft- or hard-boiled, eggs are particularly healthful because the yolk stays intact, which prevents oxidation, a chemical process in which the nutrients begin to break down (this is the same process that turns a cut apple brown). Choose eggs from free-range (not caged) chickens or "fertile" eggs, which can be found in health food stores. These types of eggs come from chickens that are able to roam instead of living their lives confined to a tiny space, where they live in their own filth and have to be fed antibiotics to prevent disease.

---

*The fastest cooking beans, lentils and split peas can be prepared in under an hour.

Fish

Deep-ocean fish have not been subjected to the hormonal and antibiotic onslaught that land animals raised as food are, and have fewer residues of human pollution than freshwater fish or shallow water seafood such as scallops, shrimp, clams, oysters, and lobster. All fish offer an easily digested protein that is also rich in minerals, such as iodine and essential fatty acids—particularly the highly beneficial but rare omega-3 oils. In general, the fattier the fish, the greater the omega-3 content. Fish oils also have general antiinflammatory qualities, reduce clotting, maintain the nervous system, and help lower cholesterol and triglyceride levels. High omega-3 sources include fish such as:

- Salmon
- Tuna (fresh is best; canned often has the fats removed)
- Mackerel
- Herring
- Sardines
- Anchovy
- Lake whitefish
- Lake trout
- Sable
- Conch
- Halibut
- Oysters
- Orange roughie
- Bluefish
- Calamari (squid)

Eat shellfish only rarely, for they live in the most polluted waters close to shore. Remember, eating deep-ocean fish is especially important if your ancestors were Scandinavian, Celtic, or Coastal Native Americans.[13]

Flaxseed Oil

Flaxseed oil contains the highest levels (52 percent) of omega-3 essential fats. Flax oil is useful for a variety of degenerative disorders, strengthens the immune response, and tones the heart and arteries.[14]

Caution: Flax oil goes rancid faster than any other oil. To assure freshness, purchase it in dark bottles and refrigerate it. Consume 1 to 3 tablespoons a day. Be sure to use the bottle within four to six weeks of opening the container.

Grapefruit

This refreshing juicy fruit is so helpful in enhancing the absorption of everything we take in that pharmacists caution customers not to eat it while taking certain medications! Grapefruit may also support us in stressful times by enhancing the effectiveness of the adrenal stress hormones.

Herbs and Herbal Teas

Herbs possess potent healing qualities. For every disease and every organ and gland, there are specific herbs that can be used to make it healthier. For example, milk thistle detoxifies and cleanses the liver, Ginkgo biloba enhances circulation to the brain, and peppermint aids digestion. You can take herbs in capsule form or as a tea—some, like peppermint, are quite delicious. You can also drink herbal teas, such as those made by Celestial Seasonings, for nonmedicinal purposes—as an alternative to water, hot or cold.

Meats (Lean)

Meat supplies a quality protein structure, iron, zinc, vitamin B_{12} and carnitine, often not present in vegetarian diets. Choose organic, free-range chickens, turkeys, and red meat, which is free of harmful antibiotics and hormones.

Rice Protein Powder

A hypo-allergenic alternative to soy, milk, and egg proteins, rice protein powder contains twelve grams of protein per tablespoon. It has a higher protein value than soy, is easier to digest, and mixes very well in a variety of foods, blender drinks, and smoothies. Ask your health food store owner about it.

Salsa

This tasty Mexican condiment makes an excellent substitute for sugary catsup. The fresher the better.

Seeds and Nuts (Raw)

Nature imbues seeds and nuts with the richest source of nutrients available. Enjoy sunflower, pumpkin, sesame, chia, and flax seeds as well as almonds, filberts, pistachios, peanuts, and cashews in their raw, unroasted, and more nutritious form. Some people find peanuts hard to digest, and some are allergic to them, but you may find them a delicious addition to your diet. Enjoy walnuts and pecans, too, but eat the unshelled variety only in the fall and winter as they go rancid quite quickly (you can enjoy them shelled any time).

Tofu (Bean Curd)

Tofu is a versatile meat substitute, used for centuries in the Orient. Derived from soybeans, tofu is a good protein and calcium source. It is bland, but will take on the flavor of whatever spices and foods it is prepared with, such as garlic (try sautéing in a little olive oil). The firm variety has slightly more protein than the softer variety, but you may want the softer one, depending on the recipe. Buy fresh tofu (watch expiration dates) and use within a week of opening (change the water daily unless it comes in a sealed package). If it smells strong or sour, do not use it. Tofu may be good for menopausal women because of its phytoestrogens, but see both sides of the story in chapter 14.

VEGETARIANISM

If you are eating plenty of vegetables, beans, and fruit, you may be healthier than meat eaters, despite these possible nutrient-deficiency risks. The National Institute for Occupational Safety and Health reported in 1989 that this kind of diet seems to protect against certain cancers. Unfortunately, most vegetarians rely more on grains, starches, and sweets than they do on legumes and vegetables. In my experience, this cancels out some, if not all, of the benefits of vegetarianism. So many of us have difficulty digesting carbos made from wheat (or white) flour, and these high starch foods, like highly sweetened foods, often provide the body with more stress than nutrition. Moreover, wheat, rye, barley, and possibly oats contain a chemical called phytate that blocks the absorption of minerals like calcium.

If you are an A blood type, you may be better adapted to a nutrient-rich (versus a low-nutrient, starch-based) vegetarian diet. But if you are an

O blood type, you may not do well at all as a vegetarian; you may need to at least eat fish and eggs.

I don't mean to make eating by your blood type a religion. It's just a guide that our clinic has found to be useful frequently, but not always. Your own body's unique responses to foods are your *best* guides by far. Just be sure to eat enough protein at every meal (average 20 grams or 3 to 4 ounces per meal: a palm-sized piece of tofu, 2 to 3 eggs). This can often put a stop to carbohydrate cravings and low energy. As a vegetarian, you also need to take supplements that supply iron, zinc, B_{12}, and L-carnitine, and if you're a menstruating, pregnant, or breastfeeding woman you will need iron supplements as well. If you are an A blood type you may need to take some hydrochloric acid, too, as you probably lack adequate amounts of this digestive aid that specifically helps with protein breakdown. This is probably the case if you feel tired and weighed down after a hefty serving of protein.

Because their diets already tend to be higher in carbohydrates, vegetarians really do need to eliminate refined carbos like sweets and starches *altogether.* It also helps if they add more vegetables, legumes (beans, peas, lentils, tofu, tempeh), nuts, and seeds to their meals. Vegetarians who can tolerate dairy products can use them to increase their protein intake. (B and AB blood types seem to be best adapted to dairy products.)

If you have a very high metabolism and are very physically active, you may need more grains than other vegetarians do. Go by your own body's response. Make them the side dish of your meals with vegetables and beans and other denser nutrient foods as your central focus.

You can come back to this chapter as a reference as often as you need to for reminders about your need to avoid some foods and work hard to get others. Remember, eat at least 2,100 calories a day and don't fast or skip meals.

I truly wish healthy eating were made easy for us all. I hope that this book will help you to keep fighting for what you need to survive and thrive.

Readings

Gittleman, Ann Louise. *The Body Knows Best* (New York: Pocket Books, 1996).
D'Adamo, Peter J. *Eat Right for Your Type* (New York: G. P. Putnam's Sons, 1996).
Tips, Jack. *Pro-Vita! Plan for Optimal Nutrition* (Austin, TX: Apple-a-Day Press, 1989).

NINETEEN

Shopping for Your Master Plan Supplies and Planning Your Meals

B y this time you know what foods and supplements you need for your individualized master plan; now it's time to go shopping. The object of this chapter is to give you suggestions on where to find these foods and supplements and how to develop new eating, cooking, and grocery shopping habits. Many of us are away from home for ten or more hours a day, so we need quick and easy suggestions for how to eat well every day, no matter how busy we are or where we are—at a friend's house, dining out, or grabbing a quick lunch before returning to the office. I'm confident that you'll find it easier than you think to stick to your master eating plan even when you're pressed for time or the choices on the menu are limited. There's so much wonderful food out there that you can enjoy that I know you won't miss the foods you're giving up. And if you're concerned about the costs of buying foods and supplements, please don't be. You are worth it. Think of all the money you'll be saving on chocolate!

MASTER PLAN COSTS

All of these supplements and organic foods may seem expensive to you, but put it in perspective. How much have you paid over the years for diet programs, prepackaged diet foods, or foods to binge on or to satisfy cravings? Have you had health problems due to your thyroid, adrenal, or hormone imbalances, or to an eating disorder that made you dig into your pocket? How much time have you lost from work because you didn't feel well enough to go in?

Some of the foods I recommend will cost more than the counterparts that you used to buy before starting your master plan. For example, organic produce usually costs more than conventional produce. But think of it as a type of health insurance—a "nutrition insurance" against future costs of poor health. Besides stopping cravings and enabling you to maintain your body's natural weight, properly balanced body chemistry can prevent cancer, heart attacks, and other debilitating or fatal diseases. This isn't another diet we are talking about. The Diet Cure is a wholistic program that will allow you to be healthy and vital for the rest of your life. You deserve that.

Besides the savings from avoiding the negative effects of eating poorly, you will often save money by buying fresh items and cooking them yourself over buying the processed equivalent. For example, potatoes are very inexpensive when bought in the produce section, but those frozen hash browns, French fries, and Tater Tots more than triple the price per pound.

EMPHASIZE EATING MORE VEGGIES

What do vegetarians, nutritionists, doctors, the Food and Drug Administration, and the average person have in common? We all know we should all be eating more fresh veggies. I know you have heard this before and it can't be said enough. There just is no better source for many of the things your body needs than fresh vegetables and lots of them. As you explore this style of eating you will find variations of some of your old favorites and many entirely new dishes that will become favorites. It's an adventure! Prepare and expect to enjoy it.

WHICH FOODS SHOULD YOU BUY?

Produce that is grown organically instead of conventionally draws a broader range of nutrients from the richer soil it is grown in. Just as junk food is made from refined sugar and flour that have been stripped of nutrients, conventional farming uses fertilizers that are refined until they contain only the minimum nutrients necessary to produce a saleable crop. In contrast, organically grown food contains the complete range of nutrients available from whole, organic compost, natural fertilizers such as

---

Food Value Continuum

Most Food Value:	Fresh, organic, naturally raised, home cooked
Next Best:	Fresh, conventionally raised meats and produce
Okay Sometimes:	Frozen, canned, dried
Avoid at All Times:	Processed, prepackaged, sugary, floury, fried, junk, or "drug" foods

---

manure, and mineral sources like kelp. Just as refined foods will eventually cause depletion of nutrients in a person, refined fertilizers result in foods with nutrient deficiencies.

In an ideal world, we would eat only fresh, raw, organic produce and naturally grown meat, poultry, and fish, and we would never touch sugar or refined carbohydrates. Lack of available sources for these preferred foods, lack of time, and price limit our ability to reach this ideal. The following suggestions are to help you work with these limitations in the real world.

Also, select foods rich in color. Your old Home Ec teacher was right: foods rich in color are highest in nutrients. Choose intensely orange carrots over pale ones, emerald green spinach over light green, and ruby red tomatoes over pink ones.

SO WHERE DO I FIND THESE FANTASTIC FOODS AND MY MASTER PLAN SUPPLEMENTS?

In Your Garden

Though organic produce is making inroads into the supermarkets in many areas, the best source is still your own garden. Growing your own leafy lettuce, mesclun, carrots, tomatoes, cucumbers, peas, or other veggies is both delicious and rewarding. You have the benefit of knowing the nutrient history of what you are eating. You also benefit from the short elapsed time from garden to plate. If you don't have the space for a big garden, try growing some vegetables in pots on your patio or balcony. Some vegetables, like the patio tomato, are especially bred for growing in pots. An herb garden takes up little room but will save you a lot of money—just snip off what you need to use. Depending on the space and time you have available, you can add other crops to your garden. Chatting with the clerk at the nursery or reading seed packages (which describe the size of the plants and the amount of space they need) will give you an idea of what is practical in your circumstances.

At the Farmers' Market

Shop your local farmers' market, if one is available to you. These are organized by farmers in a given area to give them an opportunity to sell direct to the public. They are usually held weekly and vary considerably in size. The larger markets may include hot foods to sustain you while you shop and arts and crafts vendors of all kinds. The produce is usually much fresher than the produce you find at your supermarket. Grocery store fruits and veggies may have been stored in a central warehouse for days, or even weeks, before being shipped to your local grocer. Farmers' markets often sell produce that was picked that very morning. Organic produce is more common at farmers' markets, too. You may be lucky enough to live near one of the growing number of farming cooperatives. You "invest" in the year's crops at the beginning of the season and pick up your "dividends" each week in the form of truly farm-fresh produce. Look in the phone book under "Farms" or "Cooperatives," or check the bulletin board at the health food store. It may take a little sleuthing, but the payoff in high-quality food will be worth it.

Shopping on the Perimeter of the Supermarket

Avoid the center aisles of the supermarket, which are usually filled with highly processed foods—baking mixes, packaged potatoes, canned goods, and frozen foods. These foods typically have nutrients processed out and sugar and saturated fat processed in. Instead, shop around the edges of the store, where you'll find the produce section, the meat section, and the dairy section. There you will usually find the foods needed to fulfill your master plan—fresh vegetables, fruit, meat, poultry, seafood, bulk grains, bulk beans, eggs, and milk products.

Recent years have seen the development and growth of markets specializing in healthy foods. These stores carry more organic vegetables, raw or lightly processed foods, naturally raised meats and poultry, and bulk foods like flours, grains, and beans than your traditional supermarket.

They often carry food supplements, but are larger than health food stores and stock many more food products. See the resources section for some of these markets that might have branches in your area. These markets are a boon to those of us who shop for fresh, quality meat, produce, dairy products, food supplements, and special foods for allergy sufferers.

At Your Health Food Store

Health food stores are often a good source for grains, beans, nuts, seeds, gluten-free bread and pasta, yogurt, tofu, tempeh, cheese, tortillas, polenta, organic pasta sauces, and salsa. They may also have a selection of fresh, organic produce. Many carry frozen meats and poultry raised without chemicals, or they may have fresh meats, depending on their size. But remember, just because a food is found in a health food store does not necessarily make it healthy. Use the same vigilance that you would shopping anywhere else. Not-so-healthy "health" foods include candy bars and cookies sweetened with raw sugar, concentrated fruit juice, or honey, which can be found in abundance in most health food stores. These intense carbohydrates can create cravings and deplete nutrition, just as goodies sweetened with refined sugar do.

Your health food store will have most of the nutritional supplements your master plan calls for, and may be able to order any that they don't carry in stock. When you buy supplements at your health food store, you have a better chance of finding someone to consult with personally. They can guide you to the products available in your area that contain the particular nutrients you need for your master plan. Consult with them, but be sure you do not compromise your needed nutrients when making a product decision. Check that you will be getting each nutrient in the strength suggested on your plan. You may need to go to more than one source to get all the nutritional supplements you require. See the resources section for health food stores that might have branches in your area.

Mail Order Sources

Many supplements can be purchased at discounts of 20 to 40 percent through mail order. Some of the larger companies that take orders by mail, phone, and/or Web site are listed in the resources section for this chapter. Most of these companies have people answering their phones who can help fill your particular supplement needs. Some have Web sites with information on the potencies and uses for particular herbs and supplements.

MORE TIPS FOR PURCHASING MASTER PLAN FOODS AND SUPPLEMENTS

Buying Fish

In today's world, the most healthy choice of fish is often frozen, especially if you live inland. So-called fresh fish in most supermarkets is anything but fresh. When choosing a whole fish, press the skin; if the depression remains, it's not fresh. The eyes should be clear, not frosty; the gills red and bright, not turning yellow. The nose knows, so follow your nose; if it smells very fishy, choose frozen instead. Most frozen fish today is "fresh frozen" only hours after it is caught.

Buying Spices

Add your favorite spices to a variety of foods to enhance both flavor and food value. Spices can make a boring meal interesting. Experiment: borrow a bit from a friend if you don't want to plunk down four dollars on an entire bottle, or buy in small quantities from a store that sells herbs and spices from bulk containers. It's better to buy spices in small amounts anyway, as they go bad long before you'll use up a big container. Throw them out when they no longer have a strong smell. Maintaining an herb garden is a great way to ensure you'll always have plenty of fresh herbs on hand, a great way to save money.

Buying Supplements

The cost of nutritional supplements will vary depending on your particular master plan and where you buy them. In 1998 my clients initially paid around two hundred dollars retail when beginning their programs. These initially purchased supplements run out over varying periods of time, depending on your particular master plan. The cost range for supplements for a twelve-week program at Recovery Systems was four hundred to nine hundred dollars retail in 1998. This may sound like a lot of money, but remember that you will only be taking the complete master plan nutritional supplements for a limited time. Once your body has repaired itself enough to maintain balance through a healthy diet, you will stop taking most of the supplements. Comparison shopping among local stores and mail order sources can also result in substantial savings.

Read the List of Ingredients

Wherever you shop, make sure all foods and supplements that you buy are free of hidden sugar and any other food you are intolerant of or allergic to. (See chapter 5 on food intolerance.) Read labels' ingredients lists carefully. Ingredients differ from product to product. For example, soy sauce is usually made with wheat in addition to soy, but there are a few brands made without wheat. One brand may have soy sauces with different ingredients under two different labels, one containing wheat and the other not. The only way to be sure of what you are getting is to read the ingredients list on each product.

When buying supplements, pay attention to dosages. Also, always check expiration dates. Some supplements, like flax seed oil—even in capsule form—are quick to spoil.

STAPLES OF THE DIET CURE PLAN

Many of the foods I recommend may not be staples in your household. The following are items I like to keep on hand.

Special Pantry Items

+ Bragg Liquid Aminos. A soy sauce–like product, but with twice the protein and half the sodium of soy sauce, plus amino acids.
+ Tofu. A protein substitute, with little or no taste, made from soybeans; it comes in firm, extra firm, and soft consistencies.
+ Tempeh. A soy-based product, like tofu, that contains complete protein and vitamin B_{12} and freezes well. It is usually firmer than tofu, giving it more bite, and sold in serving-size squares.
+ Hummus. A Middle Eastern spread/dip made from chick-peas (garbanzo beans), garlic, lemon juice, and spices.
+ Baba ghanouj. A Middle Eastern, eggplant-based spread.

Fruits and Veggies

These fruits and vegetables can be kept for longer periods than others, so they're good to keep on hand.

+ Apples
+ Oranges

✦ Potatoes
✦ Celery
✦ Tomatoes
✦ Carrots
✦ Onions
✦ Garlic
✦ Jicama. (A large, light brown root with a crispy white interior. The taste is somewhere between a potato and an apple.)

Canned, Jarred, Boxed, and Bottled

✦ Spaghetti (marinara) sauce. Look for organic brands with no added sugar.
✦ Extra virgin olive oil. Worth the extra price for its extra nutrients. Often available at discount warehouse-type stores (like Costco) and at Greek or Italian groceries at good prices.
✦ Canola oil.
✦ Grapeseed oil.
✦ Soy milk (unsweetened).
✦ Pasta. Whole wheat is fine if you aren't gluten-intolerant, but rice, corn, quinoa, and potato are also good choices.
✦ Canned or dry soups. Most canned soups are too salty. Look for Low Sodium, Very Low Sodium, or Sodium Free varieties, which will help you keep your daily sodium intake in the 1,800- to 2,400-milligram range. Health Valley brand canned and dry soup cups contain half the sodium of other brands.

Baking and Bread-Making Essentials

You may want to start making your own bread and other baked goods, especially if you are gluten intolerant. If so, you will find the following useful:

✦ Garbanzo bean flour (also called chana flour)
✦ Rice flour
✦ Tapioca flour
✦ Potato Starch flour
✦ Baking powder (Try the Rumford brand, which is free of aluminum, since excess aluminum builds up in the brain and is a suspected causative factor in Alzheimer's disease.)

✦ Baking soda
✦ Xanthan gum (helps give baked goods a consistency similar to gluten-containing products)
✦ Dry yeast

WHAT TO EAT

Easy Protein

It seems to take the most effort to get the protein foods, especially fish, meats, and poultry, into our diets. Here are some hints for adding protein to your meals without excessive effort.

✦ Roasting a chicken (or a turkey breast or thigh) will provide enough protein for your whole family in one meal, or for future quick, leftover meals. See chapter 20 for recipes that result in a special meal.
✦ You'll also find recipes for Easy Baked Protein, which can be used with poultry, fish, meats, or tofu to help add variety to your meals.
✦ Keep canned beans on hand (be sure there are no sweeteners listed in the ingredients, just beans, water, and salt) or cook a big batch ahead to have on hand in the refrigerator for a few days. Use beans in your vegetable salads, or add them to soups and stews. When cooking your own dry beans, pour off soak water and cook beans at low heat, to increase digestibility. If you still have a problem with beans giving you gas, try one of the commercial products such as Bean-O or AbsorbAid, which contain amylase, the carbohydrate-digesting enzyme. When using canned beans, drain and rinse them to reduce sodium and improve digestibility.

Snacking

Nuts and Seeds. For protein, healthy fats, and plenty of other nutrients, these are a sure bet. The original fast food, nuts and seeds don't require cooking or any complicated preparation. Just pop them in your mouth and chew. Remember that raw nuts and seeds contain many nutrients and enzymes that are lost during roasting. Trail mixes of nuts, seeds, and coconut flakes (with little or no dried fruit) are only slightly more complicated to prepare, or can be bought already mixed. Avoid rancid (unfresh) grains, seeds, and nuts. Eating such foods depletes the body of protective antioxidant (anti–free radical and anticancer) nutrients such as vitamin C, essential fatty acids, and especially vitamin E—the body's primary fat-soluble antioxidant. Try to buy grains in nitrogen-sealed packages (they are sold this way in many health food stores) to get them at their freshest. Discard any broken or misshapen nuts and seeds before eating; if they aren't rancid yet, they will turn rancid more quickly. Keep these foods under refrigeration once opened and use them up promptly. Discard them at the first sign of rancidity. Walnuts in particular go rancid within a month after shelling unless refrigerated or frozen. Aflatoxin, a toxic mold which grows on these foods (especially peanuts), has been directly linked to cancer.

Fresh Fruit and Veggies. Keep lots of these on hand. Yearn for an afternoon pickup? Raw veggies, celery sticks, or fresh fruit with raw nuts, seeds, or cheese will tide you over until dinner, while providing nutrition not available from a Snickers Bar or a Coke.

Simple Roasted Turkey or Beef. These can be bought at many delicatessens and market deli counters. Avoid the processed lunchmeat variety with additives and nitrates. A large salad of greens, chopped veggies, tomatoes, beans, roast turkey, and crumbled feta cheese is delicious and makes a complete meal in a bowl.

Soy Products. High in protein and needing little preparation, these essentials can be found in the refrigerator case at many health food stores. It's great to keep tempeh on hand for those last-minute meals. With luck, you'll find it already seasoned, which makes your cooking even simpler.

Dry Soup Cups. With these you make part of a quick lunch or a snack by simply adding boiling water. Some brands have more nutrition and less sodium; read the labels.

Protein Powder. A necessity for blended drinks and quick meals when there isn't time to cook. If you have intolerances or allergies, you will need to read the label carefully before you buy. Some contain wheat products and many contain milk products, such as whey. I recommend the rice-based products because they are the most digestible, but you can select any that are safe and acceptable for you. Beware of chocolate, sugar, and other sweeteners in many of the protein powders available. Twelve grams of protein per tablespoon is ideal.

Time-Saving Tips to Get More Veggies into Your Diet:

✦ Use a very sharp knife to chop vegetables. It makes the job easier and gives you more control over the final product. Food processors are fine, although I find that the extra setup and cleanup time offset any time saved in preparing the vegetables. Though veggies are most nutritious when eaten soon after being cut, you can chop them ahead of time, if necessary. Be sure to refrigerate them and use them within two to three days.

✦ Prepare a large salad, full of a variety of raw vegetables and different types of lettuces, and store it in an airtight plastic container to use for a few days in a row. Use romaine, red leaf, green leaf, or fancy mixed greens, like mesclun, because iceberg lettuce is not nutritious (and is hard to digest, too). Keep in mind when counting your daily 4 to 6 cups of vegetables that lettuce only counts as half a serving (that is, 1 cup of lettuce really only counts as a $1/2$ cup of vegetables) because of its bulk and relatively low nutritive value. Make sure your salad is chock full of other vegetables.

✦ Bake potatoes or yams five or more at a time, then use them as needed for quick snacks, soups, or side dishes.

✦ Make large quantities of vegetable soup or stew and freeze 2-cup portions for future use.

✦ Steam vegetables in a stainless steel steamer or a steaming basket.

✦ Stir-fry vegetables by putting 1 teaspoon to 1 tablespoon olive, canola, or grapeseed oil in a cast-iron skillet or wok. Heat the skillet over medium heat and add vegetables, stirring until tender, but

For more ideas, read the Foods for Special Needs section that follows. These are good foods to include in your menu even if you don't have an allergy or need to raise your serotonin level.

Foods for Special Needs

Gluten Intolerant? If you are allergic to the gluten-containing grains—wheat, oats, barley, and rye—you don't have to do without bread and pasta. Gluten-free bread and pasta are available at health food stores and natural food chains, such as Whole Foods and Wild Oats. (See the resources section at the end of this chapter.) Most are made using rice flour. One gluten-free pasta line, Pastato, is derived mostly from potatoes. Ancient Harvest makes corn and quinoa spaghetti and veggie curls. Pasta Riso still crisp. You may use the broth cubes described in chapter 20 for additional liquid.

✦ Steam-sauté veggies in a sauté pan, with a small amount of water or stock and Bragg Liquid Aminos (a nonfermented, gluten-free, soy sauce–like product made from soy beans and purified water). Heat to boiling, then remove from heat, cover, and let stand 15 to 20 minutes. You'll love the great flavor! Or sauté vegetables in water only and add 1 teaspoon to 1 tablespoon of any recommended oil after cooking.

✦ Buy vegetarian or vegetable cookbooks for help with ideas. (See the resources section for this chapter for some suggestions.)

✦ Make your own sprouts. When prepared properly, sprouts are a wonderfully rich source of enzymes, vitamins, and nutrients. Unfortunately, most store-bought alfalfa sprouts are not healthy to eat. Since 1995, U.S. health officials have traced eight outbreaks of salmonella and *E. coli* to alfalfa sprouts. The FDA has issued an advisory suggesting sprouts be avoided by the elderly, the very young, and anyone with a compromised immune system.[1] Usually, if sprouts have gone bad, you can see a yellowish discoloration at the root ends. This yellow color indicates the presence of a fungus known as damping-off. Do not eat this type of sprout. Instead, grow them at home yourself, and eat them a day or two after sprouting occurs, before the fungus ever appears. It's helpful to add a few drops of stabilized oxygen or grapefruit seed extract to the water when watering the sprouts to discourage the damping-off reaction.

and EnerG make rice spaghetti, lasagna, and other noodles that defy the wheat-eater to tell them from the usual products. Bean thread pasta is available in many markets in the section with other oriental foods.

You can also make your own delicious gluten-free bread and pasta. Arrowhead Mills Gluten Free Pancake Mix makes good pancakes and cornbread. EnerG Foods also has a line of gluten-free baking mixes available in health food stores and by mail.

See the references in this chapter for cookbooks with specific recipes for making your own gluten-free yeast breads and pastas from scratch. Many of these cookbooks have bread recipes formulated to be made in your bread machine. I have also included one of my favorite bread recipes in chapter 20.

Corn tortillas are delicious to use instead of bread or flour tortillas.

Polenta (regular, quick, or ready made) is good as a hot cereal or pasta replacement.

Rice is also gluten free. Our nutritionist, Tim Kuss, recommends basmati rice, as regular brown rice tends to go rancid rapidly during storage.

Quinoa flakes cook up like quick oatmeal, have a nutty flavor, and are gluten free.

Cider vinegar, wine vinegar, and balsamic vinegar replace, and improve on, distilled vinegar.

Trader Joe's Mayonnaise or Vegenaise (in the refrigerator case), or other brands made without distilled vinegar are a good bet.

Condiments, such as mayonnaise, catsup, relishes, and others, are a special problem because most contain vinegar and most commercial vinegar is made from wheat. Stay away from any prepared condiment (or other prepared food) listing "vinegar" or "distilled vinegar" as an ingredient. A little hunting will turn up condiments free of wheat products—including Trader Joe's Mayonnaise, Bragg Liquid Aminos (similar to soy sauce), San-J, Eden, Soken, or Chun King Soy Sauce—nutritional yeast, any miso without wheat or barley.* Look for mustards made with cider or wine vinegar instead of distilled. When you avoid these foods because of the vinegar, you get the added benefit of skipping the refined sugar many of them contain.

Lactose Intolerant? Lactose-free or -reduced milk is available at supermarkets in both 2 percent fat and nonfat. Milk with acidophilus to reduce lactose is also available at many stores.

Some people who are lactose intolerant can eat goat's or sheep's milk products. Cheeses made from goat's or sheep's milk are less allergenic. Pecorino and French feta are traditionally made with sheep's milk, but check the ingredients list on the package to be sure. Markets, delis, health food stores, and specialty stores such as Trader Joe's (see the resources section for this chapter) are carrying an increasing variety of goat cheeses.

Trying to Raise Your Serotonin Levels? Keep foods in your pantry that are high in serotonin or serotonin-raising tryptophan. Include turkey, pumpkin, milk, bananas, and sunflower, pumpkin, and sesame seeds in your menu plans. See the recipes in chapter 20 for Seed or Nut Milk Shake, which includes plenty of the serotonin-raising foods.

---

*These brands have some varieties containing wheat; check the ingredients list.

On the Anti-Yeast Diet? Bragg Liquid Aminos may be substituted for soy sauce on the yeast diet. When fighting yeast, increase the veggies you eat while you are limiting fruit. Have some celery, carrots, or other veggies prepared, ready to be eaten raw when you want a snack.

BE PREPARED FOR EATING ON THE GO

Eating on the go is one of the biggest sabotagers of a healthy eating plan. Plan ahead for meals away from home. Prepare salads and vegetables and pack them in a small cooler. Some coolers come with a refreezable ice container in the lid.

You should also make sure you always have a can opener with you: you never know when you'll be stuck somewhere and the only health food choice is a can of tuna. I also suggest you bring bottled water with you rather than relying on tap water to get your eight glasses a day. An insulated water bottle carrier is not only convenient, but can prevent the plastic bottle from overheating and leaching hormonelike chemicals into your water.

EATING AT RESTAURANTS

Restaurants present a challenge when you are following the Diet Cure Plan. Instead of ingredient lists, you are faced with menu descriptions that provide more temptation than information. Your first strategy is simple and direct. Simply say to your waitperson, "I need your help. I'm on a restricted diet, and can't have any [milk products; wheat, oats, rye, or barley; or whatever]" or "I'm trying to avoid too many carbohydrates, so could I have half the amount of rice and twice the amount of the side vegetable?" Most of the people who wait tables are happy to serve your needs. More and more, restaurant staffs are familiar with various diet restrictions and happy to help make appropriate choices. Tell them your restrictions up front, then repeat them when giving your order to be certain it's understood.

The second strategy is just as simple and direct. Be assertive about asking questions: "Are there milk products in that dressing?" "Is the (entrée) breaded or floured?" "Can I get that broiled instead of fried?" "Does the house dressing use distilled or wine vinegar?" As your experience grows you will learn the specific questions that have to be asked in your particular case. Don't be embarrassed or intimidated. Getting the information you need may mean a trip or two to the kitchen for your server, but you are paying for this meal, you are expected to give a tip for the service you are requesting, and we are talking about *your* health!

Even after you have asked for general help in avoiding dishes that contain foods off limits, explained the restrictions, and asked your questions, you still need to be careful. If you don't ask enough *specific* questions, you may be confronted with flour thickening in the clam chowder, croutons on your salad, or sugar in the Chinese food. The struggle to keep the bread and butter off your table can become comical. If, after all your efforts, your dinner arrives with unacceptable ingredients, send it back. You and your health are worth it.

Browsing the Menu

Breakfast is probably the easiest meal of the day to have in a restaurant and still keep to your program. If your cholesterol count is normal, then eggs are okay. You can even get in one of your vegetable servings by choosing an omelet with spinach, zucchini, or other vegetable offerings. The high sodium content, saturated fats, and nitrates of the ham, bacon, and sausage probably rule them out as regular fare, except for fresh sausage made from turkey or chicken. Juices concentrate the sugar of the fruit and are too sweet, but whole fruit is fine, or order vegetable or tomato juice. You are probably steering clear of the coffees and black teas because of the caffeine, but many restaurants now offer herb teas, or you can bring your own tea bags and just order hot water.

Any of the eggs and omelets listed on the menu with potatoes on the side are fine; just avoid the deep fried variety. If toast, biscuits, or a muffin is included with the entrée, ask if they will substitute potatoes or fruit for the bread. If you are gluten intolerant, you can bring a slice of your own gluten-free bread and ask them to toast it. Most restaurants will oblige. Pancakes and waffles are too high in carbos, contain gluten, usually contain sugar, and you'll be tempted to pour sugary syrup on them.

At lunchtime, concentrate on the salads, especially those with meat or poultry, such as one with grilled chicken, or a chef's salad or a Cobb salad. If you are avoiding lactose you will, of course, omit the cheeses from the salads. It will still be a very satisfying meal. All of these salads should contain some protein and mixed vegetables along with whatever lettuce is used as the base. If you can get more interesting and nutritious lettuces, great. If not, the salad is still a good bet. Chicken soup (with rice, not noodles, if you are gluten intolerant), bean or pea soup, vegetable or vegetable-beef soup, or turkey or chicken with vegetables have a good protein-to-carb ratio and are often gluten, sugar, and milk free.

If you are gluten intolerant, skip the sandwich section on the menu or order a sandwich and ask them to hold the bread; otherwise, sandwiches heavy on the protein filling can be a good choice. Most restaurants offer whole-grain breads, such as wheat or pita bread. But if you need yours gluten free, you might bring your own bread to be made into a sandwich. Skip the pasta and dessert sections unless the pasta is whole grain (which you'll find in some health food restaurants) and the dessert is a lovely fresh fruit plate most restaurants can provide on request.

Entrées that are broiled, grilled, steamed, sautéed, roasted, or stir-fried are more likely to be healthy and gluten free than fried offerings, which are often floured or breaded. Ask your waitperson to check with the kitchen, if you need to avoid gluten, because some fish, poultry, and meats are floured before being sautéed, stewed, or roasted. Avoid deep-fried entrées, which are almost always coated with wheat-flour batter and cooked at carcinogen-creating high temperatures.

Because alcohol is a super carbo, you'll need to keep your intake low, and be sure to drink only when eating a protein-rich meal. Even the non-alcoholic beers and wines are high in empty carbos and typically contain some alcohol.

Anticipating Allergy Problems You Could Have

When you consider:	You might ask the waiter to check whether:
Soup	It is thickened with wheat flour or contains any pasta, has cheese, sugar, cream, or milk added, or cheese on top?
Salad	It has any croutons on it and if the dressing has distilled vinegar; it has any cheese in it and if the dressing has milk products or sugar in it; whether it contains mostly iceberg lettuce or better quality lettuces with other vegetables, too; and how big it is (you may want to order a large instead of a side salad)?

Gravies/sauces	It is thickened with wheat flour, or if it contains sugar, or is made with milk or cream?
Entrées	The meat/fish/poultry is floured before cooking; or has breading or batter on it; or is deep fried; if it has any cheese (Parmesan is common) on it; and how large the portion size is (ideally, it will take up one quarter or more of your plate)?

The highly refined and processed foods that are so prevalent in American diets and are the source of so many of our food-related problems are largely missing from the diets in other countries. This makes ethnic or foreign restaurants promising choices when you want to eat out and stay with your plan. Comparing Diet Cure elements and culinary features shows us why.

Chinese and Other Asian Cuisines

I recommend steaming and stir-frying as preferred cooking methods. Chinese cooking features these methods in a high percentage of its recipes. Chinese restaurants can be found nearly everywhere and feature many different entrées with steamed or stir-fried vegetables with chicken or fish and various spice combinations. You will probably want to steer clear of things like Sweet and Sour Pork because it combines a particularly fatty meat with concentrated sweeteners, but there will be plenty of dishes featuring lean meat and lightly cooked veggies for you to try.

Be sure to try some of the Chinese soups. Sizzling rice soup is fun with its noisy presentation. Look for Hot and Sour soup, which is rich, spicy, and practically a meal in itself.

A few words of caution for the gluten intolerant regarding Chinese restaurants: Most of them use a soy sauce in the cooking and on the table that is made from wheat and can give you a problem. The wrappers on many foods—dim sum, spring rolls, won ton, and others—are also made from wheat. I have found the gluten-avoidance problems outweigh the benefits and have sought out other Asian cuisines where small changes in ingredients result in big increases in interesting choices.

Thai, Cambodian, Vietnamese, and other Southeast Asian cuisines usually share the attributes of their Chinese cousins—lean meats, fresh veggies lightly cooked, emphasis on steaming and quick stir-frying, for example. As an added bonus, Thai and Vietnamese restaurants usually have many gluten-free items on the menu; they tend to emphasize rice over wheat in their meals. For example, often the noodles are made from rice and therefore gluten free; ditto the spring roll wrappers. But remember, you'll still have to watch out for wheat in the soy sauce (you may want to bring your own). Milk is rare in Asian cuisines. Japanese, Chinese, Thai, and Vietnamese food seldom contain any milk products, making these restaurants' menus easy to choose from when avoiding milk.

One thing to beware of when eating Chinese food is monosodium glutamate (MSG). MSG, used heavily in Chinese food in the past, causes Chinese restaurant headache syndrome because many people are intolerant of it. Today, many Chinese restaurants forego the MSG, but some still use it. Ask. You may have to request that they leave out the MSG.

Mexican Food

This is a good choice for eating out while sticking to the Diet Cure. It is especially easy to find in cities in the western United States, where Mexican restaurants and *tacquerias* are only a few blocks apart.

Everybody's favorite appetizer in a Mexican restaurant is guacamole and chips. The good news is that the guacamole is fine, especially if it is made fresh at the table. The bad news is the deep-fried chips are on the "nonfood" list. Use the guacamole as a condiment on your entrée or on a soft, steamed corn tortilla, and enjoy.

The standard side dishes for entrées in Mexican restaurants are beans and rice, which provide a complete protein when served together. Large salads with lettuce, veggies, and grilled chicken are found in most of these restaurants. Tortilla "bowls" that salads are sometimes served in are almost always made of deep-fried flour tortillas. Ask them to hold the tortilla bowl and serve your salad in a dish instead.

If you are avoiding gluten, get corn, not flour tortillas, whether they're served on the side or as a wrap for fajitas, burritos, or some other dish. Most flavored tortillas (spinach, tomato, and others) are made from refined wheat flour. Order a burrito on a plate without the wheat tortilla wrapper, to be eaten with a fork. Ask if they will substitute rice or beans for the tortilla. Some burritos use whole wheat tortillas or soft corn tortillas. Enchiladas are traditionally made with corn tortillas, but they are sometimes made using wheat tortillas, and enchilada sauce can contain flour thickening, so ask if you are gluten intolerant.

You might also want to try tamales, which consist of meat, usually beef or chicken, or cheese, wrapped in a corn meal dough and steamed inside a corn husk wrapper. Add some salsa and guacamole if you like. Fajitas are now fashionable in almost every Mexican restaurant and represent an excellent choice. Lean beef or chicken breast are grilled and then served with warm tortillas (preferably corn), grilled veggies, salsa, guacamole, and sometimes other condiments. You assemble your own soft tacos from the array.

If you are lactose intolerant, cheese will be your main concern when you eat Mexican food because it is found in many dishes. It is usually a topping and easy for the kitchen to omit. It will sometimes be included in dishes like burritos automatically, so it is best to ask.

Italian Food

You won't have any trouble eating at an Italian restaurant, unless you don't like Italian food! After all, this is a Mediterranean cuisine using the right oils and lots of veggies. What's not to like? Well, they often feature marvelous Italian bread and pasta dishes that are out of balance with too much starch. So you'll have to leave some on the plate if you have it "as is," and concentrate on other Italian delights. Consider the usual terrific salads made with a wide variety of greens, ripe red tomatoes, a little zesty onion, and a dressing based on extra virgin olive oil. Or how about a small serving of roasted potatoes, lightly sautéed herbed veggies on a bed of al dente pasta with a nice piece of chicken or fish? Or polenta, a delicious corn meal dish formed into firm cakes, may accompany your entrée. Deep fried items are practically unheard of in Italian cooking.

There will almost certainly be salmon on the menu, which you should consider ordering. Roasted chicken with rosemary and garlic is also a frequent offering on Italian menus.

There are also wonderful vegetable dishes that appear as appetizers, such as baked eggplant with tomato, herbs, Gruyère or goat cheese, pesto and a light tomato sauce or portobello mushrooms stuffed (make sure there aren't any bread crumbs, if you are gluten intolerant) and baked. Keep your proportions in mind and you won't have any trouble finding ways to assemble a flavorful and satisfying meal.

Choices for the gluten and milk intolerant are, of course, much more limited in a cuisine built around wheat pasta and featuring lots of cheeses, but you can always order meat, chicken, or fish, or ask for a vegetable appetizer as an entrée, or order a salad (omit the croutons and grated Parmesan cheese). Most Italian restaurants will be happy to substitute polenta for pasta as a side dish, but the milk-sensitive should check to be sure it contains no cheese. Stay alert: Cheese in the polenta is something the waiter is apt to forget, even after you have told him of your allergy problem and quizzed him about other dishes. It's you who will suffer the discomfort (or worse) if a mistake is made, so always ask the extra question.

Buffets and Salad Bars

The variety of choices on a buffet or salad bar make them especially good places for eating lunch or dinner out. Try 3 to 4 ounces of one of the roast meats, some rice or potatoes, and a large salad, composed of as many different vegetables as possible. If you don't have your own salad dressing with you, your best bet is the vinaigrette, if not thickened, or simply oil and vinegar that you put on yourself. Large buffets will often have a fish entrée or two that can be good choices. Chicken is fine unless it is deep fried. Remember the balance between protein and carbohydrates and the "palm size" guide to protein serving size (3 to 4 ounces of meat will fit in your palm). Let the veggies outnumber the starches (potatoes, rice, or pasta) about three to one. Choose lots of raw veggies, skipping the mayonnaise-laden potato and macaroni salads (the mayo almost certainly contains distilled vinegar anyway, an additional problem for the gluten intolerant, and sugar). Add lots of beans, egg, or meat for protein. A baked potato is a satisfying addition available at some of the franchise salad bars. Top your potato with salsa, a little cheese or sour cream (if you tolerate milk well), butter, chopped broccoli, and/or chopped green onion. Vegetable, bean, or split pea soups are a good combination with salad and are usually gluten and milk free.

The Fast-Food Gauntlet

Sometimes you just can't avoid fast-food places. The birthday boy simply *must* go to Chuck E. Cheese. Soccer practice runs late and everybody ends up at the Burger King. Here you are in Deep Fried Sodium Heaven and so now what about your individualized master plan? Do you say, "What the heck" and order up a bacon double cheeseburger, jumbo fries, and a chocolate shake? Before we go there, let's consider some options.

If you have had some notice, you can pack up something from home to take along. This is obviously the best alternative if it is available. You will have complete control over the meal. If you are the victim of a surprise attack, your best bet is to find out what the salad offerings are. Some of the pizza restaurant chains have a salad bar where a better-than-fair meal can be assembled. If there is no salad offering and everything in sight is deep fried, sodium soaked, or worse, then all you can do is limit the damage. Even McDonald's now offers a small prepackaged salad, but it's *all* iceberg lettuce topped with American cheese and a dyed tomato slice. If McDonald's is your only choice, a grilled chicken sandwich or maybe a veggie burger (discard half of the bun) can sustain you until better fare is available. Wendy's has much better salads, heavy on the romaine, plus baked potatoes and chicken salad wraps in rather tasteless pita bread, and of course grilled chicken sandwiches as well (again, discard half the bread). Taco Bell has a lot of beans, cheese, guacamole, and some salad within the fajitas, but no side salads.

If you have intolerances, avoid the poisons. If you are gluten intolerant, tell the people at Burger King that "your way" means "No Bun." If milk is a problem, have them make your pizza without cheese. (I know it sounds odd, but lots of pizza in Italy—and New York City—is sold this way.) Just do the best you can. One meal will not be fatal to either you or your Diet Cure master plan.

EATING AT THE HOMES OF FAMILY OR FRIENDS

Most of the problems you might face while dining in other peoples' homes can be addressed by simply and politely controlling your own portions. As we have seen earlier, foods on the Diet Cure plan are mainly the foods everybody eats: It is the proportion of meat to vegetable to starch that is different. See chapter 20 for more help on visualizing proportions. Keep the ratios in mind and focus on the protein and vegetables.

If you are dealing with allergies and intolerances, your host or hostess would much rather hear your dietary needs ahead of time, before you sit down to eat the meal they've carefully prepared. Your host certainly doesn't want you to feel that you are not getting enough to eat because you are avoiding something he has cooked, or that you might chance hurting your health by eating something you shouldn't, just to please him. You might say, "I don't want to cause you to go to any trouble, but I thought you would want to know ahead of time that I can't have any _____." Give examples, to make it clear what you are saying. For example, if you are gluten intolerant, you could say, "That means no bread, flour, or pasta for me. I can have rice and corn, but wheat, oats, rye, and barley are out." Then offer to bring a dish of your own, if your special needs would inconvenience him or her. If you have mastered making your own gluten-free bread, offer to bring bread for everyone. Or offer to bring a gluten-free entrée, such as lasagna made with rice pasta, if that would be appropriate for the occasion.

Obviously, the best way to ensure that you stick to your Diet Cure plan is to prepare your own meals from fresh ingredients. While that's not always possible, in the next chapter you'll see that it's a lot easier to do than you might think.

Readings

Bailey, Janet. *Keeping Food Fresh: How to Choose and Store Everything You Eat* (New York: HarperPerennial, 1989).

Adler, Kief. *Beyond the Staff of Life* (Happy Camp, CA: Naturegraph Publishers, 1976/1980). This is an excellent wheatless and dairyless vegetarian cookbook.

———. *Without Gluten or Wheat* (New York: Henry Holt, 1996).

Cousins, Barbara. *Cooking Without: Recipes Free from Added Gluten, Sugar, Dairy Products, Yeast, Salt, and Saturated Fat* (Northampton, England: Thorsens Publishers, 1997).

Goldberg, Phyllis Z. *How to Tolerate Lactose Intolerance* (Springfield, IL: Charles C. Thomas, 1998).

Hagman, Bette. *The Gluten-Free Gourmet: Living* (New York: Henry Holt, 1990).

———. *More from the Gluten-Free Gourmet* (New York: Henry Holt, 1993).

———. *The Gluten-Free Gourmet Cooks Fast and Healthy* (New York: Henry Holt, 1997).

Kidder, Beth. *The Milk-Free Kitchen: Eating Well Without Dairy Products* (New York: Henry Holt, 1991).

Stepaniak, Joanne. *The Uncheese Cookbook* (Summertown, TN: Book Publishing Co., 1994).

Zukin, Jane. *Dairy-Free Cookbook* (Rocklin, CA: Prima Publishing, 1998).

Resources

GNC
(General Nutrition Centers)
<http://www.GNC.com>
GNC has more than three thousand stores in all fifty states and twenty foreign
countries (they are planning to expand to five thousand stores by 2002).
Their Web site includes a terrifically convenient search engine that will locate
all the stores within ten miles of your home. It also allows you to do some online shopping, but its online store doesn't carry supplements and herbs.

The Vitamin Shoppe
(800) 223-1216
<http://www.vitaminshoppe.com>
The Vitamin Shoppe has thirty-seven stores, mail order shopping, online shopping, and seventeen thousand products available at 20 to 40 percent discounts.

L&H Vitamins
(800) 221-1152
<http:www.bvital.com>
L&H Vitamins offers a broad selection of supplements at 20 percent discount
from suggested retail prices.

Whole Foods Market
<http://www.wholefoods.com>
Whole Foods Market has stores in twenty-one states under five different names.
"We're like an old fashioned neighborhood grocery store, an organic farmer's
market, a European bakery, a New York Deli, and a supermarket all rolled into
one," says Whole Foods. They also sell supplements and herbs. See their Web
site for the location closest to you.

Wild Oats
<http://www.wildoats.com>
Another of the health-conscious market chains, Wild Oats has fifty-six stores under five store names in sixteen states and British Colombia. (You can find the
closest location on their Web site.) Wild Oats offers a complete line of herbs
and supplements, plus a wide selection of Wild Oats' brand grocery items online at their Web site.

Infinity Health
(800) 733-9293
This is my clinic's order line, which has all of the supplements recommended in
this book.

NEEDS (National Ecological and Environmental Delivery System)
(800) 634-1380 Fax: (800) 295-NEED (6333)
527 Charles Ave, 12-A
Syracuse, NY 13209

Mail order source for more than 25,000 products at up to 40 percent off suggested retail. Supplements include many that are normally available only through health practitioners. You can get their 164-page catalog by writing, calling, or e-mailing their Web site.

TWENTY

Menus, Meal Ideas, and Recipes

WHAT IS THE IDEAL MEAL?

Picture a TV dinner tray with the huge section for meat, the two small ones for vegetables, and the tiny one for dessert. Or maybe a school cafeteria tray or a picnic plate with similar sections for the different parts of your meal. Or a big plate of hot macaroni and cheese or pasta primavera. Now that you will be eating differently, you will need a new visual image of portion sizes and proportions for the various elements of your meal. I will give you some guidelines to try out, and then tailor to your unique needs.

To start, take a look at the palm of your hand. The palm represents the protein portion of the meal (about a quarter of what is on your plate). Protein foods include meats such as chicken or turkey, fish, tofu, eggs, cottage cheese, and other protein choices. Next comes the low-carbohydrate vegetables portion, which ideally takes up a little over half of your plate. Low-carbohydrate vegetables include asparagus, broccoli, cabbage, celery, collards, cucumbers, kale, lettuce, scallions, and spinach, to mention a few.

The corner of the plate is for the potatoes, yams, polenta, or rice—the starchy carbohydrates or high-carb vegetables, grains, or fruits. This represents about 15 percent of your meal. Finally, allot a small percent of your plate to oils used to prepare or flavor foods, whether in the form of a pat of butter on your potato or a few tablespoons of good vegetable oil on your salad or in your cooked veggies; this is in addition to the fat in your fish, chicken, and other foods, such as nuts and avocados.

Here's an example: If your favorite dinner is a steak, potato, and salad, I encourage you to still enjoy this American favorite, but watch your proportions. Be sure your steak is about the size of your palm (takes up

Low-Carbohydrate Vegetables

- Mung bean sprouts
- Sweet red pepper
- Green bell pepper
- Chives
- Eggplant
- Spinach
- Chard
- Tomatoes
- Cucumbers
- Radishes
- Lettuce
- Cauliflower
- Cabbage
- Sunflower sprouts
- Artichokes
- Green chilies

- Celery
- Onions (raw)
- Parsley
- Leeks
- Zucchini
- Asaparagus
- Broccoli
- Green beans
- Snow peas
- Bok choy (Chinese cabbage)
- Mushrooms
- Garlic
- Brussels sprouts
- Clover sprouts
- Jicama
- Carrot

The Typical Dinner Plate

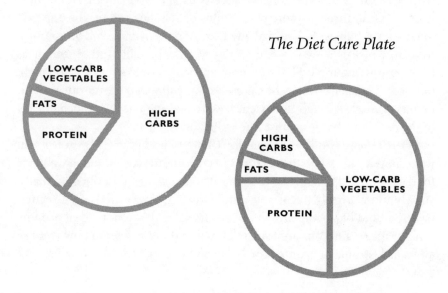

The Diet Cure Plate

High-Carbohydrate Vegetables

- Corn
- Rutabaga
- Winter squash
- Parsnips
- Celery root
- White potatoes
- Red potatoes

- Sweet potatoes
- Yams
- Beets
- Turnips
- Peas
- Jerusalem artichokes
- Onions (cooked)

almost a fourth of your plate). Don't have a little side salad. Have a salad loaded with a variety of vegetables that should be at least three to four times the size of your meat (if you have cooked vegetables, they should be about twice the size of your meat, but salad is bulkier). Have a medium-size potato. For fat, enjoy a pat of butter on your potato and dressing on your salad. Skip the bread and dessert. You'll be too full to eat them anyway.

Too Many Carbs

In America, our carbohydrate balance is usually way out of kilter. Most Americans eat three or more parts grains or starches and maybe one part low-carb vegetables. As I've explained, *excess carbohydrates are transformed into fat,* which is stored as energy reserves for possible future use, or as triglycerides in our blood. If our grain and starch intake remains too high, our body's efficient storage of calories as fat will win out over our need to maintain an ideal weight. In essence, we're fighting our own biochemistry in the process, a battle against impossible odds.

Here's some good news: You don't have to go hungry! If you feel you want more food than is represented here, you can have it. Just have more food as you need roughly in the proportions I've just described. Actually, you should eat freely but if you want extra-high-carb foods on a regular basis, without balancing protein, ask yourself "Is this a more ideal proportion for me or am I out of balance?" You'll find the answer in how you feel afterward: strong and content or heavy and dissatisfied.

Protein in Common Foods

Food	Quantity	Protein in Grams
Beans	1 cup	15
Bread	one slice	2–3
Buttermilk	1 cup	8
Cheese, firm	1 ounce	6–10
Cheese, soft	1 ounce	2–4
Corn	1 cup	4
Cottage cheese	1 cup	30
Eggs	one	6
Fruits	one (apple, banana, orange, etc.)	1
Meat, poultry, fish	3–3½ ounces (lean, no skin or bones)	17–27
Milk	1 cup	8–9
Nutritional yeast	1 tablespoon	8
Nuts	¼ cup	2–7
Oatmeal, cooked	1 cup	6
Rice, cooked	1 cup	6
Seeds	1 ounce	6
Tempeh	4 ounces	20
Tofu	8 ounces regular/ 5 ounces firm	20
Yogurt	1 cup	8–9

HEALTHY EATING AND FOOD-PREPARATION TIPS

The Best Oils for Everyday Use

For general cooking, canola and grapeseed oils are ideal choices. They both have long shelf lives, assuming they are refrigerated once opened. Moreover, they do not break down or "smoke" as quickly as other oils when heated. However, with all oils, it is best to cook at low temperatures to maintain food quality and integrity. For example, set an electric wok at 250 degrees. Do not deep fry in these oils; instead, sauté with just enough oil to coat the pan. If you like, you can add pure water or broth during the cooking process to reduce the amount of oil used.

Olive and canola are wonderful on salads. Walnut, sesame, and pumpkin seed oils are also tasty. They may be lightly drizzled over steamed

Daily Food Guide

This guide will help you to keep track of whether you are consuming enough of the right kinds of foods while on the Diet Cure.

Protein

20–30 grams per meal from fish, poultry, tofu, beef, eggs, or cheese (fish should be eaten two or more times per week)

Low-Carbohydrate Vegetables

At least 4 cups per day of zucchini, cauliflower, green beans, carrots, spaghetti squash, turnips, beets, kohlrabi, eggplant, mushrooms, chard, turnip greens, kale, or other low-carb choice.

✦ 6 spears asparagus = $1/2$ cup
✦ 1 head broccoli = $1^1/2$ cups
✦ 1 salad tomato = $2/3$ cup
✦ 3 stalks raw celery = 1 cup
✦ 1 cup raw salad greens (leaf lettuce, romaine, cabbage, spinach, arugula, etc.) counts as $1/2$ cup when calculating the 4 cups per day.

High-Carbohydrate Foods*

Legumes

Up to 1 cup per day (More for vegetarians, fast metabolizers, or in winter)

✦ 1 cup = $1/2$ can of garbanzos, kidney beans, refried beans, or navy beans
✦ 1 cup = 8 oz. split pea soup or lentil dahl
✦ 1 cup = $1/3$ cup dry beans measured before cooking

High-Carb Vegetables

1 to 2 cups (cooked or equivalent) per day

✦ 1 cup = 8 oz. cooked butternut or acorn squash, yams, Jerusalem artichoke, canned pumpkin
✦ 1 cup = 1 potato (approx. 4″ x 2″)
✦ 1 cup = 1 sweet potato (approx. 5″ x 2″)

Fruits

2–4 servings per day

✦ 1 serving = an apple, banana, nectarine, or peach
✦ 1 serving = $1/2$ grapefruit or cantaloupe
✦ 1 serving = 1 cup blueberries, cherries

Whole Grains

Up to 1 cup (cooked or equivalent) per day of rice, polenta, corn, quinoa, millet, buckwheat, etc. or other
+ 1 slice bread or 1 corn tortilla = $1/2$ cup

Raw Nuts and Seeds

Up to $1/3$ cup per day (vegetarians and fast metabolizers will need more of this rich source of protein, fats, and vitamins)
+ $1/4$ cup = $1^1/4$ oz. almonds, pine nuts, or sunflower seeds
+ $1/4$ cup = 2 oz. pumpkin seeds
+ $1/4$ cup = $2^1/2$ Tbs. tahini (sesame butter)

Additional Fats

2–3 tablespoons per day of cold pressed canola, walnut, olive, grapeseed, or sunflower oil, plus 1 Tbs. butter, if desired

Liquid

Eight or more 8-ounce (1 cup) portions of filtered water, herb tea, or mixed vegetable juice (not pure carrot)

*In winter, the intake of these high-carbohydrate foods may increase, but the stated amount per day is the maximum that we recommend for clients who desire weight loss.

vegetables after they're cooked to add more flavor. Flax oil may also be used in this way, and it comes in flavors, too. But be extra careful with it as it is fragile and will go rancid quickly if exposed to air or heat. Make sure to use all the flax oil before the expiration date on the bottle.

Fats to Avoid

Poor-quality fats and oils are the most potentially dangerous food substances in our diet. The four categories of poor-quality oils to be avoided are:

1. Unfresh oils of all kinds. Stale or rancid oils damage cells and encourage abnormal cell growth. Eating food containing rancid oil also destroys vitamins A, D, E, K, and precious essential fatty acids in the process. Keep all oils except olive oil in the refrigerator and keep them tightly sealed.
2. All hydrogenated or partially hydrogenated fats and oils. Hydrogenated oils are fried at high heat for hours without oxygen (it's replaced with

hydrogen), making the end product lifeless. Margarine and shortening are full of hydrogenated fats. Most packaged baked goods and baking mixes contain hydrogenated fats (another good reason to avoid them). All hydrogenated fats are highly reactive trans-fatty acids, which lead to detrimental free-radical activity and cause problems in heart and liver function. Avoid partially hydrogenated fats, too.

3. Fragile oils, which deteriorate quickly with age or exposure to heat or light. Such oils include corn, safflower, and cottonseed oils.

4. Oils in fried foods. These foods clog our arteries and make us feel congested, tired, and sluggish.

MEAL PLANNING

Breakfast: Don't Leave Home Without It

If you want to control cravings, breakfast is the most crucial meal for you. Too many people grab a quick muffin or bagel and coffee on the way to work, starting the cycle of craving sweets and starches that leads to blood sugar instability and more craving. Start your day right, with a nutritious breakfast. Here are some suggestions:

Smoothies Smoothies, or fruity blender drinks, are delicious and easy-to-digest meals in a glass. They can be a terrific balanced protein-carbohydrate-fat beverage. Use water, yogurt, or soy milk (not fruit juice or rice milk, because of the high sugar content), then blend in whole fruit. For protein, add nuts, seeds, or nut butters and protein powder.

Fresh fruit is best, but frozen berries are available all year round and are excellent in smoothies. However, you probably shouldn't use them frozen; let them thaw. Frozen smoothies are much too cold for the body to handle, especially in the cooler months of the year or first thing in the morning.

Other Quick and Delicious Breakfast Ideas

+ Have a large bowl of low-fat cottage cheese (1 cup) with sliced fresh fruit and a few almonds or sunflower seeds.
+ Make a base of a ¹/₂ cup rice, or a corn tortilla (heat on nonstick skillet with a few drops of water and the lid on). Top with one of the following:

+ turkey or chicken, with tomato, avocado, onion, lettuce
+ hummus (garbanzo bean spread/dip)
+ baba ghanouj (an eggplant-based spread)

✦ As an occasional meal, Cream of Rice cereal, or soft, hot polenta with a dash of cinnamon or nutmeg, plus any or all of the following sources of protein:

+ protein powder and/or nutritional yeast
+ raw nuts or seeds
+ Seed or Nut Milk (see recipe on page 319) with protein powder, yogurt, or cottage cheese (unless, of course, you're lactose intolerant), or an egg (stir in just before removing the cereal from heat, so the egg will cook)

✦ Scrambled, poached, or boiled eggs with one of the following:

+ polenta and tomato sauce
+ vegetables, scrambled with the eggs (you can use leftovers or frozen mixed vegetables, if needed, to make this faster). Sauté 1 to 5 cups (measured when raw) zucchini, tomatoes, onion, or other veggies in a nonstick pan, using a little broth, water, or oil. Then add 3 eggs and scramble. Add potatoes, or toast (gluten-free bread if you are intolerant).

Lunch Ideas

Lunches you make yourself are a sure way to get the foods you want to eat while sticking to your master plan. If you have a refrigerator available where you work, store an assortment of raw veggies, some cooked poultry or meat (not lunchmeat), cooked beans, and salad dressing to be assembled into a large salad; or bring a large mixed vegetable salad with protein from home and store it until lunch. Even if you don't have refrigeration available, you can bring your lunch to work, school, or any other outing in one of the insulated containers made for that purpose. Alternately, you could bring soup in a Thermos bottle.

Snacks

Snacks are an important part of the Diet Cure master plan. You should not go more than four to five hours without meals. Snacks can tide you over between meals. Also, snacking gives you an opportunity to work foods you might not otherwise eat, such as nuts and fruit, into your day. Carry around your own healthy snacks so you don't get stuck with convenience-store fare.

Try these healthy snacks for when you just want a bite of something.

✦ A handful of sunflower or pumpkin seeds, raw almonds, cashews, or other nuts.

✦ Pita bread, cut into triangles, topped with baba ghanouj or hummus. You can toast the pita to make it extra crispy, or substitute whole grain crackers, carrots, celery, and other fresh vegetables for your "dipper."

✦ A cup of plain, low-fat yogurt or cottage cheese with $1/2$ cup berries or a piece of sliced fruit of your choice.

✦ Vegetable sticks. Aside from carrots and celery, you can snack on red pepper strips, broccoli and cauliflower florets, cucumber and zucchini circles, jicama slices, or cherry tomatoes.

✦ A piece of fruit, with nuts or cheese.

✦ Raw almond butter or raw tahini (sesame butter) spread on crackers (Holgrain rice crackers or Trader Joe's Savory Thins are tasty, gluten-free brands). Be sure to use whole-grain crackers, not saltines or water crackers, which are just empty carbs.

Dinner Ideas

You've come home tired after a typically hectic day at work, or your afternoon has been full of running errands and cleaning up after the kids, or your energy just isn't high enough to cook big meals. Yet dinner is traditionally the biggest meal of the day, and maybe the only one when you eat together with your whole family. The following dinner suggestions are easy to prepare, nourishing, and tasty, while staying with the proportions of the ideal meal.

You could make baked fish with two or more cups of steamed veggies; a baked potato or brown basmati rice; plus cole slaw with oil-and-vinegar dressing, or cherry tomatoes and cucumber salad. Or stir-fry veggies with shrimp, chicken, or meat pieces, or tofu chunks, with ginger, garlic, and soy sauce to taste, and serve with basmati rice. Or add chicken breast, prawns, or another favorite protein prepared as you like (without breading) to whole-grain pasta (rice, corn, or quinoa for the gluten intolerant) with commercial pesto or marinara sauce; complete your meal with a large salad.

Cooking

Keep the ideal meal proportions in mind when you create a meal containing a mixture of foods, such as a chili, casserole, or soup. Put "more meat and low-carb vegetables in these dishes and decrease the starches. If the ratio of carbohydrates to protein in your casserole or soup is still too high, adjust the proportions with a side salad or side dish of protein.

For more ideas, invest in the cookbooks listed in the recommended readings for this chapter. When you use the following recipes or adjust your old standbys, keep these suggestions in mind:

+ Bake breads using extra protein items (egg; protein powder; bean, instead of wheat, flour for part of the flour; etc.) to improve these high-carbo, starchy foods.
+ Use higher-in-protein, whole-grain flours, grains, and pasta whenever possible. Good sauces and gravy can be made using rice or garbanzo flour (which is higher in protein than wheat flour). Rice flour sauces tend to get thin if reheated, so make them immediately before serving. People eating your rice flour gravy really will not be able to tell that you have done anything different. One of our Recovery Systems' staff members tells us that her turkey gravy made with rice flour is always the first gravy to go at her family Thanksgiving potluck dinner. Other thickeners such as potato starch and corn can also be used in sauces and gravies with great success.

See the resources section for gluten-free and dairy-free cookbooks.

SELECT-A-SALAD

Salads are a great way to enjoy all your food groups and get the nutrients you need. They're also easy to make, lovely to look at, and delicious when made fresh. Use the following chart for hundreds of salad variations.

For a complete-meal salad: Select items from lists 1, 2, 3, 4, and 5 and combine for a salad that is a satisfying meal.

For a side salad: For a salad to go along with a protein entrée, select from lists 1, 2, 5, and, if there's no other starchy carb in the meal, 3.

1. 2 cups or more from this list	2. 1 cup or more from this list	3. Total of ½ cup from this list	4. ¾ cup or more from this list	5. 2 Tbs. from this list
✦ green or red leaf lettuce ✦ spinach leaves ✦ romaine lettuce ✦ arugula ✦ mesclun ✦ other mixed greens ✦ cabbage ✦ *or* omit this list and use 1 more cup from list 2	✦ raw broccoli or cauliflower ✦ steamed broccoli, asparagus, green beans, or cauliflower ✦ tomatoes ✦ cucumber ✦ bell peppers ✦ avocado ✦ carrot, sliced or grated	✦ green peas ✦ black-eyed peas, lima, kidney, garbanzo, cannellini, black, or pinto beans ✦ corn, rice, or other cooked grains ✦ cooked potatoes or sweet potatoes	✦ roast beef, chicken or turkey ✦ ¼ cup nuts and or seeds ✦ cottage cheese ✦ ¼ cup feta cheese ✦ ½ cup beans or peas ✦ tofu or tempeh	✦ vinaigrette ✦ Vegetarian Caesar Salad Dressing (see recipes on page 320) ✦ other salad dressing with good oils and no sugar

CONSTRUCT-A-SANDWICH

1. On rice toast, soya bun, or other grain bread served open face
2. Mayonnaise without sugar, or Vegenaise
3. Add tuna, tofu, chicken, or turkey salad; garden burger; or hamburger
4. Top with quality lettuce
5. Stack on raw veggies (for example, cherry tomatoes, carrots, celery, cucumber, red bell peppers, or others)
6. Enjoy!

DELICIOUS VEGETABLE-PROTEIN SUGGESTIONS

✦ Rice-, tofu-, nut- and/or bean-stuffed vegetables (zucchini, squash, tomatoes, bell peppers, or some other). Be sure to use ½ cup of nuts or 8 ounces of regular or 5 ounces of firm tofu.

✦ Vegetable stew or soup (see Jiffy Soup recipe on page 321) served with a palm-size piece of meat, or ¹/₂ cup grated parmesan cheese stirred into the soup.

✦ Steamed, raw, or roasted vegetables topped with ¹/₂ ounce of melted cheddar cheese.

✦ Egg-and-Vegetable Frittata (see recipe on page 319).

✦ Stir-fry shredded veggies and 3 to 4 ounces of meat, poultry, fish, or shrimp, or 8 ounces regular or 5 ounces firm tofu, or tempeh

✦ Shish kebob and rice

SOUP SUGGESTIONS

✦ Split pea (with curry powder), Lentil (with tomato), Black Bean (add Mexican seasoning)

✦ Vegetable: Parboiled (cooked just under boiling) and puréed. (See the Jiffy Soup recipe on page 321.) Use mixed vegetables, or feature a single vegetable (leek, onion, peas, spinach, watercress).

✦ Chicken or turkey and rice or potatoes with other vegetables (see Easy Turkey or Chicken Soup recipe on page 322).

✦ Minestrone (Serve with a pasta, polenta, or rice dish from below.)

✦ Vegetarian-Stock: Blend cooked garbanzo beans with lemon rind and cumin, add Bragg Liquid Aminos and water. Use as a stock for parboiling green veggies (snow peas, snap peas, summer squash, and others).

PASTA, POLENTA, AND RICE SUGGESTIONS

✦ Soft polenta (or warmed leftover or store-bought polenta, sliced) with vegetables, tomato sauce, and meat, fish, or crumbled tofu.

✦ Pasta with vegetables, tomato sauce, and crumbled tofu.

Note: Do not use white flour pastas. Try corn, rice, bean thread, yam, or quinoa pastas, or pastas made with whole wheat flour.

TOPPINGS FOR VEGETABLES

If you aren't used to eating a lot of vegetables, you have a lot to discover about easy preparation methods that give veggies a new twist. Try these for a treat.

✦ Tomato sauce with sheep or goat feta and/or pumpkin seeds and/or crumbled tofu. Good with steamed zucchini or other squash.

✦ Olive oil. Good on everything.
✦ Veggie salt substitutes and pepper. Another reliable topping, good by itself or with oil or Better Butter.
✦ Lemon juice. Wonderful with broccoli or asparagus.
✦ Fresh herbs. Try dill on carrots, or mint with peas.
✦ Garlic. Spinach or other greens are delicious sautéed until tender in a little olive oil with minced or crushed garlic.
✦ Almond, cashew, or sesame butter. Make it into a sauce by blending it with a little water—great on green beans.
✦ Mustard or horseradish sauce. Mix powdered mustard or horseradish with a little water, or water and oil. Either is good with broccoli or asparagus, especially when served with beef.
✦ Yogurt with fresh herbs, salt, pepper, garlic. Delicious mixed with green beans, broccoli pieces, and onion.
✦ Avocado dressing. This can be made quickly in a bowl. Mash an avocado with a fork. Add about 2 Tbs. olive oil or ¼ cup yogurt, a little garlic salt, pepper, herbs (cilantro or parsley is good), and lemon juice to taste. A thinner dressing can be made by adding more yogurt and/or using a blender.
✦ Bragg Liquid Aminos and pepper.
✦ Bragg Liquid Aminos and lemon juice.
✦ Commercial oil-based salad dressing quickly makes Brussels sprouts, broccoli, cauliflower, or green beans something special.

Breakfast

N U T   M I L K   S H A K E

This shake is especially good for building up your serotonin level, and the pumpkin is good if you are hypoglycemic.

> Liquid base of I cup milk; *or* I to 2 cups Seed or Nut Milk
>   (see recipe on page 318); *or* 2 tablespoons raw tahini
>   or ¼ cup soaked seeds blended in ½ to ¾ cup water;
>   *or* I to 2 cups unsweetened soy milk
> I banana (yellow, not overripe)
> ¼ to ½ cup fruit (such as berries or apple, or cooked or
>   canned pumpkin)

I to 2 tablespoons rice protein powder
Nutmeg, cinnamon, cloves, fresh ginger, or other spices
   to taste

Place ingredients in a blender and blend until the shake reaches a desired consistency. Add more liquid if too thick.
Note: For soy milk, I recommend Yo Soy or West Soy by Westbrae, which don't have added sugar.

PROTEIN SMOOTHIE

As a base, choose one of the following:
   8 to 12 ounces of cow's milk or goat's milk; yogurt;
   or water
Pour into blender.
Add:
   1/2 banana or other fresh fruit and 1/3 to 1/2 cup berries
   Plus any or all of the following:
   I to 2 tablespoons rice or egg or whey protein powder
   I teaspoon to I tablespoon nutritional yeast
   1/4 cup raw almonds, nuts, sesame, pumpkin, and/or
   sunflower seeds
   I tablespoon flax oil and/or I teaspoon fish oil or flax
   seeds; or flax meal
   1/2 to I cup (8 oz.) plain, unsweetened yogurt

Blend well. Drink and enjoy!
Note: Do not use whey if you have milk allergies.

QUICK HOT CEREAL

1/3 cup quinoa flakes
I cup water
Pinch of salt

Add quinoa to boiling water. Return to boil and cook 90 seconds, stirring often. Makes 1 cup. You can flavor your hot cereal with tahini, chopped almonds, protein powder, cinnamon, ground flax seeds, or butter (but don't use butter and tahini together).

Note: Leftover cereal can be heated the next day by adding a little water or soy milk.

FRUIT BOWL

Place in blender:
   1/4 cup nuts or seeds soaked overnight
   1/2 piece of fruit, such as 1/2 banana or 1/2 cup berries
   1 to 2 tablespoons rice protein powder
   Your favorite spice (cinnamon, nutmeg, or some other)
   Just enough water to blend into a creamy sauce (start
      with a couple of tablespoons)

Blend everything together until the drink is as smooth as you like, adding more water, if mixture is still too thick to suit you. Pour it over pieces of fruit cut into cubes and place in a bowl.

SEED OR NUT MILK SHAKE

A half cup of seeds will usually make 1 quart of seed milk, which will keep two to three days in the refrigerator. If you like an ultra-smooth consistency, strain the seeds a second time, add more fresh water, and blend again.

   1/2 cup sunflower seeds, pumpkin seeds, pine nuts, fil-
      berts, and/or almonds

Soak the seeds or nuts overnight in enough water to cover them.

Drain off soaking water and put nuts or seeds in blender with enough fresh, cold water to cover. Blend into a cream.

Add water to the blender until the milk is a texture that you like.

EGG-AND-VEGETABLE FRITTATA

¹/₄ red onion, chopped

I cup kale or ¹/₂ cup other vegetables, chopped

I teaspoon butter

3 whole eggs, well beaten

2 tablespoons crumbled sheep milk feta

Sauté onions and fresh vegetables in the butter in a small ovenproof skillet. (If using leftovers, add them when onions are translucent.) Add the eggs and the cheese, and cook without stirring, tilting the skillet while lifting the edge of the cooked egg with a spatula, allowing uncooked egg to flow underneath. When no more uncooked egg will flow, put under a broiler and broil until top begins to brown, 1 to 2 minutes.

Variation: Use instead of the feta cheese.

✦ 1 slice rice cheese (SoyCo Rice Slice) or

✦ 2 tablespoons grated goat cheese

Lunch

PROTEIN SALAD

Place your Protein Salad on top of a collection of greens or herbs like parsley and basil, or on a piece of bread with lettuce and tomato, or on half a red bell pepper or avocado.

> **Tuna, chicken, turkey, or egg salad: Chop 3 to 4 ounces of protein (tuna, chicken breast, or roasted turkey) or 3 boiled eggs and mix with:**
>
> > **I to 2 teaspoons mayonnaise (a brand that doesn't contain sugar)**
> >
> > **I teaspoon mustard**
> >
> > **2 teaspoons mashed avocado**
> >
> > **2 tablespoons of any two or three of the following, chopped: red onion, scallion, parsley, pine nuts, red bell pepper**

Alternate ingredient suggestions for vegetarians:
+ Sheep feta and walnuts, canned organic cannellini beans
+ Garbanzos, goat cheese, mint, and pine nuts
+ White beans, sage, goat gouda, and roasted peppers

VEGETARIAN CAESAR SALAD DRESSING

This dressing can be stored in an airtight container for about a week.

In a blender, purée the following ingredients:
  1 cup olive oil
  ¹/₂ cup lemon juice (from approximately 2 to 3 lemons)
  1 teaspoon Dijon mustard
  2 teaspoons brewer's yeast
  1 teaspoon vegan Worcestershire sauce
  1 teaspoon capers
  2 teaspoons water

TAHINI YOGURT DRESSING

1 cup yogurt
3 teaspoons tahini
1 clove garlic
¹/₄ cup chopped parsley
3 teaspoons lemon juice
Salt
3 teaspoons apple juice
Fresh mint

Purée all ingredients in the blender. Add mint or any herb you like. Use this dressing on tomato slices, or cucumber and feta with arugula, or chopped romaine.

AVOCADO DRESSING

¹/₄ cup fresh lime juice
3 small avocados
1 clove garlic
2 scallions, chopped

$^1/_2$ cup water
1 jalepeño pepper, seeded
1 tablespoon fresh cilantro
Salt and pepper

Purée the ingredients in a blender. Season with salt and pepper, and store in an airtight container in the refrigerator.

LEMON-SCENTED RICE SALAD

Serves 3 to 4

Basic recipe:
  1$^3/_4$ cups water
  1 cup basmati (or other) rice
Combine the rice and lightly salted water and bring to a boil.
  Reduce the heat to low and simmer until tender, about 15
  minutes.
Cool the rice and add the following:
  2 tablespoons olive oil
  $^1/_2$ cup chopped scallions
  Zest of 2 lemons, finely grated
  1 tablespoon minced parsley
  1 tablespoon chopped basil
  2 tablespoons chopped sautéed onion
  2 tablespoons chopped pine nuts
  Salt and pepper to taste

Variations:
✦ Add 1 teaspoon curry powder or ginger with 2 tablespoons minced cilantro.
✦ Add 1 teaspoon cumin and cayenne pepper to taste for spiciness.

JIFFY SOUP

This soup is very flexible and is limited only by your imagination and what you have on hand. What follows is a basic recipe with a few guidelines that should be followed in any variation. Try the basic soup and then try minor variations, such as cauliflower instead of broccoli, or fresh basil instead of curry. Over time you will become more comfortable with trying variations on your own. Here is a beginning:

✦ Step 1: Hard Veggies. Use 2 cups (1 carrot, 1 stalk broccoli, 1/2 potato, 1 onion) cut-up hard vegetables per person. Put these in a saucepan with enough water or broth (which tastes even better) to cover, about 1 1/2 cups per serving. Bring the broth to just below a boil and cook 3 to 5 minutes. The pot will steam slightly and an occasional small bubble will rise to the surface. *Do not boil.*

✦ Step 2: Soft Veggies. For each serving, put 1 tomato and 4 summer squashes (zucchini, crookneck, or scallop) in your blender. Blend until puréed, using a little broth from the saucepan for liquid, if necessary. Add blended soft veggies to the saucepan to cook slightly from the heat of the soup.

✦ Step 3: Seasoning. Add 1 1/2 teaspoons curry powder and a few shakes of salt per serving to the saucepan. Now blend the vegetable-broth mixture in the blender in small batches until smooth. Don't fill the blender more than halfway, because too much hot liquid in the blender will cause it to spatter. The soup may have cooled a little, so return it to the saucepan to warm.

Season with miso, Bragg Liquid Aminos (decrease the salt), or other herbs like garlic, ginger, onion powder, dill, basil, or cumin.

Variations:

✦ If your goal is a one-dish meal, add 1/2 cup cubed leftover roast chicken, other cooked meat, or tofu per serving for protein.

✦ Use 1/2 cup of cooked rice or cut corn instead of the 1/2 potato

✦ Use leftover cooked veggies (green beans, broccoli, cabbage, peas, or other) in place of some of the soft vegetables.

Dinner and Beyond

EASY TURKEY OR CHICKEN SOUP

Serves 4

This meal-in-one-pot is ready in about 30 minutes from start to finish, and provides essential omega-3 fatty acids in the kale.

    I tablespoon olive oil
    I pound boneless turkey or chicken breast, cut in
       1/2-inch cubes

2 medium carrots, sliced

2 stalks celery, sliced

1 medium onion, chopped

4 cups natural chicken stock

1 1/2 teaspoons Italian herbs

1 bay leaf

2 cloves garlic, minced (or 1/2 teaspoons granulated garlic)

2 medium potatoes, diced

1 bunch of kale (clean, remove stems, and chopped fine)

Salt and pepper to taste

Heat the oil in a large pot over medium heat, then add the poultry, carrots, celery, and onion. Sauté, stirring frequently, until turkey or chicken turns from pink to gray. Add the stock, herbs, bay leaf, garlic, potatoes, and kale. Bring to a simmer. Turn heat to low, cover, and simmer until the vegetables are tender (about 10 minutes). Add salt and pepper to taste. Remove the bay leaf before serving.

Variations: You now have a basic recipe for a soup or the beginning of a stew. You can add any other vegetables you like and just adjust the liquid for desired thickness.

If you would like to add a starch, this will thicken the soup and make it more like a stew. Add one of the following:

✦ 1/2 cup split peas

✦ 1/2 cup buckwheat

✦ 1/2 cup rice noodles

✦ 1/2 cup lentils

Add 2 extra cups of water with starch.

For **Dahl-Styled Indian Stew,** omit Italian herbs and add with stock:

✦ 1/2 cup lentils

✦ 2 teaspoons curry powder

✦ Fresh chilies to taste

✦ 1 stalk lemon grass, chopped into big pieces and sautéed (used to flavor, but not eaten)

Add the following with the kale:

+ ¹/₄ cup cilantro, chopped
+ 1 can coconut milk (or light coconut milk)

For **Veggie Buckwheat Mushroom Stew,** add 2 cups halved mushrooms with the carrots, onion, and celery, and add buckwheat and 1 teaspoon sage with the stock (omit Italian herbs).

Substitute chicken sausage for the chicken and add the split peas for a hearty stew.

CORN CHOWDER WITH VEGETABLES AND SHRIMP

Serves 6

2 teaspoons butter
I onion, chopped
2 stalks of celery, chopped
I large yellow bell pepper, chopped
I pound new potatoes, diced
6 cans (12 cups) natural vegetable stock
Kernels cut from 6 ears of corn
I tablespoon chopped fresh basil
I tablespoon chopped fresh thyme
I ¹/₂ pounds cooked shrimp (about 30 shrimp per pound is
**   a good size)**
2 cups milk (optional; or 2 extra cups of stock)

In a large stockpot melt the butter and add onion, celery, pepper, and potatoes. Sauté on medium heat for about 5 minutes. Add the stock. Lower the heat and simmer until the vegetables are tender. Add the corn, herbs, shrimp, and milk, and heat through.

Variation
For **Fish Chowder,** omit shrimp and instead use 1¹/₂ pounds fish, cut in small pieces and sautéed. Add to chowder along with herbs, corn, and milk, and heat through.

ROAST CHICKEN OR TURKEY WITH LEMON, GARLIC, AND HERBS

This dish is simple and you can make extra so that you can have it for lunch.

1 head of garlic, cut in half
2 lemons, sliced in thirds
1 bunch of rosemary
1 bunch of marjoram
1 whole chicken; or 4 chicken breasts, bone in; or 1 large
  turkey breast

Preheat oven to 400 degrees. In a shallow baking dish place the garlic, lemons, and herbs on the bottom. Place the chicken or turkey on top of the other ingredients. (For the whole chicken, stuff the cavity with the garlic and lemon pieces and the herbs.) Bake until juices run clear when pierced with a fork (about 30 minutes for chicken or turkey breasts, longer for a whole chicken).

EASY BAKED PROTEIN (FISH, POULTRY, MEAT, OR TOFU)

1. Squeeze Bragg Liquid Aminos on both sides of the protein (fish, poultry, meat, or tofu).
2. Cover the bottom of a baking dish with balsamic vinegar, fresh lemon juice, fresh orange juice, or wine.
3. Place cuts of fish, poultry, meat, or tofu in baking dish and turn them to coat both sides (tofu and some dryer cuts of meat may need a little rub of olive oil).
4. Sprinkle the protein with one or two herbs: oregano, parsley, cilantro, thyme, dill, basil, rosemary, garlic or onion powder, cumin, etcetera. Parsley, onion powder, and garlic powder can be used by themselves or in combination with one or more other spices. Thyme, marjoram, oregano, and rosemary go well together (they are the basis of the "Italian Seasoning" herb combination sold in stores). Curry and dill seem to be best on their own. Cilantro and cumin make a nice combination. Look on spice labels. They often suggest companion spices.

5. Bake at 400 degrees for 20 to 30 minutes (time depends on the type and thickness of the protein).

BLACKENED TEMPEH

You can use this spice rub for more than just tempeh; it's also good for fish, poultry, and meat.

1 package of tempeh
Spice rub ingredients:
    2 teaspoons crushed coriander seeds
    2 teaspoons cumin
    2 teaspoons paprika
    1/8 teaspoon cayenne pepper
    1 teaspoon allspice
    1 teaspoon cinnamon
    1 teaspoon ground ginger
    1/2 teaspoon ground clove
    1/2 tablespoon olive oil

Combine the spice ingredients and rub on the tempeh. Heat the olive oil in a nonstick skillet. Cut tempeh in half and then in half again down the middle so you have four square pieces. Pan sear (cook over high heat) the tempeh pieces on each side until very dark and cooked through.

STEAMED SALMON

Serves 1

1 slice lemon
1 bay leaf (optional)
3 to 5 ounces salmon fillet

Put the lemon slice and bay leaf (if used) in a pot. Put a stainless steel steamer basket in the pot and add water to come up to, but not cover, the bottom of the basket. Bring the water to a simmer over medium heat. Place the salmon fillet in the basket and cover the pot with a lid. Steam the salmon just until it looks pink and no longer red inside when flaked with a fork (check after about 5 minutes). Serve with lemon, salt, and pepper to taste. Can also be served with Roasted Red Bell Pepper Butter (page 330), or dill mayo (1 tablespoon sugar-free mayonnaise blended with ¹/₂ teaspoon dried or minced fresh dill). Remove bay leaf before serving.

JOE'S SPECIAL

Serves 4

Gluten free and milk free, Joe's Special is a nutritious standby for a quick meal.

4 ounces (I cup) sliced fresh mushrooms
I onion, finely chopped
2 tablespoons butter
I pound lean ground meat (turkey or beef)
I bunch spinach, cleaned and chopped (other greens, such as kale, can be substituted, but will take longer to cook)
I teaspoon garlic (2 cloves, minced)
Salt and pepper
6 eggs, beaten

Sauté sliced mushrooms and onion in the butter until lightly browned, then add ground meat and cook until it has browned. Stir in the spinach, garlic, salt, and pepper. When spinach has cooked down, pour in the eggs and stir, scrambled-egg style, until done and lightly set. Turn over once with a spatula and cook a minute or so longer. Serve very hot.

TURKEY BURGERS

Serves 4

I pound ground turkey
I teaspoon cumin
¹/₂ onion, chopped
¹/₄ teaspoon salt
Pepper to taste
I teaspoon canola or olive oil

Mix the first five ingredients in a bowl. Form this mixture into four patties. Heat oil in skillet over medium heat, add patties, and sauté until cooked through and not pink.

ZUCCHINI WITH CHERRY TOMATOES

Serves 2

2 teaspoons olive oil
4 cups sliced zucchini (about 6 zucchini)
4 ounces mushrooms, sliced
2 to 3 cloves garlic, minced
8 ounces cherry tomatoes, halved
Salt and pepper to taste

Heat olive oil in a heavy pan or skillet on medium heat. Sauté zucchini, mushrooms, and garlic until zucchini are just tender. Add the cherry tomatoes, and salt and pepper to taste. Heat just until the cherry tomatoes are warm, and serve.

PAN-SEARED GREENS

Serves 2

1 tablespoon canola or olive oil
1 teaspoon garlic (2 cloves finely minced)
4 cups of any of the following, chopped (listed in approxi-
    mately the order of time they take to cook, from
    fastest to longest):
Spinach
Bok choy
Broccoli rabe
Purple cabbage
Kale
Collard greens
Salt to taste

Heat the oil in a large nonstick or cast-iron skillet or pan until hot. Add the garlic and greens to the oil and sauté, tossing until wilted. Add little sprinkles of water to keep the greens from burning, until they are cooked through. Add salt, if needed.

OVEN-ROASTED VEGETABLES
AND POTATOES

Root vegetables are good for roasting in the oven. Squash and eggplant slices are also delicious roasted.

2 cups high-carbohydrate vegetables along with 2 cups low-carbohydrate vegetables, cut in large pieces.
  Here are some suggestions:

High	*Low*
Jerusalem artichoke	**Leeks**
Onions	**Carrots**
Potatoes	**Mushrooms**
Winter Squash	**Turnips**
Parsnips	**Kohlrabi**
	Eggplant
	Summer Squash

I to 2 tablespoons olive oil
Salt to taste
I teaspoon garlic (2 cloves, minced)
2 teaspoons chopped rosemary

Preheat oven to 400 degrees. Toss the vegetables with the oil and salt, and place them on a baking pan. Bake until veggies are almost cooked. Add the garlic and rosemary, and continue to roast just until they "open up," but don't brown (about 5 minutes). Toss the veggies once more, then remove from the oven.

CREAMY POLENTA

6 cups water
2 cups polenta
Salt and pepper
2 tablespoons butter or Roasted Red Bell Pepper Butter
  (see page 330)

Bring the water to boil in a large pot and slowly stir in the polenta. Lower heat and cook, stirring almost constantly, until polenta forms a very thick mass. Add salt and pepper to taste. Stir in butter, if desired. You can put the leftover polenta in an oiled loaf pan, cover, and put in the refrigerator. When it's cool, slices can be cut and warmed in a lightly oiled or buttered pan for a few minutes, then served with breakfast or dinner.

ROASTED RED BELL PEPPER BUTTER

Use this butter wherever you would use plain butter, from polenta or hot cereal to baked potatoes or vegetables. You can also toss it in rice or with rice noodles. Roasted bell peppers can be bought in jars at Trader Joe's or other stores.

> I cup roasted red bell peppers
> ¹/₂ pound (2 cubes or I cup) butter, softened
> Squeeze of lemon (optional)

Purée the peppers with the butter and lemon in a food processor or blender at lowest speed until smooth. Place in a container and refrigerate. It will become firm when cold.

BREAD MACHINE YEAST BREAD

Dry ingredients:
I ¹/₄ cups chana (garbanzo bean flour)
I ¹/₄ cups rice flour
¹/₂ cup tapioca flour
¹/₂ cup buttermilk powder, or ¹/₂ cup nondairy substitute
2¹/₂ teaspoons xanthan gum
I ¹/₂ teaspoons salt

Wet ingredients:
I ²/₃ cups water
4 tablespoons (¹/₂ stick) butter, melted
I teaspoon apple cider vinegar
3 eggs, beaten

I tablespoon dry yeast granules

Combine the dry ingredients in one bowl and the wet ingredients separately in another bowl.

Combine the dry ingredients, the wet ingredients, and the yeast in the baking pan of the bread machine according to the manufacturer's directions.

Use the white bread setting at medium brownness, if you have this selection.

SAMPLE MENUS

Here are sample menus for two weeks to help you get started:

WEEK ONE

Day 1

Breakfast
Egg-and-Vegetable Frittata (page 319)
1 orange, sliced
Lunch
Two chicken or beef tostadas or soft-shell tacos, with beans (no rice, the tortillas provide enough grain carbohydrates), avocado, lettuce, and salsa. (Steam corn tortillas, if you want them soft, or bake them in an oven until crisp, instead of frying.)
Dinner
Top 1/2 cup soft Creamy Polenta (page 329) with 1 cup vegetables (sautéed onions, bell peppers, and mushrooms with garlic would be good); 4 to 6 ounces of meat, fish, or crumbled tofu; and a commercial marinara sauce
Side salad (Select-a-Salad, page 313)

Day 2

Breakfast
Protein Smoothie (page 317)
Lunch
Complete-Meal Salad (Select-a-Salad, page 313)
Dinner
3 to 5 ounces of baked fish (Easy Baked Protein, page 325) with lemon and dill
1/2 cup brown basmati rice
1 cup steamed asparagus with a pat of butter
1 cup cherry tomato halves and cucumber slices dressed with a mixture of 1/4 cup yogurt, 1/4 teaspoon cumin (or 1 tablespoon minced fresh cilantro), a dash of paprika and salt

Day 3

Breakfast
> ¹/₂ cup soft, Creamy Polenta (page 329) with ¹/₂ cup of chopped apples, peaches, or berries; a dash of cinnamon or nutmeg; and ¹/₄ cup of Seed or Nut Milk (page 318)
> 3 turkey or chicken sausage

Lunch
> Tuna salad Protein Salad (page 319)
> Side Salad (Select-A-Salad, page 313)

Dinner
> 3 to 5 ounces Blackened Tempeh (or chicken breast) (page 326)
> Pan-Seared Greens (4 cups raw) (page 328)
> ¹/₂ cup small boiled potatoes with Roasted Red Bell Pepper Butter (page 330)

Day 4

Breakfast
> 3 eggs, scrambled, boiled or poached
> 1 piece of rice toast or a corn tortilla
> ¹/₂ grapefruit or ¹/₂ small melon

Lunch
> Complete-Meal Salad (Select-a-Salad, page 313)

Dinner
> 5- to 7-ounce steak or lamb chop (with bone), cooked in a skillet or broiled
> 1 cup steamed broccoli with 2 teaspoons butter
> 1 cup carrots steamed with 2 teaspoons butter and 2 teaspoons balsamic vinegar
> ¹/₂ ear corn on the cob

Day 5

Breakfast
> Fruit Bowl (page 318)

Lunch
> Jiffy Soup (page 321) with ¹/₂ to ¹/₄ cup leftover meat or poultry added

Dinner
> 1 Turkey Burger (page 327)
> 1¹/₂ to 3 cups Oven-Roasted Vegetables (only ¹/₂ cup should be potatoes, sweet potatoes, yams, or winter squash) (page 329)
> Side Salad (Select-A-Salad, page 313)

Day 6

Breakfast
Large bowl of low-fat cottage cheese (1 cup or more) with 1/2 cup sliced fresh fruit and 1/4 cup almonds and/or sunflower seeds
Lunch
Complete-Meal Salad (Select-a-Salad, page 313)
Dinner
Joe's Special (page 327)
Side Salad (Select-a-Salad, page 313)

Day 7

Breakfast
Nut Milk Shake (page 316)
Lunch
Open-faced roast turkey sandwich, with tomato and lettuce
1 cup carrot, celery, and bell pepper sticks
Dinner:
Steamed Salmon (page 326) with dill mayo
Pan-Seared Greens (page 328)
1/2 cup Lemon-Scented Rice Salad (page 321)
1 to 2 cups coleslaw with oil and vinegar or Vegetarian Caesar Salad Dressing (page 320)

WEEK TWO

Day 1

Breakfast
1 cup chopped vegetables (mushrooms, green onions, red peppers, or others) sautéed until just tender, then add 3 eggs, and scramble until cooked to your liking
1 corn tortilla with 1 teaspoon butter or Roasted Red Bell Pepper Butter (page 330)
1/2 cup fresh fruit or berries
Lunch
Complete-Meal Salad (Select-a-Salad, page 313)
Dinner
4 to 6 ounces Easy Baked Fish (page 325) brushed with garlic, olive oil, lemon juice, and Bragg Liquid Aminos
2 cups Zucchini with Cherry Tomatoes (page 328)
1/2 cup baked sweet potato or yam

Day 2

Breakfast

$^1/_2$ cup cream of rice cereal or Creamy Polenta (page 329) with an egg beaten in (while hot, so egg will cook) and 1$^1/_2$ tablespoons protein powder (or omit egg and increase protein powder to 2 tablespoons, if desired)

$^1/_2$ cup fresh fruit

Lunch

Construct-a-Sandwich (page 314) with chicken salad, tomato, and lettuce

1$^1/_2$ cups raw veggies (celery, cherry tomatoes, carrots, cucumber, or some other)

Dinner

Easy Turkey or Chicken Soup (page 322)

Side Salad (Select-a-Salad, page 313)

Day 3

Breakfast

3 scrambled, poached, or boiled eggs with $^1/_2$ cup Creamy Polenta (page 329), all covered with salsa or a commercial marinara sauce

1 orange, sliced, or $^1/_2$ grapefruit

Lunch

Complete-Meal Salad (Select-a-Salad, page 313)

Dinner

Roast Turkey (3 to 5 ounces) with Lemon, Garlic, and Herbs (page 325)

$^1/_2$ to 1 cup basmati rice

Pan-Seared Greens (page 328)

1 cup sliced tomatoes and cucumbers with Avocado Dressing (page 320)

Day 4

Breakfast

$^1/_2$ cup cream of rice cereal with $^1/_2$ cup berries, and 1$^1/_2$ to 2 tablespoons protein powder or nutritional yeast

Lunch

Boca burger (vegetarian) on $^1/_2$ soya bun, open faced, with mayonnaise or mayo substitute (get a brand with no sugar) and lettuce

1$^1/_2$ cups raw veggies (cherry tomatoes, carrots, celery, cucumber, red bell peppers, jicama)

Dinner

Steak, lean, 3 to 5 ounces

Side Salad (Select-a-Salad, page 313)

Baked potato with butter (1 pat) and chopped green onion

Day 5

Breakfast

3 scrambled, poached, or boiled eggs

$^1/_2$ cup sautéed sweet potatoes

$^1/_2$ grapefruit or $^1/_2$ small melon

Lunch

Complete-Meal Salad (Select-a-Salad, page 313)

Dinner

4 to 6 ounces Roasted Chicken with Lemon, Garlic, and Herbs
(page 325)

1 potato mashed (using chicken stock for liquid, 1 teaspoon butter,
salt, and pepper)

$1^1/_2$ cups steamed broccoli

$^1/_2$ cup cherry tomatoes

Day 6

Breakfast

$^1/_2$ cup cream of rice or Creamy Polenta (page 329) with $^1/_2$ cup
yogurt or $^1/_2$ cup cottage cheese (substitute Seed or Nut Milk
[page 318] and 1 tablespoon protein powder if you're lactose intolerant), and $^1/_2$ cup fresh fruit

2 turkey or chicken sausage links or patties

Lunch

Jiffy Soup (page 321), with leftover roasted chicken

Dinner

Stir-fry 3 to 5 cups of veggies plus 1 cup tofu chunks (or 3 to 5 ounces
chicken chunks), with ginger, garlic, and soy sauce to taste

$^1/_2$ cup basmati rice

$^1/_2$ cup fruit salad with 3 to 4 tablespoons yogurt

Day 7

Breakfast

3 eggs, scrambled, boiled, or poached

1 piece of rice toast or a corn tortilla

$^1/_2$ grapefruit or $^1/_2$ small melon

Lunch

Complete-Meal Salad (Select-a-Salad, page 313)

Dinner

Corn Chowder with Vegetables and Fish (variation, page 324)

Side Salad (Select-a-Salad, page 313)

Readings

Eades, Michael and Mary Dan. *Protein Power* (New York: Bantam Books, 1998).

Fallon, Sally. *Nourishing Traditions* (San Diego: Promotion Publ., 1995).

Fielden, Joan and Stan Larke. *From Garden to Table: A Complete Guide to Vegetable Growing and Cooking* (Toronto: McClelland and Stewart Limited, 1976).

Okamoto, Sam. *Incredible Vegetables* (New York: Pelican, 1993).

TWENTY-ONE

Essential Support

Exercise, Relaxation, Counselors, and Health Care Resources

While supplements and the right foods are, as you have seen, at the core of the Diet Cure, I'd like you to have all the additional support you need to make your cure as successful as possible:

+ For a lifetime cure, exercise and relaxation are a must. And I think that what I have to say about these topics may surprise you.
+ Counseling will be essential for some of you and just plain helpful for others.
+ Without a wholistic health professional, some of you will not be able to pull off important features of your cure, such as getting blood tests or prescriptions.
+ You and your M.D. or D.O. will need to know where to get special tests and how to contact compounding pharmacies to fill medical prescriptions.

FINDING SUSTENANCE IN EXERCISE

You're in a lovely, long meadow leading to some low curving hills near the ocean. Do you feel like walking along the trail, running across the field, sitting on a bench enjoying the view, riding a bike, or taking a nap in the high grass and flowers nearby?

Did you think about which choices would burn the most calories? If you did, then try again after taking several deep breaths. This time imagine you will burn just as many calories no matter which choice you make. So you can choose what you honestly want to do or not to do.

I asked these questions of Kim in a family session that took place early in her recovery from bulimia and not long after an abortion. Kim kept saying, "I've got to exercise hard every day. I've just been going for walks, and it's not enough." (She'd been a star athlete in college.) Then I asked her what she would do if she could do anything she wanted, anywhere. She smiled for the first time in the session and said, "I'd go to the south of France. And I'd lie on the beach and just go into the water to cool off every once in a while. And I'd have a dog with me." Her answer revealed how much she needed rest and comfort above everything at that point in her life.

Exercise can be invigorating, strengthening, and *fun*. Healthy bodies naturally like, or even love, to "get out there." But are you, like so many people who come to Recovery Systems, feeling guilty and lazy because you don't exercise enough? Please don't.

I actually should be the one feeling guilty, because I used to chide clients who were not exercising, or not exercising up to our standards. Eventually, I realized something that I should have suspected from the start. In the San Francisco Bay area, probably anywhere in California, everyone knows how to exercise and why to exercise, and feels lots of pressure to do so, particularly if they are not thin. The main reason my clients weren't exercising was because they didn't have the energy. When treating their imbalances solved that problem, they were delighted to be able to get moving. If you are too tired to exercise, you probably need to read about adrenal and thyroid burnout in chapters 3 and 4. Another possibility is that foods like wheat and sugar are dragging you down (see chapter 5).

If you hate exercise, I'll bet money that your body is being sapped of its natural vitality by dieting or some other physical imbalance. However, if you want to exercise, and love it when you do, but just "can't find the time," then you probably don't have an energy problem (or maybe you have both a time problem and an energy problem!).

Ask yourself, is it really that I don't have the time, or do I choose not to make the time? If you think exercise means a big production of dragging yourself to a crowded gym and sweating it out on a stationary bike as you stare at a wall, then no wonder you are avoiding exercising. Exercise can, and should, be fun. Enjoy the outdoors as you bike, hike, or ski. Make going to the gym a social event—have an exercise partner. Work out on a mini trampoline or a NordicTrack at home in front of your favorite television show, use an aerobics video, or dance in your living room to your favorite music tapes. When exercise is a pleasure, it's easier to find the time for it.

Exercise Addicted?

Do you get depressed or anxious, or both, if you can't exercise hard almost daily? See chapter 1 on amino acids to permanently elevate your mood so that you can exercise for strengthening, stress reduction, and good health, not for keeping you sane. I want you to be able to break your leg and not fret even though you can't be exercising for a period of time.

Kari was a prime example of an exercise addict. She was training for a triathlon when she came to our clinic. She'd always been "a jock," but her exercise regimen had never been so obsessive. She had just cracked her pelvis, but kept on training, so her therapist sent her to us. Kari was afraid to stop overtraining because she had become an addictive carbo-loader. Like many athletes, she ate lots of starch: *pasta*, cereal, granola, *pasta*, bagels, and *pasta*. She was so addicted that she could not cut her carbs to match a reduced exercise program.

On the supplements, she lost her carbo cravings and quit overexercising with no anxiety. For the first time, Kari began to realize how much time she had wasted on excessive exercise. She began to date more, read, write letters, and rethink her career. Blessed with this new insight into herself, she was happier than she'd been in years. When she went back to exercise, her performance was better, even without the constant workouts.

Your Exercise May Be Too Stressful for You

Many clients who come to us are too tired to exercise, but they force themselves anyway. Usually they feel worse afterward: more tired, drained, sometimes emotionally "down," too. They usually turn out to have exhausted adrenal glands (see chapters 3 and 11 for information on adrenal exhaustion). One of our clients (a fitness trainer!) finally started losing weight when she cut her own workouts in half!

Creating Your Exercise Plan

Think of it this way: Imagine you've been given a darling pony that means the world to you and your family, but it's a lot of work. It needs good regular feedings. And it needs to be exercised—a lot. Otherwise it gets depressed and sluggish and weak and sick. You love it, so you take care of it. Well, I want you to take the same kind of loving care of your body.

There are three important facets to exercise: strengthening, stretching, and maintaining heart function by steady movement. Getting exercise of some kind at least four times a week seems to correlate best with staying healthy long term. So make it your goal to exercise four times a week until you sweat a bit for fifteen or twenty minutes or more at a session. It may take a while to reach that goal, so be patient with yourself.

What kind of exercise animal are you? Are you a pony that needs to run and stretch its neck? A fish that lives to swim? A dancing dolphin? A stretching, meditative cat? Are you more of a stallion than a pony, with a capacity and need for really arduous exercise—a natural athlete? One way to identify your best personal exercise style is to look at your blood type. O blood types can, and usually love to, exercise hard. A blood types seem to do better with gentler, shorter workouts, like yoga and walking. B blood types are somewhere between O and A, doing well in a variety of types of exercise. AB types may lean either toward gentler exercising, like A's, or more vigorous, like B's.

At the very least you can usually walk, preferably outside (or inside—your local shopping mall may be open for exercise walking before the stores are open). Walking is a great exercise because it's always available, and you can walk any distance you like. You may want to start easy by walking just a few blocks and add a block a week. Add hills when you can, and stairs. Try to walk away from traffic and off the pavement as much as you can. And get good shoes with cushioning and traction so that you can walk anywhere in comfort.

Other exercises that have been shown to benefit people of all ages are simple stretches and home weight lifting. Nancy began lifting five-pound dumbells in a routine because she used to get backaches carrying groceries or anything heavy (she played electric guitar in a band and every time she carried her sixty-pound amplifier she'd pull a muscle). It was easy to do in front of the TV and the best reward is that by keeping this up, she never, ever pulls muscles in her upper body now—it's incredibly practical for women for that reason if no other.

Stretch videos (such as tai chi and gentle yoga) or classes can teach you to do the simple stretching that will keep you physically relaxed and protect you from damaging yourself from stiff, pulled muscles. It doesn't take long to do—just a few minutes a day.

FINDING SUSTENENANCE IN REST AND RELAXATION

I'm going to give you some specific suggestions about relaxation in this chapter, but there may not be anything on my list that you haven't already thought about or even done. The problem is that it's so hard for most of us to find the *time* to relax. We seem to be running out of time. In surveys about what people would most like to have more of, time is now valued over money. So here you have very little time and I'm already suggesting that you take more time to eat and prepare food, take supplements, get exercise, and find a health professional.

Let me explain. I'm not just advocating relaxation to make you feel extra good for a little while. I'm imploring you to make the time to relax because I think that it can save your life and make your Diet Cure a bigger success. If you need a Diet Cure, you have been under more than the usual external stresses from work, family, friends, financial problems, pollution, traffic, and a host of other problems. You've also been under *internal* stresses from not enough food or too much toxic food (or both), from an eating disorder or an addiction, from food allergies or yeast overgrowth. These are all serious and usually long-term assaults. Meanwhile, you can rarely take time to relax and you may have been too anxious and mentally obsessive to have been able to relax effectively. And if your internal stressors (for example, yeast, a food allergy) were at work against you, rest would not have done you much good anyway.

But now you can be free of internal stressors by identifying them and going after them with supplements, good foods, and whatever other strategies you'll need, so it's time to make the time for relaxation.

Relaxation: What Is Relaxing to *You?*

Techniques that will provide sustaining rest in a hectic world:

+ Close your eyes and rest during the day, even if just for five or ten minutes.
+ Take breaks at work, and just clear your mind with a short walk or lie down. Get out and get some air, particularly if you work in an office building with closed windows.
+ Don't let more than four or five hours go by without consuming protein-containing meals, which will provide you with energy. In between have snacks.
+ Get plenty of rest, eight hours of sleep a night (although some people require slightly more or less—listen to your body), and try to get to bed by three hours after sunset for optimum health.
+ Eat within one hour after awakening.
+ Use hot water bottles on tense or chilled spots on your body. You'll be

---

What Is It That Really Needs to Rest, and How Can You Rest It Most Effectively?

There is only one part of you that sallies forth to meet all of life's challenges on your behalf. Actually there are two parts—your two adrenal glands.

The adrenals were designed for the simple life. Like the rest of our body's design, the adrenals haven't changed much in a hundred thousand years. They were designed to kick in and provide adrenaline to keep you going in times of famine and danger (such as during the "hunt" or warfare). But a hundred thousand years ago there were long periods of R&R just naturally. No one had to work at making time for R&R then. When it was dark, they went to sleep. When it was light, they woke up. Their winters were very long, restful months when they couldn't do much but sleep. In other words, the adrenals only had to perform their emergency services occasionally. Not anymore. Especially if you have inherited weak adrenals that wear out extra easily, modern times are an adrenal nightmare.

If you just can't relax and seem to be permanently wired and stressed out, and the relaxation techniques here don't help, please turn to chapter 3 and read the adrenal exhaustion section, if you haven't already.

---

surprised at how relaxed you get. Let the bottle conform your body—don't overfill it. Put another one at your feet, if they are cold. (You may become addicted to this luxury.)

+ Take long hot baths with relaxing essential oils like lavender.
+ Take vacations. Choose destinations that don't require too much air flight or tight scheduling. Take long weekends off and go away, or even hunker down in your own home with the phone off and your feet up.
+ Meditate and pray. These practices can be tremendously regenerative. There are many books and audio tapes available on how to meditate and pray.
+ Walk. Walks, especially in nature, are very relaxing. Appreciate your surroundings, whether it's the scent of pine as you walk through the woods or the myriad faces you see while walking in the city.
+ Plant and work in a garden. For many people, gardening is regenerating, bringing one back in touch with nature, the earth, and the seasons.
+ Practice stretching, yoga, and tai chi: Try classes that are slow and sensual, not athletic (such as hatha yoga instead of Iyengar yoga).

✦ Get massages. There are several types of massages available. A masseuse can concentrate on your neck, shoulders, back, or feet, or he can work on your full body for an hour or two.

✦ Indulge in body pampering. Get a facial or a manicure. At first it might seem uncomfortable having someone fuss over you, but you'll get used to it quickly!

✦ Listen to relaxation tapes. Progressive relaxation tapes step you through the process of relaxing every part of your body, or send you on a guided fantasy to relaxing places.

✦ Sing or play a musical instrument. Forget about sounding perfect. If you can sing or play an instrument just a little, have fun with it.

✦ Listen to music. For some, quiet music such as New Age or traditional Japanese is relaxing, while for others, listening to rock-and-roll oldies or dramatic classical pieces do the trick.

✦ The following Instant Calming Sequence, developed some years ago by Dr. Robert Cooper at his Institute of Health and Fitness Excellence, minimizes the negative effects of stress *before* your body reacts, making all of the above relaxation efforts more effective.

Step 1. Keep Uninterrupted Breathing. When faced with the first stress cue (that is, your boss comes up to your desk, fuming), continue breathing—smoothly, deeply, and evenly.

Step 2. Keep a Positive Facial Expression. Even a slight smile can "reset" your nervous system to react less to a negative stress. Flash a slight smile "just at the corners of your eyes" the moment stress strikes.

Step 3. Maintain a balanced postural stance in the face of stress. Keep your chest high, head up, neck long, chin in, pelvis and hips level, back comfortably straight, and abdomen free of tension. Imagine a sky hook gently lifting your whole spinal column upward from a central point on top of your head.

Step 4. Wave of Relaxation. Scan all your muscles quickly to locate any tension. At the same time, send a "wave of relaxation" through your body, as if you're standing under a waterfall that washes away all tension. Allow your mind to remain alert while your body stays relaxed and calm.

Step 5. Acknowledge reality. Try to break the pattern of negative thinking, wishing the situation weren't happening. Instead, think something like, "What's happening is real and I'm finding the best possible solution right now."

FINDING A COUNSELOR

At our clinic, we always make sure that whoever comes in gets whatever counseling and education they need along with their nutritional therapy. I learned the value of individual, group, and family counseling many years ago when I became a counselor myself. I have never gotten over the thrill of seeing my clients balanced out emotionally as well as nutritionally. You may have already had years of counseling, or have no problems that you really need to talk about. But please consider counseling if any emotional problems do continue to affect you. For example, maybe you now realize you want to quit dieting and obsessing about your body; if so, look for a counselor who is experienced in eating disorders and/or women's issues. Ask if she has a group. Interview your prospective counselor carefully. Will she support your working with this book? Is she aware that there's a physical basis for many psychological problems? Does she understand that lack of discipline is not the issue if you have a weight or overeating problem? Does she know that weight gain and health deterioration do not normally go hand in hand? Do you like her? Can she stand up to you without being intimidating? You must find a counselor if you have an eating disorder or an addiction to a drug or alcohol (see chapter 18). Please explore twelve-step programs, such as Overeaters Anonymous and A.A., as well.

Some people do need therapy for issues beyond simple (though crucial) body-image education and diet-mentality deprogramming. Sexual abuse can have deeply affected your body image. I have had two clients who had to stop our program because they weren't ready to lose weight and feel vulnerable, powerless, and sexually more attractive. They needed to stop and do some therapy first. Most of my other clients have been able to follow the Diet Cure and do therapy at the same time, quite successfully.

I have had a few clients who found that once they were in biochemical balance, issues that had been repressed came up, which caused them to need therapy. When you are no longer eating foods that numb and distort your feelings, when you can think about something besides food and your body, you may become aware of issues within yourself and in your relationships that need some attention. You'll need a counselor to discuss your new feelings with. A side benefit of getting physically healthy is that it becomes more possible to be emotionally healthy, too.

One of my clients was sent to us by her therapist, who had been unable to help her with her depression and anger. After a few weeks on the program, she discovered that she did not hate her job or her mother-in-law after all. Her brain chemistry deficiencies had produced negative feelings that had no real basis. When her negativity was neutralized by amino acids, she discovered she was actually a contented person with a pretty good life. Several marriages have been saved by this same process, "Oh, I do like him. It was me after all!" these women say.

I like to see chronic dieters get counseling, because they have a tendency to undereat no matter what, and that sabotages any weight loss they might actually need and the benefits of their total program. With a counselor, they can look at the old patterns and work their way out of them. But again, the counseling must not compete with the nutritional program. They're both important. Sometimes a counselor can help you to find the time to set up your new life—how to eat, buy, and prepare food; exercise; relax; and still work and have a family and social life, without more stress.

Ask family and friends for referrals, or look in your Yellow Pages under "Counseling," "Marriage and Family Therapists," "Psychologists," "Psychotherapists," or "Eating Disorders." If you need consultation on medication, look under "Psychiatrists" in the "Physicians" section.

FINDING THE RIGHT HEALTH PROFESSIONALS

In a well-publicized 1993 survey, more people went to wholistic health practitioners than went to conventional medical practitioners: 400 million visits. I would like to see you find your own wholistic health practitioner, one who agrees with the general approach of the Diet Cure, is experienced with helping people correct the eight key imbalances, and can order tests and prescribe medications, if you need them. The only practitioners that I know of who can do all of this in every state are wholistic M.D.s and D.O.s (doctors of osteopathy).

Wholistic health practitioners focus on the whole person: the physical, mental, emotional, and spiritual aspects of the individual. Ideally, the relationship with a practitioner involves cooperation and respect for a patient's wisdom and knowledge of themselves. You will want him or her to consider both conventional and complementary therapies when making a treatment plan, but also lean toward the least toxic therapy first. Always ask your practitioner how toxic the treatment is, what the side effects are, and whether there are treatments available that have fewer side effects.

The Differences Between Various Health Professionals

Ordering Tests. Any health professional can order urine, stool, and saliva tests. M.D.s and D.O.s can order blood testing and skin prick testing. But keep in mind that the way many health insurance policies are written these days, often the doctor is financially punished for ordering too many tests, hence their reluctance to perform them. Be up front with your doctor about why she/he doesn't want to order particular tests. Perhaps you can pay for them out of pocket.

Advising You on Nutrition. Whether you consult your local health food store expert, or a private nutritionist, acupuncturist, chiropractor, naturopath, D.O., or M.D., ask what their nutritional experience and approach is. They are all potentially good candidates, but you'll need to ask good questions. (In some parts of the country, you'll be lucky to find any wholistic practitioners at all, unfortunately.)

Providing Medication. Wholistic M.D.s and D.O.s are the only health practitioners that can order any test in any state and prescribe medications as well as advise you nutritionally. Find one if you possibly can. Or, if you really like your chiropractor or acupuncturist, ask him or her to help you get whatever medical services you need, beyond what he/she can do. Most will usually have a working relationship with a cooperative M.D. or D.O.

How Do You Know What Kind of Wholistic Practitioner You Should See?

Within different wholistic specialties are many schools of thought. Ask potential practitioners how they would treat your condition and you'll probably get different answers from each one. To keep it simple, show them *The Diet Cure* and see if they are open to the recommended plans.

Holistic Medical Doctors (M.D.s). A medical doctor has four years of graduate training and specializes in a particular area of medicine. Endocrinologists, for example, specialize in disorders of the thyroid and other glands, but are not usually wholistic. Until recently, medical doctors have received very little training in nutrition. A wholistic medical doctor can take additional training from a certified wholistic medical school of naturopathy or osteopathy. Many doctors research wholistic medical treatments on their own and through various conferences or workshops, but don't have a formal certification in wholistic medicine. The American Holistic Medical Association requires its members to be state certified in wholistic medicine.

Doctors of osteopathic medicine (D.O.s). An osteopath has medical training, but is also trained to correct structural problems in the body with adjustment techniques that predate chiropractic. This is an old and highly respected form of treatment in Europe. In fact, the British royal family's physician is an osteopath. Some are more nutritionally and wholistically oriented than medical doctors, but many are not.

Licensed naturopathic physician (N.D.s). A naturopath attends a four-year graduate level naturopathic medical school and is educated in all of the same basic sciences as an M.D. They also study holistic and nontoxic approaches to health with a strong emphasis on disease prevention and optimizing wellness. Even though they are not medical doctors, they are licensed in Washington State and Oregon and practice with many of the same freedoms, including ordering blood tests and prescribing.

Unlicensed naturopathic physician (N.D.s). A naturopathic degree can also be obtained from correspondence courses. Students who complete a correspondence course are not eligible to sit for the naturopathic exam, required by states that offer licensure. Most states do not license naturopaths at this time. Even though unlicensed, these naturopaths can be helpful regarding your nutritional and health needs.

Chiropractors (D.C.s). A chiropractor practices spinal manipulation and structural adjustments. There are two schools of thought within the chiropractic profession. "Straight Chiropractic" practices structural adjustments exclusively, while the other school of thought includes other wholistic modalities in their practice. Most chiropractors have some nutritional expertise, and chiropractic is usually covered by insurance. Some states allow chiropractors to order blood and other tests and others do not. You will have to ask what tests they can order for you. They cannot prescribe medication.

Acupuncturists (L.A.C.s). Acupuncture has more than a 2,500-year history. They use thin needles that penetrate the skin to stimulate energy and healing systems in the body. They also use Chinese herbs and sometimes supplements, depending on their orientation. Typically, American edu-cated acupuncturists will incorporate the use of nutritional supplements and other treatment options, while traditional Chinese acupuncturists use only herbs along with their needles. Acupuncturists are generally licensed for diagnostic and treatment procedures pertaining to "Oriental medi-cine" only. In a couple of states they can order Western, biomedical clini-cal tests, but in others they cannot. Insurance often covers acupuncture. Acupuncturists cannot prescribe medication.

Nutritionists (R.D.s, C.N.S.s, C.N.s, N.C.s, C.N.C.s, C.C.N.s)— Look for one in the Yellow Pages under "Nutrition." A registered dietitian (R.D.) has an undergraduate degree and has taken American Dietetic Association–approved course work in dietetics with an additional six or twelve-month internship in a hospital. Most dietitians believe you can get what nutrients you need from the food you eat and often do not approve of the use of supplements. Nutritionists, on the other hand, have a different approach that actually emphasizes the use of nutritional supplements. Their train-ing and certification varies tremendously. (There are still very few wholis-tically oriented nutritional training programs. You will need to ask the nutritionists you interview if they believe in the use of supplements and what their experience is in using them.)

After working with many R.D.s for six years, I finally found a certified nutritionist and the real success of our program began. We do not usually find R.D.s helpful because they are only now beginning to update their profession regarding the use of nutritional supplements. (Even worse, they are the ones responsible for hospital food!) But they are starting to learn from the constant flow of research confirming the effectiveness of nutri-tional supplementation and from their work with AIDS patients how beneficial a wide range of supplements can be.

Still, certified nutritionists aren't usually perfect either. Find out if they have received any formal training in the use of supplements. Avoid nutri-tionists who are enthusiastic about fasting or have any other very narrow eating philosophy that does not match the philosophy of the Diet Cure. For example, do they advocate low-fat, low-calorie, or strictly vegetarian diets? Ask what their approach is to your imbalances, which nutrients they use, and what kind of dietary guidelines they generally advocate. Be sure that they have been counseling people for a while and try to get a reference, as you should on all practitioners.

How to Find a Wholistic Practitioner in Your Area

If you want to find a good wholistic practitioner that you can work with, start asking for referrals from friends, family, or colleagues. The next best source is the Yellow Pages under "Wholistic" or "Alternative Medical Practitioners," or look up the type of practitioner you need: physicians (medical doctors), acupuncture, chiropractic doctors, to name a few. Not all Yellow Pages have a heading for "Wholistic Practitioners," so you may have to look for key words in the practitioners ads, like *wholistic, holistic, alternative, nutrition, complementary, integrative, wellness, prevention, nontraditional, natural,* and *food allergy.* In ads or brochures, wholistic practitioners might say that they treat the whole person (body, mind, and spirit), that they believe in patient education, that they include you as part of the treatment team, and trust your knowledge and wisdom about your own body.

You can visit your local health food store bulletin board or ask the store manager how to find a wholistic practitioner in your area or to recommend one to you. To find a health food store in the Yellow Pages look under: "Health and Diet Foods Products" or "Health Foods."

There are also many resources on the Internet for finding health practitioners in your area. Most professional organizations offer referrals by phone, on the Web, or through a referral directory. Remember that practitioners usually pay to be listed or are members of that association, so the lists do not include every practitioner in your area. If you don't have access to a computer, some libraries will allow you access to the Internet for a limited period of time, usually thirty minutes.

I hope that you'll be able to find all the support you need, whatever it is, more easily after reading this chapter. The resources below will lead you to additional sources for wholistic testing and medication, as well as organizations.

Readings

Most of these books are available through the Gurze Catalog (800-756-7533).

EXERCISE

Nelson, Miriam, Ph.D. *Strong Women Stay Young* (New York: Bantam Doubleday Dell, 1998).

COUNSELING

Hall, Lindsey, ed. *Full Lives: Women Who Have Freed Themselves from Food and Weight Obsession* (Los Angeles: Gurze Designs and Books, 1993).

Shepperd, Kay. *Food Addiction: The Body Knows* (Health Communications, 1993).

OVEREATERS ANONYMOUS
Miller, Caroline Adams. *My Name Is Caroline* (Los Angeles city: Gurze Designs and Books, 1991).

RELAXATION
Davis, Robbins Eshelman, and R. McKay. *The Relaxation and Stress Reduction Workbook* (Oakland, CA: New Harbinger, 1998).

Resources

The following list includes wholistic professional organizations and health-related consumer organizations to call for practitioner referrals in your area:

MEDICAL
The Broda O. Barnes M.D. Research Foundation
(203) 261-2101 ($10 charge for list of M.D.s and D.O.s in your area)

American College for Advancement in Medicine
(949) 583-7666 (800) 532-3688
<www.acam.org>
An organization for educating physicians (D.O.s and M.D.s) in complementary and alternative medicine. Referrals can be found through a search page on their Web site.

American Holistic Medical Association (AHMA)
(703) 556-9245
To order the Referral Directory, phone (703) 556-9728; or write 6728 Old McLean Village Drive, McLean, VA 22101-3906; or fax (703) 556-8729.

The International Society for Orthomolecular Medicine
(416) 733-2117
<www.orthomed.org>

CHIROPRACTIC
American Chiropractic Association
(800) 986-4636
<www.amerchiro.org>

International Chiropractor Association
(800) 423-4690
<www.chiropractic.org>

HOMEOPATHIC
Homeopathic Educational Services
21248 Kittredge St.
Berkeley, CA 94704
(510) 649-0294
fax (510) 649-1955

e-mail: mail@homeopathic.com
Directory of U.S. practitioners, study groups, pharmacies, and resources will be sent for $5. They are a mail-order source for homeopathic books, tapes, home medicine kits, and software. On Web page see "How Do I Find a Homeopath?"

ACUPUNCTURE
National Acupuncture and Oriental Medicine Alliance
(253) 851-6883
<www.acuall.org>

American Association of Oriental Medicine
(610) 264-2768
<www.aaom.org>

MISCELLANEOUS HOLISTIC
The American Holistic Health Association
(714) 779-6152
<www.ahha@healthy.net>

American Association of Drugless Practitioners
(888) 764-AADP
<www.netins.net/showcase/aadp/>

NATUROPATHIC
The American Association of Naturopathic Physicians (AANP)
(206) 298-1025
<www.naturopathic.org>
This organization has a searchable database of N.D.s online.

NUTRITION
National Institute of Nutrition Education
(800) 530-8079 (press 0)
<www.nines.com>

International and American Association of Certified Nutritionists (IAACN)
Referral source and certifying board: (972) 407-9089

National Health and Healing
(888) 817-5566
<www.hhc.com>

The Society of Certified Nutritionists
(800) 342-8037

FIND WHOLISTIC PROFESSIONALS ON THE NET
✦ Check the Web sites of any of the above organizations that give referrals.
✦ Check the AOL browser <www.aol.com/netfind> Select "Yellow Pages" for

U.S. listings* (results give address, phone number, map, and directions) Input "holistic" or "alternative" in Business Category. (You may input a city name, but this will limit the search to that city.) Select your 2-letter state abbreviation. Hit "Enter." Skim results for medical centers and call those that sound promising for more information on what problems they treat and their philosophy of treatment.

*Note: Select "International Listings" for U.K., Australia, Canada, and many other countries directory listings.

✦ Check the HeatingLinks Web site:
<http://healinglinks.com/links/directory.htm> for Practitioner Directories in U.K., Australia, Canada, and the United States.

✦ Check Health World Online <www.healthy.net/referral/> for alternative and wholistic practitioners by categories.

SALIVA TESTING LABS

You can order saliva and other tests yourself through these resources, or you can ask your health practitioner to contact them for you. All can provide adrenal, reproductive hormone, and melatonin testing. Most provide additional tests as well.

Bio Health Diagnostics, San Diego, CA
(800) 570-2000

Tests, educates, and consults with all individuals and health professionals, as well as provides holistic treatment recommendations and products based on specific test results. Professional training. Saliva testing for gluten, milk protein, and yeast testing also done.

Madison Pharmacy Associates
Women's health specialists (800) 558-7046

They will consult with you directly or with M.D.s and D.O.s about testing. Provide natural hormones by prescription, designed according to your specific test results. They will refer you to wholistic doctors in your area.

Great Smokies Laboratory
For practitioners orders, call (800) 522-4762
Or for you directly, call (888) 891-3061
Wholistic referrals made by phone.

Diagnos-Techs, Inc.
U.S. (800) 878-3787
fax: (425) 251-9520
U.K. 179-246-4911
fax: 179-247-2466

Saliva testing plus written interpretation of results and recommendations for treatment primarily for professionals (no M.D. required). Gluten and milk protein and other tests also available.

TESTING FOR OSTEOPOROSIS

A simple urine test, the Dpd test, will tell you if, and at what rate, your bones are *now* breaking down.

Madison Pharmacy will arrange for you to order the test personally or through your health practitioner, or it can be ordered by your physician through other labs.

COMPOUNDING PHARMACISTS

There are many excellent compounders in and beyond the United States. They work primarily by phone with M.D.s and D.O.s from any state.

Madison Pharmacy Associates
(800) 558-7046
Specializes in women's hormonal and health issues. Their staff works closely with M.D.s and D.O.s on testing and prescribing to correct reproductive and adrenal hormone imbalances.

Professional Compounding Centers of America, Inc. (PCCA)
9901 S. Wilcrest
Houston, TX 77099
(800) 331-2498
<www.thecompounders.com>
The company has more than 2,200 retail pharmacists/customers in the United States, Canada, Puerto Rico, South America, Australia, and New Zealand.
Referrals: Web page has pharmacy links, a list of pharmacies in the United States, and related associations.

International Academy of Compounding Pharmacists (IACP)
P.O. Box 1365
Sugarland, TX 77484
(800) 927-4227
fax: (281) 495-0602
<www.iacprx.org>
Referrals: Refer by phone, not on Web site.

BLOOD TYPE HOME TEST KITS
Recovery Systems Clinic
order line: (800) 733-9293

ALLERGY TESTING, WHOLISTIC SKIN PRICK OR PROVOCATION AND
NEUTRALIZATION (P/N) TESTING:
The American Academy of Environmental Medicine
For wholistic allergy testing and treatment (215) 862-4544

Contacting Julia Ross and the Recovery Systems Clinic

WEB SITE
<www.dietcure.com>
For updates on the use of supplements, food, and other resources, supplement order line, and Julia's personal and media appearances

ADDRESS FOR CONTACTING JULIA ROSS BY MAIL
The Diet Cure
775 E. Blithedale #402
Mill Valley, CA 94941

CLINIC PHONE CONTACT
Because the clinic cannot continue to function effectively with the number of calls that sometimes come in, an informational number was set up to let you know more about the clinic and how to consult with us. (415) 458-8446

TWENTY-TWO

Your Master Plan in Action

The Diet Cure from Day One to Week Twelve

Now that you have worked your way through this book, you're ready to put all that you've learned into action. Read this chapter now and plan to read it again when you actually start your first day of detox. In this final chapter I'm going to tell you everything I typically tell my clients as they go through their twelve-week programs. After that point, they usually don't need much from me, though they may be working on long-term projects such as major weight changes or thyroid medication adjustments. By then they have determined just what foods and supplements work for them. They are well established in their new way of eating—and feeling. They've often forgotten, until I remind them, how overpowering their food cravings and negative moods used to be. I'd like to see you develop the same amnesia.

Let's look at what you need to do before you start your master plan.

+ Review the Quick Symptom Questionnaire. Even a few yes answers, if they indicate significant symptoms, may need to be explored, either now or later, if you continue to have these symptoms. Each of the first eight chapters contains a much more complete list of symptoms than the first quick symptom questionnaire did, so that you can do more exploring if any of the imbalances is in question in your mind.
+ Study pertinent chapters in parts 1 and 2, and all the chapters in part 3.
+ See a health professional and start interviewing counselors, if needed.

✦ Get testing done, if needed.

✦ Think through and plan your first week of meals (at home and out).

✦ Get the nonfoods and druglike foods out of the house, if possible.

✦ Buy your supplies of supplements and foods.

✦ Organize your supplements so that you will be equipped all day. Get a watch with an alarm to remind you about taking supplements, if you'll tend to forget (or set your computer to remind you). Get a vitamin-organizing system that will work for you. Buy several daily pill boxes and fill them all up at once to make your life simpler.

✦ Take your time. Don't get overwhelmed. If you are due for PMS or your period, wait until afterward to begin the full eating changes program. You can start taking your supplements immediately, though. If you've been misled before about quick cures, and you're afraid you're being misled again, keep in mind that in just twenty-four to forty-eight hours you will definitely notice an improvement in how you feel.

Now you are ready for Week One.

WEEK ONE: DETOX WEEK

Days 1 to 4

In your first day or two your food cravings should disappear (unless you start during PMS, which I don't recommend). You should lose your food cravings entirely by Day 5, at the latest. If they have not decreased dramatically by Day 2, gradually increase the amounts of the supplements that are intended to reduce your cravings. The aminos, especially L-glutamine, 5-HTP, and DLPA (or DPA) are the usual helpers here. Open an L-glutamine capsule under your tongue if you get a sudden carbo craving; this often works within five minutes. If you eat for an energy lift and really need your caffeine, try some extra L-tyrosine.

If you forget to take your supplements at any point, or do not eat as planned (for example, if you don't get protein at all three meals), you can expect your cravings to return briefly. But bumps like this should quickly smooth out and you'll be craving free again. What does it mean to lose your cravings? It means you'll be indifferent to old favorites; that you wouldn't even cross the room to get formerly irresistible foods; that you might have brief thoughts about old eating habits, but that you really won't care to act on them. The old food fantasies will really be gone. My clients call us every day of their first week on our program, to give progress

---

Troubleshooting Note

If you are doing everything right and you still have cravings, turn to chapter 7, page 93, and take the long questionnaire to make sure that you don't have a yeast overgrowth, if you haven't already done so. This is a common but sneaky problem.

---

or problem check-ins. I love taking these calls, because I get such happy reports. Typically, clients say, "I didn't believe you when you told me that I was going to stop wanting chocolate in twenty-four hours, but it's true! I really don't care about it now. I'm really satisfied without it. I can't believe it! Amazing! It's a miracle!" You can imagine how I feel on the other end of the phone getting these kinds of calls.

Even my problem calls are rarely real stumpers. Usually the trouble is easily solved by increasing the amounts of amino acids to completely eliminate any cravings that may be hanging on. The other minor problem that comes up occasionally is loose bowels, usually caused by too much magnesium. If you should suddenly get loose bowels, just cut back on any supplement that contains magnesium until it stops. More rarely, loose bowels are a short-term detox symptom that does not feel debilitating or draining, but more like a good cleaning out. (This is also typical at the beginning of a yeast "kill off" process.)

You may lose your appetite, or even get a bit nauseated in your first four days on the Diet Cure. One of our food-addicted clients, a 50-year-old psychotherapist, told me during her check-in on Day 2, that until now she'd never *not* wanted to eat before in her life. If any nausea continues past two days, it may be that the supplements are bothering you. (If you take your with-meal supplements without food, the same thing can happen.) Very rarely, the aminos cause an overly acid feeling. If they do, try them with a bit of vegetable or fruit, which is naturally antacid. Or stop all supplements and gradually reintroduce them to identify the culprit.

Expect some other withdrawal symptoms in the first two to four days. Many people feel tired, though you may already be so tired that you won't notice. The other top detox symptom is headache. If you are prone to migraines, you may get one in the first few days of your detox. At lease a quarter of my clients who are migraine sufferers do. But it may be the last migraine you ever have!

Troubleshooting Note

Please do not now, or ever, use the fact that the supplements have relieved you of food cravings as an opportunity to undereat. Even if you feel guilty about a final binge the night before Day 1, eat something with protein in it for breakfast on your first day and again at lunch and dinner. Unless you really are too nauseated to eat for a day or two, eat well at least three times per day from the start to make sure you get the benefits of the Diet Cure right away. Smoothies with protein powder will do if you feel queasy in detox, as a temporary lunch or dinner meal until you get a healthy appetite in a few days. *But undereating is our enemy.* It will cause the cravings to come back and keep your weight static. If you aren't used to eating breakfast, a big omelet may be unappetizing. In that case, make the breakfast Protein Smoothie on page 317. It will go down easily and keep you happy until lunch. If you have trouble even swallowing a smoothie in the morning, you're probably still drinking coffee when you wake up. Caffeine kills your appetite, so it will have to go. If you are tapering off of caffeine, wait until after your smoothie to have a cup of decaf (which has a little caffeine but much less than regular coffee). Even decaf can disrupt your blood sugar and appetite. Get off it as soon as you can.

To treat these symptoms, feel free to take whatever over-the-counter painkillers you need during this week. Alka-Seltzer Gold is a helpful antidote to detox discomfort, which is largely due to your system becoming very acidic. Two tablets of Alka-Seltzer (Gold only) will de-acidify you, as will baths with 3 cups of Epsom Salts. By Day 5, you should feel very good.

Detox Symptoms

+ Headache (May be severe if you have a history of migraine)
+ Low energy
+ Depression
+ Muscle aches
+ Cravings
+ Irritability
+ Panic feelings (anxious, sweaty, clammy)
+ Diarrhea
+ Teary state

The Food-Mood Log

Every day, pay attention to how you feel and to how food, or the lack of it, changes how you feel emotionally (for example, irritable) as well as physically (for example, tired, craving sweets). You should do this for several months until listening to your body and moods becomes second nature. After that, use your log at the end of any problem days to help you figure out what went wrong. Think back: Did the problem actually start a few days or weeks before, for example, with a trip out of town when you started eating foods that unbalanced you?

By keeping the food-mood log, you will discover much interesting nutritional information about your own body and its likes and dislikes. This information will allow you a measure of health and personal freedom you may never have known before. Your body must be the final authority in choosing what is right for you. The process of recovery is really the process of establishing a relationship with your body, free of the damaging foods and drugs (like caffeine) that have alienated you from yourself.

In any relationship the most important element is communication. True communication is the ability to listen and to respond. Your food-mood log will help you reestablish real communication with your body. You will have the opportunity to see how your body feels and begin to discover what your body really needs and wants, and what it does not want, and when. In my experience, any cravings occur primarily because true nutritional needs are not being met, although external stresses can play a part, too. Please keep this log until your body is functioning without problems. Without knowing what you have done, and how you felt, you cannot make the appropriate choices and changes necessary to recovery. I like calling this record a log—part of the process of successfully navigating your ship into safe waters. In your Food-Mood Log, record the following information:

+ All food and beverage intake, and approximate time of intake. Note whether you ate the recommended amounts of protein and vegetables and the protein/carb ratio.
+ Any supplement that you did *not* take according to your plan. This includes any supplement that you took more of or less of, that you took with food when you should have taken it without (and vice versa), or that you forgot altogether. Note the time you should have taken the supplement.
+ Do you have any cravings? For what and at what time of day?

> ✦ How you felt throughout the day, emotionally and physically (bloated, depressed, energetic, cheerful, constipated, or some other.).
> ✦ How you slept the night before.
> ✦ Your temperature. (You only need to do this if you're checking your thyroid, and then you only need to do it three days a month—during your period if you're premenopausal.)
> ✦ Your exercise time and intensity. Record how you felt before and after you exercised.

✦ Constipation
✦ Restlessness
✦ Too much sleep
✦ Mental confusion
✦ Difficulty sleeping (nightmares)
✦ Cramping
✦ Respiratory problems
✦ Repulsed by food
✦ Skin rash

Possible Emotional Reactions During Detox Week One

✦ Overwhelmed
✦ Unfamiliar feelings/memories emerge
✦ Grief, loss (of old food friends, habits)
✦ Deprived
✦ Fearful (of change)
✦ Envious of "normal" eaters

Check In with Yourself. It is crucial that you check in with yourself or with a buddy *daily* during the first week of your program, and that you keep the food-mood log.

Reactions of Family and Friends

Mostly, you can expect interest and support in your Diet Cure efforts. Maybe you can launch your Diet Cure plan along with some friends or relatives to keep each other motivated, share ideas and meals, and have fun with it. Check in with each other often (daily during Week One).

Some friends and family members may not support this effort. The changes involved may be threatening to them. Have they been eating buddies for years? Sharing a latte every afternoon? Their initial negativity often passes or improves, as they see that you really transform. If not, you'll need to detach from them for a while, at least until you are firmly on your own feet and know how to handle the temptations that they represent. Don't let them make you feel like a prude because you've stopped eating junk food.

If you live with someone, ideally he or she would share the benefits of the Diet Cure with you. See if you can help them design a supplement plan for themselves to make it easy for them, too, to give up junk foods. If they won't, I hope that they will at least agree to keep junk food out of the house and eat it elsewhere, and that you won't be expected to make both their food and yours, too.

Losing Weight

In the first week, it is not unusual to lose more weight than you ever do again at any one time. If you are giving up foods you've been allergic to, you'll probably lose water weight—up to seven pounds of it. One of the doctors that consults with us was on a very healthy diet and exercised regularly, but could not get rid of twelve pounds of mysterious weight. At my suggestion she went off gluten-containing grains and lost it all, most of it in Week One.

Men have the fastest weight loss, because, once free of burdensome foods, their higher testosterone levels and greater muscle mass burn calories like crazy. One of our favorite clients practically disappeared in the first three weeks on the Diet Cure, and he was eating plenty of food.

Women usually lose slowly and steadily. This is best, to avoid the health consequences of quick weight loss and to ensure that the weight stays off. Usually they also lose their obsession with weight loss and are so thankful to be free of compulsive eating and mood swings that they move along serenely. If you continue to fret about not losing weight fast enough, you'll need to do two things: reread chapter 2, and try taking a serotonin booster like 5-HTP, L-tryptophan, and/or St. John's Wort. Low serotonin states breed negativity, worry, obsessiveness, and low self-esteem. (See chapters 1 and 9.)

Food-Mood Log

DATE	TIME	FOOD, DRINK, OR DRUGS CONSUMED

TIME	SUPPLEMENTS TAKEN AT WRONG TIMES, WRONG DOSAGE, ET CETERA, OR NOT TAKEN AT ALL	TIME	CRAVINGS; PHYSICAL; MENTAL; EMOTIONAL SYMPTOMS; BODY TEMERATURE; EXERCISE

What if you stop overeating and start feeling on an even keel emotionally, but do not lose weight? Ask yourself:

✦ Am I eating enough (more than 2,100 calories) to speed up my metabolism?
✦ Am I looking and feeling better in my clothes? Many people who begin to lose fat, build muscle at the same time. Muscle, being heavier than fat, can keep you at the same weight, but change your body a lot. Sometimes your dress size will change, but not your weight. That's one of the reasons I hate the scale—the scale and the mirror both take you out of yourself. In evaluating how you are, your inner eye is what's most accurate
✦ Am I eating enough protein in relation to carbohydrates?
✦ Do I have symptoms of stress exhaustion? If so, see chapters 3 and 11. Adrenals burned out by stress cannot send the message to burn fat. (See chapter 21, too, for good stress-reduction techniques.)
✦ If your metabolic rate is too slow, you can't lose weight.

These last two issues are often twin causes of really stubborn weight retention. The adrenals and thyroid usually work together, or fail to work together, to keep your metabolism active. Follow the directions in chapters 11 and 12 for correcting one or both of these imbalances, if your answers to the first three questions here were yes.

Please don't get frustrated and jump into a low-cal diet if your weight loss is slow. Slow is safe. You now have the opportunity to find out why it is slow! And, better yet, to repair any underlying problem once you find it. If you have low adrenal and/or thyroid function, you will need to spend a few months of your life attending to it, because it is serious. Restoring these glands to full function will benefit you for the rest of your life, far beyond (but including) any weight considerations.

WEEK TWO

Are you stuck in a rut, eating the same foods because it was all so new, unfamiliar, and intimidating at first that you just picked a few dishes that you liked and kept repeating them? If so, you're probably sick of them. That's why I've included lots of quick and tasty eating ideas in chapters 19 and 20. Take the time to use these chapters. Talk the problem over with friends. Find solutions, because you can't afford to get bored. Get food delivered. Hire a cook. There are lots of good cooks doing to-order meals to go now. Pick up freshly made food at good delis or restaurants. Be sure that you are taking enough supplements: Boredom is sometimes craving in disguise—"I'm so bored with this food, I think I'll just go back to the old food." Check your food diary. Have you been eating enough? Are you taking enough amino acids? Some people forget them when things start improving. Or do you have an adrenal or thyroid problem making you too tired to prepare or plan appealing food?

Don't forget: This is a diet *cure,* not a diet! You may have gone into "diet mode" without even realizing it when you started this program, undereating and expecting just another short-term weight loss, at best. No! Relax. Eat well. You won't have to white knuckle your way to the eventual surrender this time. Don't fear that dreaded "permanent maintenance" phase. The hard part will be to keep eating, and eating *well,* not trying to count and minimize calories.

Try to forget about calories, fat grams, and pounds. Please stop weighing yourself. I have seen more binges triggered by weigh-ins than any other single cause. Now that you are free from cravings for the kinds of foods that put on unneeded weight, why would you gain weight? The foods that you are eating are safe and healthy, not binge foods. Remember, the more safe foods you eat, the better off you are, because your metabolism responds to freedom from sweets and other junk foods and steady doses of *plentiful* and nutritious food.

You may feel that "It's so much food. I'll never be able to eat that many vegetables." Just keep working at it. Don't get overwhelmed, you'll get the hang of it.

Slips

If you do find yourself eating sweets or other nonfoods, you'll probably find it's surprisingly hard for you to binge on them. But if you do it often enough, you'll unbalance yourself again and be back where you started. But please do *not* go into the usual broken-diet/self-blame/oh-what-the-hell-eat-more-junk routine. Either outer pressure or inner imbalances, or both, are at fault, not your intentions. Instead, look at what actually happened. Did you miss lunch and then have to go to a cocktail party with hors d'oeuvres? Fatal. Did you have too light a breakfast and then go out to lunch at a restaurant that brought bread to your table? Fatal (especially if you have allergic cravings triggered by bread). Skipping or undereating really is the most common problem, so be clear—you *have* to think through your day ahead to be sure you can get *enough* of the right foods at least three times a day. Did you experience emotional trauma or stress? A terrible week at work, a marital problem, or the revisiting of a childhood trauma can set off a need for druglike foods. Counseling and Overeaters Anonymous can both provide support and better techniques for handling these kinds of upsets.

WEEK THREE

Test Results Are Back

If any results are abnormal, it's time to add new supplements or medications to your master plan, depending on what needs correction. Take this book to your session to compare its suggestions with whatever your practitioner's suggestions might be. Be sure to review and mark the pertinent sections in the book, or copy them for your practitioner. This will make your discussion and planning really productive. If your practitioner cannot prescribe medication, and I have indicated that you might need it, make copies of your test results to take to an M.D. who can prescribe. I hope you're either already seeing an M.D. or D.O. or you will be referred to a wholistic M.D. with whom your practitioner has been able to collaborate on other prior cases.

WEEK FOUR

Mild afternoon or evening cravings sometimes start to crop up around this period. There is typically one cause. If you are not eating enough food at your three-plus meals, the supplements won't protect you from cravings. These kinds of cravings are inevitable when you undereat. Even if they're turning you toward eating the wrong foods, their basic message, "eat more," is right on. As soon as you add more protein and/or fat and/or whole-food carbos to your meals, any yen for sweets will disappear again. One of our clients said she was eating "so well" that she couldn't understand why the same foods she'd been eating successfully for two and a half weeks weren't still "working." It turns out that when she said "eating so well" she meant "*under*eating so well." She had dieted so often that she only had two ways of eating: undereating or overeating. She had cut back too far on carbos. This is a common mistake. I suggested she eat more generous portions, of all three kinds of foods (protein, fats, and carbos). It worked right away, with no weight gain.

If you are skimping on calories, add a potato with butter or olive oil, or a cup of brown and wild rice pilaf to your salad with chicken breast, or to your steamed veggies with broiled salmon steak. Sometimes just adding an oil and lemon juice or vinegar dressing makes all the difference, allowing you to feel full and satisfied. Fats will often turn off your appetite at just the right point, the point of real body satisfaction. Your body can't be satisfied without a certain amount of fat.

WEEKS FIVE THROUGH SIX

Going Out to Dinner

Frank was a tall, friendly man who owned a local restaurant. He was a recovering alcoholic who had become a compulsive eater in sobriety. He came to us miserable from eating too many pastries and other goodies from his own restaurant for too long. He responded beautifully on the supplements, dropping some weight right away (as men, with their higher testosterone and muscle mass, tend to do). But the date finally arrived to go to a long-scheduled business banquet. He called the caterer ahead and found that the main course would work for him (chicken breast stuffed with spinach and mushrooms, rice pilaf, and sautéed vegetables with a side salad). He began to look forward to the evening, until he arrived and was reserve-seated within reaching distance of the dessert buffet! He broke out into a cold sweat, knowing that he was doomed to reach over all night long, as he had done so often before, and wreck his successful new program. Ten minutes later, he realized that he'd forgotten that he was sitting next to all those desserts. It turned out not to be a real problem for him at all, because he had naturally become immune to dessert. He just wasn't interested anymore.

While it's important to keep trigger foods out of your home entirely (if possible), you, too, should be able to manage well around former temptations when you are out to dinner after the first month, if you take precautions. Ask ahead about the menu, and bring food or eat something before you go, so that you won't get hungry and eat something that will throw you off. Discuss your strategy with your hostess or host, if you can, so that she will understand when you don't eat her best recipe lasagna or black forest cake. If your hostess entices you, saying "You've got to try this, it's so good," or, "It's my birthday, you've got to have at least a tiny piece," just say, "Oh, I wish I could," and quickly change the subject.

The hardest thing tends to be your own inner nostalgia about going to occasions where everyone is expected to have a good time by eating and drinking things that you can't. A long time successful O.A. member once told me something I've never forgotten: "My feeling is, I don't *have* to eat that stuff anymore, not 'I don't *get* to.' I feel relieved, not deprived."

Consider this: You've already tested just about every interesting food that you're going to avoid now. It's not like you've never had any. I think you'll find you won't miss that stuff once you start eating the foods that make you feel terrific.

Why not quit dieting by just eating whatever you want? I don't advocate the feminist approach that Geneen Roth and others have developed to end dieting through free eating of any and all foods. For people who are still relatively well balanced, that approach can be great. But for the many people whose biochemistries have been seriously unbalanced by dieting and other problems, this approach can be dangerous. One of our clients developed some minor food cravings five years after using our clinic's nutritional techniques to stop a twenty-year problem with compulsive eating and major depression. She had gone back to college where she was inspired by her feminist instructors. She decided, rather than revisit us to figure out why she was having these cravings, that she'd just try to end them by giving in to them (though it had never worked in the past). She came to us a year and 125 pounds later, still bingeing. This is a story I've heard many times from people, like our former client, who make their already existing imbalances much worse by eating toxic foods in large quantities.

Plan, Plan, Plan

Just like you couldn't leave the house without the right clothes on, don't leave the table without the right food on. Whatever you do, please don't leave the table after *any* meal without your protein on. I can offer you a deal. Go ahead and eat a high-carb dessert occasionally, as long as you get a "dessert" of extra protein, too. A side of chicken breast with your crème brûlée, anyone? Be sure not to leave lunch or dinner without considering how you're going to get your four cups of vegetables that day. If you don't get some vegetables at lunch, you'll need to plan on a big salad or a medium salad and some cooked veggies at dinner, or you can have a huge helping of steamed veggies with lemon butter for a fast, easy, and yummy solution to your veggie needs. Don't go to bed without your veggies on. But if you have some days when you can't get them all, don't be too hard on yourself. Just be sure to get them the next day, not go into a long low veggie slump.

Weekends, or Longer, Away

If you plan to eat out every meal because you're going away, you'll need to be prepared. In California we have no problem getting the foods we need in restaurants because there is so much fresh food available, but in other areas it may be more difficult to customize your orders. Breakfast is always easiest: fresh fruit, eggs, omelets, potatoes. Many restaurants have "light" menus for all meals with cottage cheese and tomatoes, breadless sandwiches, and other appropriate selections. Do not go hungry trying to keep to the Diet Cure. If you plan to make at least some of your own meals on a trip, take a cooler. They come in all sizes with blue ice packs. Or pack a blender and make your own breakfast smoothies.

Do Not Forget Your Supplements! Forgetting your supplements is a real danger. You don't want to start those cravings for nonfoods and junk foods again. And don't feel that nonfoods are your only choices. Here are some ideas for what you can eat in away-from-home situations.

On a Plane Ride. Take substantial snacks to substitute for whatever they serve on the plane that you won't want to eat. Drink lots of hot water and cold water. Avoid the sodas or juices, and caffeinated drinks. Bring your own tea bags everywhere if you like hot drinks. Note: melatonin can really help with jet lag.

In a Convenience Store. Is there any food at a gas station or convenience store that you can eat? Yes. A package or two of pistachio nuts (which are not roasted in lots of rancid oil), a Balance Bar, or a 30,40,30 bar, a can of chili (always leave a can opener and plastic knives, forks, and spoons in your car), a pop-top can of tuna or chicken—anything but high sugar or starch foods, or junk fats, will see you through to a real meal.

Hospital Food. Here is where a wholistic doctor can be so helpful in backing you up to get the healthiest food possible. Hospitals are set up to deal with dairy and gluten allergies and diabetic diets. If you are planning a stay, call and speak to the dietitian and ask how you can get what you need. Ask your family members or your doctor to do it for you, if you are feeling too weakened to take the job on yourself. Your family can also help by bringing food in and making sure that you get whatever supplements you are allowed. (Hospital rules on this can vary a lot.)

If you haven't been able to stay on your Diet Cure while on your trip to friends, family, a vacation, or to the hospital, don't worry too much, you'll be home soon and right back to your eating and supplement plan.

WEEKS SEVEN THROUGH TWELVE

Cutting Back on Supplementation

Chapter 17 advises you on gradually reducing your special supplements until you're just down to the basic supplement plan. Be sure to keep some of your old favorite supplements around, especially the amino acids and antistress supplements for hard times: If you get cravings after an illness, when you've been traveling, or during a major stress, you may have become depleted and unbalanced again. But your supplements will shore you right back up. Review the amino acid chart on page 120 (chapter 9), if you've forgotten or want to be sure that you're taking the right doses, or to explore to see if there is a mood-lifting supplement that you need now that you did not need to take before, when your life was different. You'll need to regularly review the sections in chapters 3 and 11 on how to recognize and repair the damage to your adrenals caused by stress, because you never know when too much of it will hit you, or build up too high.

AFTER WEEK TWELVE

How will you be doing in a year or in five years? Six of the most impaired clients we ever had were interviewed nine months to three years after working with us for, at most, ten sessions. One was male, three were anorectic, and three were overeaters or bulimics. Their nutritional counseling had been paid for through a scholarship arrangement with a county agency. The agency required the follow-up interviews as a way of determining if it should continue funding low-income county residents who wanted our clinic's help.

The interviews showed that all six had made major improvements early on in their work with us. Of the six, one anorectic had done poorly later. But all five of the others had not only sustained their original gains, they had gone on to make even more progress. The results of this small follow-up reflect the same success rate that I have found in every study that I have seen on nutritional therapy for addiction problems: approximately 80 percent success. (You can find the details of our followup in the appendix.)

*   *   *

You can save yourself from a life of dieting, moodiness, and ill health, and this book is a very good start. But we are learning more every day about new nutritional tools that will make your Diet Cure even better. Keep your eyes open. Read wholistic health magazines. Keep taking good care of yourself, now that you know how, for good and all. I wish you the very best diet-free life.

A Follow-up of Six Recovery Systems Clients

Six independently selected follow-up subjects were interviewed nine months to three years after their last session in Recovery Systems' outpatient eating-disorder treatment program. All subjects were severely disabled by anorexia, bulimia, and/or compulsive overeating when they were admitted. The subjects received *only* nutritional counseling (including dietary supplements); most had already received extensive psychotherapy and 12-step group support. Within two months, all subjects made dramatic initial improvement in mood, relief from obsessive eating, and weight normalization. At follow-up, five of the six had sustained or exceeded all the benefits they had received from the program.

The following section describes each client's symptoms as they appeared on admission, at discharge, and as they were reported in the follow-up interviews with psychotherapy graduate student Denise Heiden.

DANA S.

First visit: June 1, 1992. Dana was age 30, five feet seven inches, and had been anorectic since age 15. Her weight fluctuated between 87 and 92 pounds. She had twice been hospitalized for treatment. She had had three years of psychotherapy. Although she had graduated with honors from an Ivy League school, she was unable to work except as a babysitter. She ate nothing all day; milk and sweets at night. She was terribly anxious and depressed and was addicted to laxatives. She suffered constant negative obsessive thoughts about her body shape, weight, and about herself in general.

Dana started supplements on June 12.

By June 18, Dana was much more relaxed (which we attribute to GABA supplements) and less depressed (L-tyrosine supplements). She was able to eat two meals a day. B vitamins in nutritional yeast gave her energy. She drank this in water several times a day in the first few months. She stopped using scales and was less obsessed with weight. She gained three to four pounds (by our scale).

By July 20, she was eating three meals a day. Thyroid support (Gf Thyroid) helped increase her appetite.

July 30: Dana reported feeling "much clearer in the head." Her abdominal bloating was finally decreasing due to digestive enzymes and an herbal antiparasite protocol to treat parasites she picked up in South America at the age of 15.

August 13: Dana reported feeling "so much less insecure" and able to see things differently, clearly.

August 17: Her bowels were now working better on their own (aided by aloe vera juice, magnesium, and flax oil).

By August 2, 1992, Dana S. had gained ten pounds and her anxiety and depression were much reduced. Together with our medical consultant, we identified several major physical problems, including candidiasis, amebic cysts, and gluten intolerance, dating back to age 15, which had caused much of her digestive dysfunction and bizarre appetite.

By August 30 she had gained five more pounds. Her parents said she looked good when she arrived back home to start teacher training (which she had been unable to do one month earlier). After that we had two final appointments.

Follow-up: June 1995. Dana has no negative obsessions about her body, has maintained her weight gain, and is not depressed. She's had no sugar binges and has learned to enjoy eating good food. She is working full time, in graduate school completing an M.A., living on her own, "None of which I could have done prior to Recovery Systems," she said. She had not been able to afford counseling, but had used Overeaters Anonymous successfully (another thing she previously had been unable to do).

ANDREA J.

First Visit: June 22, 1992. Andea was 34. She had lived through a traumatic childhood. Her eating disorder began when she was 15 and using diet pills. Her food bingeing started at 16 and was out of control by 17. By 24 she was using cocaine, sugar, and diet soda daily to control her appetite. This drug use continued until she entered a treatment program at St. Helena Hospital. Her compulsive eating and depression continued. By age 29 she had made two major suicide attempts.

When she came to us she had been in weekly therapy and Overeaters Anonymous for six years, yet her compulsive eating was so out of control that she was afraid she would die soon. After bingeing she frequently drove along the cliffs in West Marin trying to make herself drive off. An O.A. member brought her to us. She had been unable to work for some time and was living with friends. She could only afford the most minimal supplement program.

She withdrew from sweets, gluten-containing grains (foods containing wheat, rye, oats or barley), and NutraSweet in Week One. By the end of the week she had become binge free, and mostly craving free on GTF Chromium and L-glutamine three times a day.

By **July 30** she was depression free and energetic on L-tyrosine three times a day. She cleared further mentally and became healthy physically by December 10. She had met with us five times initially then five more times over the course of the next two years. She had no relapses.

March 25, 1993. Andrea reported "I have never binged again, though I had struggled all my life with sugar bingeing. I went through an eating disorders treatment program and years of therapy and O.A. with no results. Now I am craving free, depression free, earning a living, present and healthy."

On follow-up in June 1995, she had maintained all of her improvements. She had been able to sustain a stable relationship and was going to college in addition to having developed her own successful business. She was still active in O.A.

G R E G   E .

November 9, 1992. Greg (age 51) came to Recovery Systems with life-long depression and an alcohol and drug addiction history starting at age 16. He had been in alcohol/drug recovery for ten of the prior twelve years after receiving intensive addiction treatment. But his depression and other compulsive behavior (food cravings, smoking, sexual obsessions) had continued. He was unable to concentrate or work and complained of a constant burning sensation across his temples, insomnia, and anxiety.

In the next twelve months, although he only came for two and a half of his six follow-up visits (four and a half visits total), his depression and anxiety reduced dramatically. He cut his smoking from two and a half to a half a pack per day and he started school in a rehab program and loved it. His concentration improved and the burning sensation disappeared. Although he continued to have some food cravings, he was not overeating.

On follow-up (August 20, 1995) he was gainfully and happily employed for the first time in years. His depression had improved even further as had his ability to concentrate. He was sleeping well and had little anxiety. He was not overeating. He continued to have mild sweet cravings. His sexual obsession continued (at that time, L-tryptophan and 5-HTP was not available, which we would use today to treat anyone with obsessive behavior).

CARLA V.

On February 18, 1993, Carla came to Recovery Systems with lifelong depression, too despondent even to fill out our intake forms. Her mother had committed suicide and alcoholism ran throughout her father's side of the family. She had been anorectic in the past and still ate very irregularly since eating made her so tired and she associated it with lifelong constipation. She was chronically fatigued and craved sugar constantly. On **May 1, 1993,** she wrote about her progress to the funding agency, saying that her depression was gone and her energy much improved. She no longer needed naps and was alert until ten P.M. instead of being exhausted by six P.M.

On May 12, 1993, Carla reported that she had stopped taking the nutritional supplements after two months. (We usually recommend taking them for three to six months.) Her energy dropped after she stopped them, so we agreed that she would come back in to address low thyroid and other issues, and to get back on the supplements, but she had never returned to do so.

At follow-up, February, 1995. Her depression had continued to improve, her bowels as well. She had no food cravings. But her energy had remained low. Stress and anxiety had become much worse, precipitating a nervous breakdown in 1995. She was undereating again in reaction to her stress and anxiety. She was finding psychotherapy helpful.

NATALIE G.

April 7, 1994. Natalie, age 25, was brought in by her mother because she had anorexia that had begun six months previously. She was low weight (thirteen-pound loss from a naturally slender frame), unkempt, weak, and very depressed. She was unable to leave the house. Her periods had stopped. She was obsessive and her sleep was disturbed. Her mother and medical doctor were planning to hospitalize her if she did not respond to our program because blood work showed alarming evidence of malnutrition.

For a few days she was too frightened to take the supplements, but on April 10 she called to say she felt much better on them. Her mother confirmed that she was indeed eating again and feeling less depressed. Recovery Systems saw her three times. Grief counseling was recommended, which she refused. Her last visit was **April 21, 1994,** although we continued to monitor her program through her mother by phone.

On follow-up in February 1995, Natalie was free of the extreme depression. She had regained ten pounds, her energy was "excellent," her sleep was much better, she was worrying much less, was able to go out, was using makeup and keeping clean again. She was menstruating regularly. She was eating regularly. She had continued to explore nutritional supplements on her own very successfully. (Natalie's mother confirmed all of the above sustained improvements.)

JANICE C.

1993: Janice came to Recovery Systems at age 45. She had been obese since age 3. She had been addicted to alcohol and marijuana from adolescence until 1990 (age 42) when she began using 12-step programs successfully. She was the victim of violent and protracted childhood sexual abuse and had been working hard in therapy for several years to recover from it. She craved and overate sugar uncontrollably and was chronically exhausted. She became depressed and anxious, to the point of having panic attacks, when she tried to go without sugar. She weighed over 300 pounds. (At age 16 she had weighed 380 pounds.) She was emotionally dissociated much of the time, a state that the bingeing promoted. She had irregular periods.

During her twelve-week program at Recovery Systems, Janice stopped craving and overeating foods, her energy rose, her period started again, her energy and mood rose and stabilized. She was much less dissociated, which made her psychotherapy more effective. (She attributed this directly to her normalized eating.) She said that she was processing her traumatic past emotionally and moving on (her previous dissociation had made this level of psychotherapeutic work impossible). Her weight began to decrease, although she refused to weigh herself, and her clothes became loose and had to be replaced.

On follow-up, February 1995. Janice C. had sustained all of the above improvements! She had continued to lose weight.

SUMMARY OF FOLLOW-UP

Of the six clients interviewed, six received dramatic benefit from the nutritional program within two months. At follow-up ten months to three years later, only one (Carla V.) had lost any benefits. Eighty-three percent had achieved and sustained a remarkable level of recovery.

NOTES

Chapter 2. Malnutrition Due to Low-Calorie Dieting

1. Cincinnati Grammar School Study Results, *Eating Disorders Review*, 1993.
2. Frances Berg. "Health Risks of Weight Loss," *Healthy Weight Journal*, 1995.
3. R. Garrison and E. Somer. *Nutrition Desk Reference* (New Canaan, CT: Keats, 1985).
4. K. S. Kendler, K. S., C. MacLean, M. Neale, et al. "The genetic epidemiology of bulimia nervosa," *American Journal of Psychiatry*, 148 (12) 1627, 1991.
5. A. Schauss and C. Cossin. "*Anorexia and Bulimia: A Nutritional Approach to the Deadly Eating Disorders*" (New Canaan, CT: Keats, 1997).
6. Ibid.
7. *Behavioral Therapy*, 7:463, 1976.
8. R. Garison and E. Somer. *Nutrition Desk Reference* (New Canaan, CT: Keats, 1995), pp. 560 and 573 re a national government health and nutrition (NHANES) survey.
9. *New York Times* re M. Fava, M.D., *Massachusetts General Hospital Study*, Boston, May 28, 1993.
10. K. Smith, C.G. Fairburn and P.J. Cowen. "Symptomatic Relapse in Bulimia Nervosa Following Acute Tryptophan Depletion," *Arch Gen Psych*, 1999; 56:171–176.
11. Forrest Tennant, M.D., Ph.D. *Carbohydrate Dependence, Is This Why I Can't Lose Weight?* Veract Handbook Series, 1995.
12. H.J. Roberts, M.D. *Aspartame, Is It Safe?* (The Charles Press, 1990, p. 142).
13. Dennis Remington, M.D., and Barbara Higard. *The Bitter Truth About Artificial Sweeteners* (Vitality House International, 1987), p. 29.
14. S.E. Benson, and K.A. Englebert-Fenton. "Nutritional Aspects of Amenorhea in the Female Athlete Triad," *Int. Jrnl Sports Nutrition*, 1996, 6, 134–145.

Chapter 3. Unstable Blood Sugar

1. Larson '97, M, M&P (549).
2. Health Appraisal Questionnaire; *Solved, The Riddle of Illness*; M&P.
3. Stephen Langer, M.D. *Solved: The Riddle of Illness* (New Canaan, CT: Keats, 1984), p. 75–84.
4. "Americanization a Health Risk, Study Says," *L.A. Times*, September 15, 1998 pp. A1 and A19. Study released September 7, 1998 by the National Research Council and Institute of Medicine.
5. Carey Goldburg. "The Simple Life Lures Refugees from Stress," *New York Times*, September 21, 1995, B1 and B6.
6. Susan Mitchell, Ph.D., and C. Christie, *I Could Kill for a Cookie* (New York: Penguin, 1998) p. 17; from a survey conducted by the authors).

7. Linda Rector Page, N.D., Ph.D., *Healthy Healing: A Guide to Self-Healing for Everyone*, 10th ed. (Healthy Healing Pub, 1997), p. 439.

Chapter 4. Unrecognized Low Thyroid Function

1. P. Chomard, et al, "Serum concentrations of T$_4$, T$_3$, RT$_3$, and free T$_4$, T$_3$ in moderately obese patients," *Ilum Nutr Clin*, September 1985, 39(5):371–8.
2. Stephen Langer, M.D. *Solved: The Riddle of Illness* (New Canaan, CT: Keats, 1984), p. 156.
3. R. Marcchaud, "Low T$_3$ Syndrome," *Rev Prat*, November 15, 1988, 15; 48(18):2018–22.
4. Broda O. Barnes, M.D., *Jour Amer Med Assoc*, 1942, 119:1072.
5. Sacher and McPherson, *Widmann's Clinical Interpretation of Laboratory Tests* (Salam, MA: F.A. Davis, 1991) p. 583.
6. L.E. Braverman and R.D. Utiger, eds. Werner & Ingbar's *The Thryoid: A Fundamental Clinical Text*, 6th ed. (Philadelphia: J. B. Lippincott, 1991), p. 1331.
7. Steven Langer, M.D. *How to Win at Weight Loss* (Rochester, VT: Thorsons, 1987), p. 199.

Chapter 5. Food Addictions and Allergic Reactions

1. Kathleen Des Maisons *Potatoes Not Prozac* (New York: Simon and Schuster, 1998).
2. C. R. Ziovdron, Strearly, and W. Klee, "Opiate peptides derived from food proteins: The exorphins," *J Bio/Chem* 1979: 254:2379–2380; cited by Garrison, p. 625.
3. A study published in the April 1996 issue of *Gastroenterology* found the prevalence in the United States of celiac disease is 1:250. This is similar to that reported from countries in Europe. They concluded that CD is not rare in the United States and may be greatly underdiagnosed. See T. Not, K. Horvath, I. D. Hill, A. Fasano, A. Hammed, and G. Magazz, "Endomysium antibodies in blood donors predicts a high prevalence of celiac disease in the USA," *Gastroenterology*, April 1996.
4. Doris Rapp, M.D. *Is This Your Child?* (New York: William Morrow, 1991), p. 547.
5. NIH National Digestive Diseases Information Clearinghouse.
6. Carl Pfeiffer, *Nutrition and Mental Illness: An Orthomolecular Approach to Balancing Body Chemistry* (Inner Traditions International, Ltd., 1988).
7. Theron Randolph, *An Alternative Approach to Allergies* (New York: HarperCollins, 1989).

Chapter 6. Hormonal Havoc

1. Michael Murray, N.D. *Premenstrual Syndrome* (Rocklin, CA: Prima, 1997), p. 9.
2. Susan Love, M.D. *Dr. Susan Love's Hormone Book* (New York: Random House, 1997), p. 40.
3. Debra Waterhouse *Outsmarting the Midlife Fat Cell* (New York: Hyperion, 1998), pp. 18–19.
4. Michael Murray and Joseph Pizzorno. *Encyclopedia of Natural Medicine* (Rocklin, CA: Prima, 1988), pp. 744 and 910.
5. Vliet, Elizabeth L., M.D. *Screaming to Be Heard: Hormonal Connections Women Suspect and Doctors Ignore* (M. Evans & Co., 1995), p. 88.
6. *Ibid.*, p. 326.
7. *Ibid.*, p. 84.
8. *Ibid.*, p. 143.
9. *Ibid.*, p. 181.
10. *Ibid.*
11. G. B. Phillip, M.D., "Relation between serum sex hormones and the glucose-insulin-lipids defect in men with obesity," *Metabolism*, January 1993, 42 (1). 116–120.
12. Jonathan Wright, M.D. *Natural Hormone Replacement For Woman Over 45* (Smart Publications, 1997), p. 56.
13. Love, op.cit., p. 123.
14. Love, op.cit., p. 48.

Chapter 7. Yeast Overgrowth

1. Michael Murray, N.D., and Joseph Pizzorno, N.D. *Encyclopedia of Natural Medicine*, 2nd ed. (Rocklin, CA: Prima, 1998), p. 300.
2. Luc De Schepper, M.D., *Full of Life* (Los Angeles: Tale Weaver Publishing, 1991), p. 81.
3. Elaine Gottschall *Breaking the Vicious Cycle* (Kirkton, Ontario: Kirkton Press, 1994), p. 10.
4. De Schepper, *Full of Life*, p. 72.

Chapter 8. Fatty Acid Deficiency

1. Artemis Simopoulos, M.D. *The Omega Plan* (New York: Harper-Collins, 1998), p. 29.
2. Ibid., pp. 79–80.
3. H. Okuyama, "Dietary fatty acids—the n-6/n-3 balance and chronic elderly diseases. Excess linoleic acid (n-6) and relative n-3 deficiency syndrome seen in Japan," *Progress in Lipid Research*, Vol. 35, No. 4, 1997, pp. 409–457.
4. Charles Bates, Ph.D. *Essential Fatty Acids and Immunity in Mental Health* (Life Sciences Press, 1987), p. 110.
5. Joan Mathews-Larson, Ph.D. *Seven Weeks to Sobriety* (New York: Ballantine, 1992), p. 109.
6. Tim Kuss, Ph.D. *A Guidebook to Clinical Nutrition for the Health Professional* (Institute of Bio-energetic Research, 1992), p. 87.
7. Udo Erasmus, *Fats That Heal, Fats That Kill* (Blaine, WA: Alive Books, 1997).
8. Peto D'Adamo, M.D. *Eat Right for Your Type* (New York: G.P. Putnam's Sons, 1996).

Chapter 10. Nutritional Rehab for the Ex-Dieter

1. Gaesser, Glen, Ph.D. *Big Fat Lies* (New York: Ballantine, 1996); all of the "facts" on page 134 are from this source.
2. *Consumer Reports*, 6/93 p. 350.

Chapter 11. Balancing Your Blood Sugar

1. R. Anderson, et al., "Dietary Chromium Intake Freely Chosen Diets," *Institutional Diet and Individual Foods*, January 1992, pp. 117–21, in *Biological Trace Element Research* 1992; 32:10–24.
2. Robert C. Atkins, M.D. *The Vita-Nutrient Solution: Nature's Answer to Drugs* (New York: Simon & Schuster, 1998).
3. Michael T. Murray, N.D. *Hypoglycemia and Diabetes* (Rocklin, CA: Prima Publishing, 1994).
4. Ibid., p. 97.
5. Artemis Simopoulos, M.D. *The Omega Plan* (New York: HarperCollins, 1998).
6. James Balch, M.D., and Phyllis Balch, C.N.C. *Prescription for Nutritional Healing* (Garden City, NY: Avery, 1997).
7. William Timmons, N.D. *Practitioners' Manual* (San Diego, CA: BioHealth Diagnostics, 1999), p. 48.
8. William Jeffries. *Safe Uses of Cortisol* (Springfield, IL: Charles C. Thomas Pub, 1996).

Chapter 12. Thyroid Solutions

1. Jeffrey Bland, Ph.D., from an article published in *The Journal of Clinical Endocrinology and Metabolism*, vol. 56, 1993, as quoted in "Keep Your Thyroid Healthy for Peak Energy," *Health and Nutrition Breakthroughs*, January 1998.
2. Broda Barnes. *Hypothyroidism: The Unsuspected Illness* (New York: Thomas Y. Crowell Co., 1976), p. 98.

Chapter 14. Hormone Help

1. Michael Murray, N.D., *Premenstrual Syndrome* (Rocklin, CA: Prima, 1997).
2. J. Chen and J. Gao. "The Chinese total diet study in 1990 Part II: Nutrients," *Jrnl of AOAC Int*, Institute of Nutrition and Food Hygiene, Chinese Academy of Preventative Medicine, Beijing, China November-December 1993, 76 (6): 1193–1213.
3. Joseph Pizzorno, N.D., and Michael Murray, N.D. *The Encyclopedia of Natural Medicine* (Rocklin, CA: Prima, 1998).
4. J. Suzuki, H. Yoshida, and T. shizaki (Dept Epidemiology, Tokyo Institute of Gerontology), "Epidemiology of osteoporosis: incidence, prevalence, and prognosis," *Nippon Rinsho*, 6/98;56(6):1563–8.
5. C.Y. Hsieh, R.C. Santell, S.Z. Harlan, et al., "Estrogenic effects of genistain on the growth of estrogen receptor-positive human breast cancer (MCF-7) cells in vitro and in vivo," *Cancer Research*, 1998 September 1; 58(17):3833–8.
6. D.F. McMichael-Phillips, C. Harding, M. Marton, et al., "Effects of soy-protein supplementation on epithelial proliferation in the histologically normal human breast," *Am Jrnl of Clin Nutr* 12/98; 68(6 suppl):1431S–1435S.
7. A.M. Duncan, B.E. Marz, X. Lu, et al., "Soy isoflavones exert modest hormone effects in premenopausal women," *Jrnl Clin Endocrinologic Metabolism* 1/99; 84(1):192–197.
8. Jane E. Benson, Kathryn A. Engelhart-Fenton, and Patricia A. Eisenman, "Nutritional aspects

of amenorrhea in the female athlete," *Triad International Journal of Sports Nutrition,* 1996, pp. 134–145.

9. R. Vettor, G. DoPergda, C. Pagano, et al., "Gender differences in serum leptin in obese people: relationships with testosterone body fat distribution and insulin sensitivity," *European Jrnl of Clinical Investigation,* 1997 Dec: 27(2): 1016–24.

Chapter 15. Repairing the Damage Caused from Yeasts

1. Timothy Kuss, Ph.D. *A Guidebook to Clinical Nutrition for the Health Professional.* (Pleasant Hill, CA: Institute of Bioenergetic Research, 1992), p. 31.

Chapter 16. The Fatty Acid Fix

1. Artemis Simopoulos, M.D. *The Omega Plan* (New York: HarperCollins, 1998), p. 124.

2. D. Rudin, M.D., and Clara Felix. *Omega-3 Oils: A Practical Guide* (Garden City, NY: Avery, 1996), p. 22.

3. Timothy Kuss, Ph.D. *A Guidebook to Clinical Nutrition for the Health Professional* (Pleasant Hill, CA: Institute of Bioenergetic Research, 1992), p. 92.

4. Ibid.

5. Charles Bates, Ph.D. *Essential Fatty-Acids in Immunity and Mental Health* (Tacoma, WA: Life Sciences Press, 1987), p. 69.

Chapter 17. Your Master Nutritional Supplement Plan

1. A. E. Czeizch, "Prevention of congenital abnormalities by periconceptional mutlivitamin supplementation," *Brit Med Jrnl,* vol. 306, June 19, 1993, pp. 1645–48.

2. Norra Macready, "Vitamins associated with lower colon-cancer risk," *The Lancet,* November 15, 1997, p. 1452.

3. Krispin Sullivan, C.N. *Nutrition for the 90's,* (Woodacre, CA: Middle Marin Labs, 1999), pp. 15–16.

4. J. Lazarou, M.Sc., B. H. Pomeranz, M.D., Ph.D., and P. N. Corey, Ph.D., "Incidence of Adverse Drug Reactions in Hospitalized Patients: A Meta-analysis of Prospective Studies," *JAMA* April 1998;279:1200–1205 (No. 15).

5. *Nutritional Desk Reference,* 1995, pp. 597–8.

Chapter 18. The Best Foods for Your Special Biochemistry

1. Colin Campbell, J. Chen, and J. Gao, "Study of Chinese diet and cancer rates," *The Chinese Total Diet Study,* Institute of Nutrition and Food Hygiene, Chinese Academy of Preventative Medicine, Beijing, China, November–December 1993, 76(6):1193–1213.

2. "Post prandial integrated amounts of insulin and glucagon over 4 hours as a function of carbohydrate to protein ratio." *J. Clin. Nutrition* 52:267–272 (1990).

3. *The Supplement Review* (Pittsburgh, PA: Douglas Laboratories, vol. 1, no. 4), p. 1.

4. Elizabeth Somer, *The Essential Guide to Vitamins and Minerals* (New York: HarperPerennial, 1995), p. 3.

5. Tim O'Shea, "Minerals, Part I: Essential Minerals" in *Dynamic Chiropractic,* October, 5, 1998, p. 14.

6. Timothy Kuss, *A Guidebook to Clinical Nutrition* (Pleasant Hill, CA: Institute of Bioenergetic Research, 1992), p. 78.

7. Brenda Biondo, "Is There Poison in Your Produce?" *USA Weekend,* August 15, 1997, p. 10.

8. L. Christensen, "The Roles of Caffeine and Sugar in Depression," *The Nutrition Report:* 9; 3, pp. 17 and 24.

9. Michael Jacobson, "Liquid Candy," *Nutrition Action Health Newsletter,* Nov. 1998, vol. 25, no. 9, p. 8.

10. James F. Balch, and Balch, Phyllis, *Prescription for Cooking and Dietary Wellness* (Greenfield, IN: P.A.B. Publishing, 1987), p. 196.

11. Andrea Widener, "Study Warns of Danger in Meat," *Contra Costa Times,* Oct. 31, 1998.

12. Ron Kotzsch, and Frances S. Goulart, *Whole Life Times,* Dec. 1983, p. 20.

13. Jean Carper, *Jean Carper's Total Nutrition Guide* (New York: Bantam Books, 1987), p. 44.

14. Paul Pitchford, *Healing with Whole Foods* (Berkeley, CA: North Atlantic Books, 1993), p. 493.

Chapter 19. Shopping for Your Master Plan Supplies and Planning Your Meals

1. "Interim Advisory on Alfalfa Sprouts," Food and Drug Administration Talk Paper, JN8–47, August 31, 1998.

INDEX